Reproductive Technologies as Global Form

Eigene und fremde Welten

The series »Eigene und fremde Welten« is edited by Jörg Baberowski, Vincent Houben, Stefan Beck, Thomas Mergel, and Gabriele Metzler in connection with the Collaborative Research Center no. 640 »Representations of Changing Social Orders: Cross-Cultural and Cross-Temporal Comparisons« based at Humboldt-Universität, Berlin (Germany).

Volume 19

Michi Knecht, PD Dr., is a senior researcher and lecturer at the Department of European Ethnology and the Collaborative Research Center no. 640, »Representations of Changing Social Orders. Cross-Cultural and Cross-Temporal Comparisons« at Humboldt-University, Berlin.

Maren Klotz is a research fellow and PHD candidate at the Department of European Ethnology at Humboldt-University, Berlin.

Stefan Beck, Dr., is professor for European Ethnology at Humboldt-University, Berlin.

Michi Knecht, Maren Klotz, Stefan Beck (eds.)

Reproductive Technologies as Global Form

Ethnographies of Knowledge, Practices, and Transnational Encounters

Campus Verlag
Frankfurt/New York

Bibliographic Information published by the Deutsche Nationalbibliothek.
The Deutsche Nationalbibliothek lists this publication in the Deutsche Nationalbibliografie; detailed bibliographic data are available in the Internet at http://dnb.d-nb.de
ISBN 978-3-593-39100-7

Cover design: Campus Verlag, Frankfurt-on-Main
Printing office and bookbinder: CPI buchbuecher.de, Birkach
Printed on acid free paper.
Printed in Germany

This book is also available as an E-Book.
www.campus.de
www.press.uchicago.edu

Contents

National Styles of Reproductive Governance and Global Forms

Tracing Transnational Scapes of Reproductive Technologies: Emergent Forms and Domains of Regulation

Transnational Reproductive Mobilities, Materialities, and Agencies

Acknowledgments

This volume is the product of a collective effort and many discussions during the workshop »IVF as Global Form. Ethnographic Knowledge and the Transnationalization of Reproductive Technologies,« organized by Michi Knecht, Maren Klotz and Stefan Beck for the research project »Kinship Cultures and Reproductive Technologies« as part of the Collaborative Research Center no. 640 (SFB 640), »Representations of Changing Social Orders. Cross-Cultural and Cross-Temporal Comparisons« at Berlin's Humboldt-University, June 12 – June 14, 2008. The workshop received financial support from the German Research Foundation (DFG), for which we are truly grateful. We wish to express our special thanks to Sarah Franklin for accepting our invitation to hold the keynote lecture. The workshop also profited enormously from the contributions by Willemijn de Jong, Bernhard Hadolt and Elizabeth Roberts. We much regret that for a number of different reasons it was not possible to include their papers in this volume.

The discussions during the workshop benefited greatly from the commitment and the investments of our chairs and commentators Christine Bischof, Tanja Bogusz, Jeanette Edwards, Babette Müller-Rockstroh, Ferhunde Özbay, Shalini Randeria, Carmel Shalev, Michael Schillmeier, and Shahana Schmidt. Their thoughtful comments, stimulating analyzes and advancing questions have found their way into this book via the process of developing and rewriting the earlier versions presented at the workshop into full papers. During the workshop, participants and organizers alike could always rely on the support from our student assistants Feray Halil and Franziska Wegener and on the management and organizational skills of our colleague and PhD student Sulamith Hamra. As editors, we have benefited greatly from the intellectual and academic environment provided by the Collaborative Research Center ›Representations of Changing Social Orders: Cross-Cultural and Cross-Temporal Comparisons‹. Warm thanks are extended to all our colleagues there. Finally, we owe thanks to Xenia Krüger for helping to organize the workshop, to Kareth Schaffer for language-assistance, to Robin Cackett for final editing and to Anika Kreft and Sascha Stingl for their scrutiny in preparing the manuscript.

Stefan Beck, Maren Klotz and Michi Knecht, Berlin, May 2012

Reproductive Technologies as Global Form: Introduction

Michi Knecht, Maren Klotz, Stefan Beck

A few years after the British Government had made ova and sperm donation non-anonymous in 2005, one of the editors of this volume spent a series of rainy summer afternoons in a sperm bank in Northern England. Maren Klotz was shadowing the practices of the two young female biologists working in the laboratory and the administration office. She was shown how to count sperm cells under the microscope following WHO standards to determine semen quality. The staff told her that the interlaboratory testing rounds to establish a high level of standardization within these quality measurements, existent both in Germany and Great Britain, were »fun in a geeky scientist kind of way.« And she tried to understand how the minute guidelines of the British Human Fertilisation and Embryology Authority (HFEA) were actually playing out in the English clinic. When biologists Rose Daffyd and Canelle Ukwu quizzed her about the German regulatory situation they could not believe that in Germany ova donation was illegal while sperm donation was allowed and actually hardly regulated at all. One afternoon Ukwu, who was mainly in charge of donor recruitment and administration and who was spending a gap year before going back to a prestigious university to pursue postgraduate studies in cell biology, showed this editor how to centrally register sperm donors with the HFEA. The main bulk of information was filled into an Electronic Data Interchange (EDI) document and electronically transferred to the HFEA computers. »How is that handled in Germany?,« Canelle Ukwu asked. »We have also had a change in regulations,« Maren Klotz said. »It is non-anonymous donations in Germany now as well, but what kind of data needs to be stored and how it could actually become accessible is quite unclear to German experts.« Klotz added she would next be interviewing British donor-conceived persons who had used the service

UK Donorlink to potentially find half-siblings and donors via DNA testing. Ukwu shook her head and said that she did not understand at all what was motivating these searches or why the HFEA should make available the information she was just punching into her keyboard in 18 years: »My family is from Cameroon and my father, the man who raised me, my mother's partner, also isn't my biological father. Why should I care about that?« Ukwu asked. »Where my family is from,« she added, »it's normal that children are raised away from their biological parents. Don't people in Britain have more important things to do than look for their sperm donor or half-siblings they have nothing to do with?« She shook her head in a gesture as if she viewed such endeavors as English extravagance. Then she offered her view as a biologist: »Medical histories of family members have become less important nowadays anyhow; you can simply use genetic testing if you want to know something about risk susceptibilities.« The donor-conceived adults Maren Klotz met later that night were of a different opinion: They mourned the absence of identifiable donor information for them and cursed that they had been born before the comprehensive regulations on reproductive technologies had come into force in Britain. One of them had spent years being monitored for a hereditary condition prevalent on her father's side before finding out she was donor-conceived.

Ukwu's casual commentaries in the ethnographic vignette above capture quite pointedly some of the contemporary questions raised through reproductive technologies within a period of increased globalization, questions which have motivated the compilation of this book: Reproductive technologies have spread across various kinds of boundaries and into socially and culturally diverse settings, situations and regions. However, while people, technologies, human gametes, knowledge and ideas about appropriate regulation circulate widely, the legislation of reproductive technologies is still primarily implemented in territories, whose borders are duly policed by a nation state. Furthermore, local articulations of assisted reproduction in their uneven technological spread across the globe never take place in a social or economical vacuum: They instead become part of emergent national styles of reproductive governance[1]

1 Lynn M. Morgan & Elizabeth F.S. Roberts, »Rights and Reproduction in Latin America«, in: *Anthropology News*, March 2009, pp. 12, 16.

shaped in interaction with local understandings of kinship, the role of »biologies and the biological«[2], legitimate family forms, prevalent gender asymmetries and economic considerations. As a result, the proliferation of reproductive technologies into different contexts of appropriation does not lead to homogenous forms of deployment. Rather, it has led to a wide range of very different forms of regulation, bans, and approvals as well as to considerable differences in clinical practice, public or private financing, and moral or ethical reasoning. A multi-local configuration has emerged from the multitude of practices that are generating, transferring, acquiring, imagining, and regulating reproductive technologies across and beyond regional and national borders: a transnational or even global »assemblage«[3] that constantly re-defines and re-produces reproductive technologies and its contexts, both locally and globally.

During the interaction in the British sperm bank described above the participants level out a number of differences they collaboratively detect and evaluate. The short vignette is exemplary for the broad range of very different rationalities, practices, and legal regulations that can be observed within a single situation or institution »doing« reproductive technologies and even more so when comparing different settings. The field observations described are part of a collaborative research project, established in 2005 at the Department of European Ethnology at the Humboldt-University in Berlin[4], which focuses on the nexus of knowledge, kinship, regulation and reproductive technologies, generating comparative longi-

2 Sarah Franklin, »Biologization Revisited: Kinship Theory in the Context of the New Biologies«, in: *Relative values: reconfiguring kinship studies*, ed. by Sarah Franklin & Susan McKinnon (Durham, NC: Duke University Press, 2001), pp. 302–328.

3 Cf. Stephen J. Collier & Aihwa Ong, »Global Assemblages, Anthropological Problems«, in: *Global Assemblages. Technology, Politics, and Ethics as Anthropological Problems*, ed. by Aihwa Ong & Stephen J. Collier (Malden, MA et al.: Blackwell, 2005), pp. 3–21; Helen Watson-Verran & David Turnbull, »Science and Other Indigenous Knowledge Systems«, in: *Handbook of Science and Technology Studies* (rev. edition), ed. by Sheila Jasanoff, Gerald E. Markle, James C. Petersen & Trevor Pinch (Thousand Oaks, London and New Delhi: Sage Publications, 1995), pp. 115–139; George E. Marcus & Erkan Saka, »Assemblage«, in: *Theory, Culture & Society* 23 (2006), 2/3, pp. 101–106; John Phillips, »Agencement/Assemblage«, in: *Theory, Culture & Society* 23 (2006), 2/3, pp. 108–109.

4 For further information about this research project see [http://www.sfb-repraesentationen.de /teilprojekte/c4/english].

tudinal ethnographic data over a period of up to ten years. The project aims to »map« reproductive mobilities across European borders (internal as well as external) and to understand reproductive medicine as a tool for making, re-making and re-inventing kinship as a central »organizational apparatus«[5] of societies to order the social. Kinship in its Euro-American variety produces persons who consider themselves to be a product of nature and culture, as having come into being through »biological« as well as »social« processes: fused gametes merge and recombine generational pasts while love and care, socialization and education guarantee an individual future. Kinship is an imaginary institution of society – as Cornelius Castoriadis defined the term. As an apparatus for producing social forms and orderliness it is leaning »on the natural stratum which is [… conceived as being] internal to society.«[6] It is imaginary in providing enough vagueness and openness for cultural interpretations of the »facts of nature« and at the same time makes these interpretations invisible through naturalization: social facts appear as natural facts.

Our project comparatively investigates local and national modes of using and appropriating reproductive medicine – what we tentatively call IVF-cultures – in Turkey, Great Britain, and Germany. The research project traces the emerging transnational forms of mobility, competition, inequality, and collaboration in the domain of reproductive medicine. Doing so, we take reproductive medicine to be a prime field-experiment within modern societies, an experiment that challenges existing imaginaries of kinship through affording the manipulation and intervention into the »facts of nature.« We interpret reproductive medicine as an experimental system »in the wild,« not confined to laboratory settings and fertility clinics, that allows the reinterpretation of »social facts,« destabilizing or undermining the conventionally unquestioned naturalization of kinship. But reproductive medicine is also an experiential system, affording new experiences, producing new subjectivities, new objectivities, new moralities, and social obligations. Reproductive medicine thus can also be used as a sort of natural experiment for anthropology: It implements

5 Fredrik Barth, »Analytical Dimensions in the Comparison of Social Organizations«, in: *American Anthropologist* 74 (1972), 1/2, pp. 207–220.

6 Cornelius Castoriadis, *The Imaginary Institution of Society* (London: Polity Press, 1987), p. 230.

tools and concepts in modern societies and introduces an experimental mode of producing biological and social kinships across a diverse number of social and cultural contexts. As reproductive medicine opens up a space for defining and experiencing relations held to be based on »nature« in a new way – be it on the level of individuals, families, or societies – it offers rare analytical opportunities to comparatively observe the remaking of kinship as an imaginary institution and a generator of social orders.

In this book, the idea of reproductive technologies as constituting an experimental set-up is further elaborated. The contributions assembled here use their analyzes of such field experiments not only to look into the contemporary renegotiations of the made and the given, they also provide us with empirical insight into the ambiguous phenomenon of »globalization.« Some of the articles depict reproductive technologies as they are practiced and lived in very diverse settings, not only in Great Britain, Germany and Turkey, but also in Sri Lanka and Mali, in Middle Eastern Countries, India and Spain, in public and private hospitals, families and concerned groups, and along the brim of affluence that separates East and West, North and South. Other contributions chart the mobility of experts, substances, patient-consumers, practitioners, and bioethical discourses across fuzzy terrain or focus on transnational arrangements of ova »donation« or »surrogacy« – often against a grim backdrop of increasing global inequality and depleted agency and control through women. The ensemble of these ethnographic case studies is not so much comparative as such, but rather focuses on the question, how dense and detailed ethnographic knowledge – interactively produced in widely different situations and regions, mobilized by multi-sited research, and reconnected in new forms of research cooperation or in publications such as this – can enhance the understanding of the globalization of biomedical technologies. How can such knowledge invigorate the analysis of global forms? How can ethnographic work contribute to an understanding of global forms as »not simply agglomerations of brief encounters« but structures which develop their own temporalities?[7] Karin Knorr-Cetina has described global forms as providing »an enhanced environment or laboratory for the study of contemporary extensions and reconfigurations of interaction order prin-

7 Karin Knorr Cetina, »The Synthetic Situation: Interactionism for a Global World«, in: *Symbolic Interaction* 32 (2009), 1, pp. 61–87, in particular p. 83.

ciples.« Global forms in her view »define the order of things on which such principles become further articulated and thrive (...).«[8] By addressing emergent transnational junctions and disjunctions, the uneven global distribution and accessibility of reproductive technologies, and a broad spectrum of localizing articulations from the perspective of ethnography, the contributions demonstrate in how far reproductive technologies can been seen as an experimental set-up for the reconstruction of late modern topologies (see Beck in this volume) and of a contemporarily emerging order of things.

Reproductive Technologies as Global Form

In this volume, reproductive technologies such as in vitro fertilization (IVF), different forms of insemination, intra-cytoplasmic sperm injection (ICSI), so-called »surrogacy« arrangements, and conception via »donated« ova are conceived of *as a global form*. By using this term *we* refer to three distinguishable, but interconnected dimensions. *First*, it is a conceptual move following Aihwa Ong's and Stephen Collier's suggestion to rethink global phenomena beyond notions of mapping, spread and space. It is certainly true that during the last 40 years reproductive technologies have moved at high speed across borders and domains so that they have become increasingly well-known in many parts of the world.[9] But spatial

8 Loc. cit.

9 Anthropologists have investigated, charted, and in many ways accompanied these developments since the 1990s; for surveys and important landmark volumes see e.g. Marcia C. Inhorn & Daphna Birenbaum-Carmeli, »Assisted Reproductive Technologies and Cultural Change«, in: *Annual Review of Anthropology* 37 (2008), pp. 177–196; Carole H. Browner & Carolyn F. Sargent (Eds.), *Reproduction, Globalization, and the State* (Durham, NC: Duke University Press, 2010); Daphna Birenbaum-Carmeli & Marcia C. Inhorn (Eds.), *Assisting Reproduction, Testing Genes: Global Encounters with New Biotechnologies* (New York and Oxford: Berghahn Books, 2009); Lorraine Culley, Nicky Hudson & Floor B. van Rooij (Eds.), *Ethnicity, Infertility and Reproductive Technologies* (London: Earthscan Books, 2009); Willemijn de Jong & Olga Tkach (Eds.), *Making Bodies, Persons and Families. Normalising Reproductive Technologies in Russia, Switzerland and Germany* (Münster: LIT-Verlag, 2009); Marcia C. Inhorn (Ed.), *Reproductive Disruptions: Gender, Technology, and Biopolitics in the New Millennium* (New York and Oxford: Berghahn Books, 2007); Aditya Bharadwaj (Ed.), »Divine

distribution and spread are only one, and not even one of the most telling features of their globalization. Arjun Appadurai's concept of »scape«[10] has done important work in theorizing the proliferation of global entanglements, of spaces and forms emerging out of continuous acts of border crossing and transnational connections. However, spatially colored concepts such as »scape« tend to define global forms in analogy to relatively coherent spaces, often modeled on the idea of a landscape. They are less helpful for capturing the more discontinuous and schizmogenetic qualities of these emergent phenomena, the plethora of fissures and countercurrents, in which they are entailed. More to the point and analytically fruitful might be Aihwa Ong's and Stephen Collier's observation that global forms are characterized by a »specific capacity for decontextualization and recontextualization.« [11] Because of their standardized features – ranging from cryopreservation protocols, best practice guidelines, ISO-norms, and evidence based medicine to paper technologies, medical statistics, and universal concepts in international bioethics – reproductive technologies travel and arrive in various destinations; but in being reappropriated in different contexts, they also generate new alterities. They are »designed to produce functionally comparable results in disparate domains,«[12] but they also effect a proliferation of differences in working and living with

---

Intervention and Sacred Conceptions: Religion in the Global Practice of IVF«, special issue of *Culture, Medicine, and Psychiatry* 30 (2006), 4; Maya Unnithan-Kumar (Ed.), *Reproductive Agency, Medicine and the State. Cultural Transformations in Childbearing* (New York and Oxford: Berghahn, 2004); Marcia C. Inhorn & Franz van Balen (Eds.), *Infertility around the Globe. New Thinking on Childlessness, Gender and Reproductive Technologies* (Berkeley and Los Angeles: University of California Press, 2002); Jeanette Edwards, Sarah Franklin, Eric Hirsch, Frances Price & Marilyn Strathern, *Technologies of Procreation: Kinship in the Age of Assisted Conception*, 2nd edition (London: Routledge, 1999); Faye D. Ginsburg & Rayna Rapp (Eds.), *Conceiving the New World Order. The Global Politics of Reproduction* (Berkeley and Los Angeles: University of California Press, 1995).

10 Cf. Arjun Appadurai, »Global Ethnoscapes: Notes and Queries for a Transnational Anthropology«, in: *Capturing Anthropology: Working in the Present*, ed. by Richard G. Fox (Santa Fé, NM: School of American Research Press), pp. 191–210. For a more detailed and pronounced discussion of the concept of »scape« with regard to reproductive technologies see also Inhorn and Hörbst (both in this volume).

11 Collier & Ong, »Global Assemblages«, op. cit. (note 3), in particular p. 11.

12 Ibid.

these technologies[13] and generate new constellations and frictions. The contributions to this volume share a common concern to make visible the ways in which reproductive technologies replicate standards and at the same time create differences. By describing this double effect of reproductive technologies as global form in finely grained ethnographic detail they trace the emerging new orders of sameness and difference in the context of their uneven global distribution.

A *second* understanding of reproductive technologies as global form is introduced most elaborately by Sarah Franklin in the opening paper of this book. Franklin chronicles the history and prehistory of in vitro fertilizations and embryo-transfers in animals and humans in order to understand their significance for current and future concepts of »the biological.« »The biological« entails both living matter itself and the biological sciences.[14] Franklin uses the term »global biological«[15] to refer to developments and processes that potentially affect all human beings independent of their concrete involvement, for example, in in vitro technologies. Her analytic angle is genealogical. It was in vitro fertilization, she argues, and not later, more spectacular genetic experiments like Dolly, the sheep, that has fundamentally altered concepts of human reproduction and biological relationships. By explicating how biological facts in general belong to multiple transferable logics and by normalizing technological interventions into human cells and gametes, in vitro fertilization according to Franklin functioned like a precursor for further interventions and subsequent technological developments. In her astute analysis Franklin shows that the most important implications of in vitro technologies for social relations do not consist in their close connection with infertility. Rather, their impact is considerable because they paved the way for a more general acceptance of hybrids, for the culturing of biology in a glass, and for the blending

13 Margaret Lock, Allan Young und Alberto Cambrosio, *Living and Working with the New Medical Technologies: Intersections of Inquiry* (Cambridge: Cambridge University Press, 2000).

14 Sarah Franklin, »Stem Cells R Us: Emergent Life Forms and the Global Biological«, in: *Global Assemblages. Technology, Politics, and Ethics as Anthropological Problems*, ed. by Aihwa Ong & Stephen J. Collier (Malden, MA, and Oxford: Blackwell, 2005), pp. 59–48.; Sarah Franklin, *Dolly Mixtures. The Remaking of Genealogy* (Durham and London: Duke University Press, 2007); Sarah Franklin, »Embryonic Economies: The Double Reproductive Values of Stem Cells«, in: *BioSocieties* 1 (2006), pp. 71–90.

15 Franklin, »Stem Cells R Us«, op. cit. (note 14).

of technology with biology. Reproductive technologies then constitute a global form not so much because they directly affect many involuntarily childless women, men, and couples all over the world, but rather because they introduce »new models of biological relationships among parts as well as wholes« that might matter for all humankind, as Franklin writes in her contribution.

A *third* understanding of reproductive technologies as a global form charted in this volume refers to the ways in which such forms in their diverse localizations, transnational conjunctions and global dimensions directly challenge ethnographic modes of knowledge production. This touches on a problem which has been intensely discussed in contemporary social and cultural anthropology and on which a fair amount of research[16] has already been undertaken and published: What kind of conceptual and methodological innovations are necessary in order to do justice to the complexity of global forms?

The problem has preoccupied social and cultural anthropology for at least two decades now. Conventional concepts of the local, focusing on bounded entities and emphasizing what is shared by members of a certain group, have been just as much criticized as the assumption of a territorial culture, which makes recourse to an a priori congruence of space, language and identity. Meanwhile there is an entire arsenal of terminologies to capture and analyze the increasing entanglement of widely different and remote phenomena and to illuminate the interaction between local diversifications and supra-local influences. Some of these conceptual approaches, like the research on cultural transfers, primarily focus on the aspect of mobilization through such entanglements.[17] A second group of research more strongly focuses on practices and processes of appropriation,

16 See for example Jonathan Xavier Inda & Renato Rosaldo (Eds.), *The Anthropology of Globalization.* A Reader (Malden: Blackwell, 2005); Michael Burawoy, »Introduction: Reaching for the Global«, in: *Global Ethnography. Forces, Connections, and Imaginations in a Postmodern World,* ed. by Michael Burawoy (Berkeley and Los Angeles: University of California Press, 2000), pp. 1–40; Thomas H. Hylland Eriksen (Ed.): *Globalisation – Studies in Anthropology* (London and Sterling, VA: Pluto Press, 2003).

17 Thoma Keller, Kulturtransferforschung. Grenzgänge zwischen den Kulturen. In: *Kultur. Theorien der Gegenwart,* ed. by Stephan Moebius and Dirk Quadflieg (Wiesbaden: VS Verlag für Sozialwissenschaften, 2006), pp. 101–114.

acculturation, and enculturation.[18] A third approach tries to conceptualize the results of continuous exchange with respect to the transformations of the social and cultural fabric: here transculturation, syncretism, hybridization, and creolization figure as key themes.[19] Most of these concepts imply a more or less extensive theoretical reflection about the simultaneous production of localizations and transnational connections and the emergence of global patterns/orders and problems.

The present volume is especially concerned with the methodological path an anthropology of global forms can choose and with the specific knowledge it produces. In recent years, perhaps the most influential attempt to introduce a new dynamic into contemporary ethnography has been George Marcus' program of »multi-sited« research.[20] However, the great success of this program by now has led to an overemphasis on mobility and on the spatial aspects of emerging patterns/orders. In contrast, as early as the 1990s Marilyn Strathern already stressed that it was of minor importance whether researchers did enter their field at one particular site only, whether they placed themselves in multiple sites, whether they kept themselves permanently mobile and followed their topics and subjects or whether they entered the field via online communication and with the help of their laptop.[21] According to Strathern, the crucial axis of difference and distinction nowadays is in time rather than space. What distinguishes

18 For a survey on ideas of »entering or growing into« another society, group or culture from the point of view of historical anthropology see Peter Burke, *Cultural Hybridity* (Oxford: Polity Press, 2009), in particular p. 9–40; Gerd Baumann, Riva Kastoryano, Werner Schiffauer & Stephen Vertovec have described »enculturation« as a »dynamic process of growing into« society as opposed to »acculturation« and »integration«, which they both see as tainted by ideas of assimilation; cf. Werner Schiffauer et al., *Civil Enculturation: Nation-State, Schools and Ethnic Difference in Four European Countries* (New York and Oxford, 2004).

19 For an overview see Phillipp W. Stockhammer (Eds.): *Conceptualizing Cultural Hybridization. A Transdisciplinary Approach* (Heidelberg: Springer, 2009).

20 George Marcus, »Ethnography in/of the World System: The Emergence of Multi-Sited Ethnography«, in: *Annual Review of Anthropology* 24 (1995), pp. 95–117; James D. Faubion & George E. Marcus (Eds.), *Fieldwork Is Not What It Used to Be. Learning Anthropology's Method in a Time of Transition* (Ithaca and London: Cornell University Press; 2009).

21 Marilyn Strathern, »The Ethnographic Effect I«, in: *Property, Substance and Effect. Anthropological Essays on Persons and Things* (London and New Brunswick, NJ: The Athlone Press), pp. 1–26, in particular p. 1.

the ethnographic moment from other ways of knowledge production is the idea of »immersion,« and immersion needs time.[22] The specific facility of ethnography is, that it is a »method for ›finding‹ the unlooked for.«[23] Attempts to update the program of »extended case studies,« developed by Max Gluckman and the Manchester School, focus on the temporal dynamics of translocal orders and try serial ethnography by »following cases over extended periods of time.«[24] Like restudies, such experiments with recurrent forms of participant observation are methodologically concerned with capturing gradual change and the long-term development of global assemblages. Some of the contributors to this volume use a modified form of serial ethnography in analyzing the development of reproductive technologies in different settings over a time of several years – either systematically or in a more »opportunistic« way. Apart from the dimensions of time and space of field-sites many contributions have been inspired by the proposals of James Clifford and Anna Tsing, to conceptualize ethnographic sites as places of encounter[25] and emergent contact zones[26]. Finally, the problem of how ethnography should research global forms like reproductive technologies can also be tackled by developing new forms of cooperation – this at least was one of the topics that very much concerned us during the workshop »IVF as Global Form. Ethnographic Knowledge and the Transnationalization of Reproductive Technologies,« which took place at Humboldt-University, Berlin in 2008 and which was the departure for this book. How can we design forms of international cooperation that will allow ethnographers of emergent global forms to in-

22 Loc. cit.

23 Ibid., p. 3.

24 Cf. Max Gluckman: *Analysis of a Social Situation in Modern Zululand* (Manchester: Manchester University Press, 1958); Michael Burawoy, *The Extended Case Method and Theoretical Tradition. Four Countries, Four Decades, Four Great Transformations* (Berkeley and Los Angeles: University of California Press, 2009), T.M.S. Evens & Don Handelman, *The Manchester School. Practice and Ethnographic Practice in Anthropology* (New York and Oxford: Berghahn, 2006).

25 Anna Lowenhaupt Tsing, »Conclusion: The Global Situation«, in: *The Anthropology of Globalization. A Reader*, ed. by Jonathan Xavier Inda & Renato Rosaldo (Malden, MA: Blackwell), pp. 453–486; Anna Lowenhaupt Tsing, *Friction. An Ethnography of Global Connection* (Princeton, Oxford: Princeton University Press, 2005).

26 James Clifford: *Routes. Travel and Translation in the Late Twentieth Century* (Cambridge, MA and London: Harvard University Press, 1997).

creasingly share and jointly analyze data without limiting the openness and process orientation so essential for anthropological research by a premature fixation on certain topics and approaches? How can positioned and partial insights of particular ethnographers be coordinated without totalizing claims? And how can new types of team research and cross-border collaborations be established within and across existing academic research structures?[27]

Practice, Knowledge and Transnational Encounters

The ethnographies brought together in this collection analyze local articulations as well as transnational entanglements of reproductive medicine; and they raise questions about the emergence and tentative stabilization of global forms. They ask how reproductive technologies are related to aspirations and ideas of Western and other modernities and demonstrate how they contribute to the reproduction or renewed constitution of boundaries of knowledge, agency, access and distinction. Rather than simply demonstrating diversity these case studies work towards a broader contextualizing of reproductive medicine and try to interrogate perspectives on unwanted childlessness concerning their entanglements with topics like abortion, demographic policies, gender, power relations, legal regimes, and economic conditions.

The chapters in the first section, *Localizing In Vitro Fertilization: The Cultural Work of Encounters with Medical Technologies,* explore the production of differences[28] by closely focusing on the actual work of localization. Instead of starting with a dichotomous view on global force and local response[29] they seek to trace the coproduction of the local and the translocal, of in vitro technologies and societies in diverse settings. Following Anna

27 Cf. Matsutake Worlds Research Group, »A New Form of Collaboration in Cultural Anthropology: Matsutake Worlds«, in: *American Ethnologist* 36 (2009), 29, pp. 380–403.

28 Akhil Gupta & James Ferguson, »Beyond culture: Space, identity, and the politics of difference«, in: *Cultural Anthropology* 7 (1992), 1, pp. 6–23.

29 Tsing, »The Global Situation«, op. cit. (note 25), p. 472.

Tsing's suggestion to carve out »the cultural work of encounters,«[30] they detail the emergence of »national« IVF cultures developing out of localized interactions with reproductive technologies.

Bob Simpson chronicles the arrival and dissemination of IVF since the late 1990s in Sri Lanka, a country riddled by political conflict, where regulation of in vitro technologies is weak, public attention limited, and access is restricted to a small elite. Focusing on practitioners in reproductive medicine and ethicists, Simpson reconstructs the struggles entailed in cultivating a »nationally appropriate« regulation of reproductive technologies. It must be compatible to local sensibilities and socialities and at the same time capable of demonstrating the country's participation in global scientific advance. Like Simpson, Zeynep B. Gürtin focuses on the localizing work done by professionals but her research is situated within the developed and flowering Turkish IVF sector. Gürtin portraits practitioners as interface agents simultaneously committed to negotiating local as well as transnational credibility. She particularly shows how constant practices of comparing, of defining and assigning variability and sameness are contributing to the establishment of something like »Turkish IVF,« which is simultaneously seen as »same as« and »very distinct from« global IVF forms elsewhere. Maren Klotz's contribution takes a double perspective on how families-by-sperm-donation in Germany make and maintain (transnational) connections and how her own research is implicated in this. Here, the analytical strategy centers on the complex connections between the regulation of reproductive technologies and the reflexive practices and experiences of actors in the field. Klotz raises the issue how contemporary practices of anonymous donation might be threatened by what she calls the »convergence between telecommunication or IT-based networks and kinship.« This convergence potentially undermines anonymity by making kinship knowledge »uncontainable.«

Contributions to Part II, *National Styles of Reproductive Governance and Global Forms*, focus on different styles of reproductive governance emerging out of the interaction with assisting reproductive technologies as global form. Aditya Bharadwaj points to the lack of theoretical work and critical research about transnational surrogate motherhood in India. He combines a historical perspective on sexual genealogies and gendered

30 Tsing, »Friction«, op. cit. (note 25), pp. 1–18.

asymmetries with a political anthropology of the involvement of the state. His contribution offers new interpretations of what it means to be »the other mother« in transnational surrogacy today. Viola Hörbst provides a detailed case study of the local and transnational articulation of assisting reproductive technologies in Mali, one of the poorest nations in the world. There, a limited array of reproductive technologies is available for a small urban, often transnationally oriented, elite only. Her work chronicles how the local governance of reproductive technologies in Mali is deeply entangled with trans- and international reproductive institutions. These center on poverty, high Malian birth rates, the dangers of »overpopulation« and development; leaving almost no space for a political awareness of the plights of the involuntary childless. Equally targeting the conjunctions of transnational institutions and local subjectivities and agencies, Nurhak Polat presents results from her ethnographic study of a concerned group of patient-consumers in and around Istanbul. Her perspective on this new actor in the field of reproductive governance is particularly concerned with the knowledge practices of this group and their narrative, economical, and political interventions in regulation, markets, and medical practice.

Transnational Reproductive Mobilities und Figurations

Whereas the chapters in Part I and II of this volume are more concerned with the localizing pole of global forms, contributions to Part III and IV give their empirical and theoretical attention to transnational entanglements and reproductive mobility. Ethnographic research along the routes of reproductive travel – of users and practitioners, standards and equipment, hormones and other bodily substances – or within transnational clusters of intensified clinical cooperation in infertility treatment has been taken up only recently. Six essays in this volume empirically investigate transnational reproductive mobilities and figurations in different world regions. Their dynamics and structures are not easily mapped and cannot be explained by center and periphery patterns alone. In Section III, *Tracing Transnational Scapes of Reproductive Technologies: Emergent Forms and Domains of Regulation,* Marcia Inhorn introduces the Middle East as a »key site for understanding current intersections of technoscience, religious morality, and modernity.« Focusing on the experiences and movements of involuntarily childless couples from a number of Middle Eastern states, Inhorn provides an analysis of the complex legal topography of bans on third-party gamete donation in Sunni Muslim-majority countries and on the permission of donor technologies in Shia Muslim-majority countries, particularly in Iran and Lebanon. This constellation has considerably intensified transnational reproductive mobility across the Middle East. Eva Maria Knoll charts in a similar way the border crossing activities and grey zones generated by the national ban on egg donation in Austria and follows women and couples in search of female gametes to Hungary. Under-regulation, half-hearted firewalls drawn up against the commercialization of human ova or embryos and a certain degree of elbowroom have made available very different, sometimes antagonistic policies and practices in three researched Hungarian IVF-clinics. Maren Klotz and Michi Knecht in their joint contribution focus on the unintended consequences of the implementation of the EU-tissue directive – a transnational piece of regulation – in a German sperm bank in 2007. Their case study is concerned with a conceptual rethinking of the ethnography of Europeanization as an exemplary transnational process and with the way in which not only laws, but also standards and often neglected infrastructural details have far reaching effects on how reproductive technologies allow to do kinship.

Section IV, *Transnational Reproductive Mobilities, Materialities and Agencies,* continues the exploration of transnational reproductive mobilities and figurations, but foregrounds reflections on research practice and politics, analytical tools and conceptual questions. Michal Nahman opens this part of the volume with a case study situated in an Israeli ova extraction clinic in Romania. Difficult encounters, antagonistic aspirations of clinic operators, young Romanian ova sellers and Israeli ova recipients, and the awareness of conflicting ethical regimes – global forms of their own – all prompt questions on the politics of (public) anthropology in such a setting. They also raise questions on the possibilities and potentials of ethnographic knowledge as a contribution to the situation itself. In his analysis of reproductive mobility at fertility clinics in Spain and the Czech Republic, Sven Bergmann points to emerging transnational »cultures of disguise« and the practices of anonymity and fabricating resemblance, that are connected with them. Again taking the trade in egg cells as ethnographic example, he analyzes matching strategies, synchronization practices, and the production and safeguarding of supply and demand in situations of starkly-stratified transnational interaction and encounter.

In the final contribution to this volume, Stefan Beck reconstructs the reflexive practices of diverse actors that generate the transnational spaces of reproductive technologies and a new *body cosmo-politic*. Taking as his examples a Cypriot patient organization, and different forms of collaboration and *knowledge-franchising* between Turkish clinics and their international partners, Beck in his descriptions and interpretations experiments with a vocabulary that no longer takes nation states as blueprint for the analysis of transnational conjunctures and global forms.

Outlook

The articles brought together in this volume demonstrate the strength of ethnographic accounts to analyze the diverse local articulations as well as the transnational entanglements of reproductive medicine. In vitro-fertilization and other related medical technologies like for instance the biobanking of gametes, pre-implantation genetic diagnosis etc. together constitute a global form, an assemblage of knowledge and technologies that is enacted in quite diverse social and cultural contexts; that is used by a range of actors for quite divergent purposes; and that raises different questions for different actors. Reproductive technologies have challenged kinship as a central »imaginary institution« of Western and non-Western modernities alike – and they will do so in the near future as new technologies and procedures will be developed and be made available on a global scale. The task of anthropology will not simply be to demonstrate that reproductive medicine is implemented and put to use quite differently in diverse socio-cultural contexts, but to use this field-experiment to inquire how demographic policies, gender- and power-relations, legal regimes, and economic conditions shape and are shaped by this global form.

Five Million Miracle Babies Later: The Biocultural Legacies of IVF

Sarah Franklin

Introduction

Accompanying the birth of approximately five million babies worldwide through IVF over the past 30 years, in what is arguably one of the largest human reproductive experiments ever undertaken, has been the ongoing effort to understand and characterize the biocultural legacies of this technique's success »in man.«[1] The effort to understand these legacies traverses a range of disciplines – from politics and ethics to anthropology and economics – and this volume represents a significant contribution to the documentation of IVF's global proliferation and diversification. The question of what it means to be »after IVF« has at least two different meanings. One is historical: humanity now exists after the fact of successful human IVF (since 1978 or 1969, depending on whether IVF is taken to refer to the fertilization of a human egg or the birth of viable human offspring). This new biological fact of human existence is now part of the human condition, a »fact of life.« A second sense of »after« describes the somewhat more complicated project of re-engineering human biological futures that is now to a certain extent modeled on IVF. The question here is one of style: to what extent are biological systems increasingly refashioned and restyled »after« IVF, in the sense that IVF »modeled« a technologically assisted *in vitro* replica of conception that became at once synonymous with and different from »the real thing«?[2] This could be called life's imitation

1 This chapter is a rewritten version of the keynote address to the conference on which this volume is based. My thanks to the organizers of this event and the editors of this volume who very kindly invited me to participate in both projects.

2 Perhaps one of the most dramatic examples of this modelling effect is the extent to which earth is compared to a microorganism in the work of prominent climate change theorists such as James Lovelock, whose Gaia model is closely based on the symbi-

of life, and effects its doubling, or supplementation, as life and »biolife.« If one of the most revolutionary features of IVF, paradoxically, is how unremarkable this form of bespoke human life has become in the relatively short period of three decades since its highly controversial debut in Greater Manchester, what does this tell us about the cultural status of biological facts more broadly – indeed the »facts of life,« or »biolife« – that are newly modeled upon, and literally reproduced through, human in vitro culture systems? Arguably one of the possibilities this rapid normalization of IVF suggests about the future of biological control is that *the fusion of biology and technological control* has somewhat ironically »naturalized« a condition we could describe as that of being *biologically relative*. Increasingly, the biological exists *relative to* technological control. And this, in turn, has become a condition that throws into question what »human biology« refers to »itself.«[3]

A biocultural history of IVF enables us to engage these questions empirically, as well as ethically and politically. Such a history must consider the genealogical legacies of IVF in the double sense of »genealogical«: how we inherit them in direct, or proximate, historical time, and in the more diffuse Foucauldian sense of the often paradoxical unfolding of interwoven events that opposes singular or ultimate origins.[4] It is the combination

---

otic theories of evolution of the microbiologist Lynn Margulis. »Re-engineering« the earth's future survival along the lines of the positive and negative feedback systems and loops proposed by Lovelock, among others, epitomizes the »earth as a Petri dish« model that constitutes the paradigm of biolife. See James E. Lovelock & Lynn Margulis, »Atmospheric Homeostasis by and for the Biosphere: The Gaia Hypothesis«, in: *Tellus*, 26 (1974), 1/2, pp. 2–10; Lynn Margulis & James Lovelock, »Biological Modulation of the Earth's Atmosphere« in: *Icarus* 21 (1974), 4, pp. 471–489.

3 In respect of Foucault's (1973) famous declaration that life »itself« was only conceivable as a result of the emergence of modern biology (»itself« in turn the result of the emergence of the evolutionary view of life's emergence), we might, in the wake of cloning and the human genome project, now argue that there is no such thing as either life »itself« or biology »itself.« Both life and biology are now analyzed under a looser set of definitions, closely bound up with technology, in a manner closer to their classical enunciation as *physis* – as physical form – or as chemistry. We might say, for example, that all of life is the same as »chemistry itself« – except that this does not really say anything. Michel Foucault, *The Order of Things: An Archaeology of the Human Sciences* (New York: Vintage, 1973).

4 Foucault was particularly interested in genealogy as a means of tracing power, or power as it constituted subjects. He was also concerned to provide a history for elements of

of these two that I refer to as the »thick genealogies« of biotechnical innovation.[5] In this sense, IVF itself can be analyzed as a »culture medium« – a continuous history of biotechnical innovation that derives from deliberate human intention, but which also changes the terms of such aspirations, as it also changes the conditions of human life.[6] This approach enables us to examine the histories that have helped to shape human IVF and their dialectical relationship to the post-IVF imaginaries that in turn have reconstituted reproductive hopes and reproductive choices, while giving birth to new reproductive technologies and transforming the science of reproductive biology.[7] A question we might prioritize is what the history of IVF in both animals and humans can tell us about the changing meanings of biological reproduction, reproductive biology, or the biological more

human life that are often imagined as ahistorical, such as sexuality or biology. Reproduction, of course, fits into this model very »naturally.«

5 Sarah Franklin, *Dolly Mixtures: The Remaking of Genealogy* (Durham, NC: Duke University Press, 2007).

6 In contrast to the presumption in much 20th century philosophy that *techne* exists in tension with humanity (e.g. Heidegger, Habermas, Marcuse, or Arendt), anthropological accounts of technology more closely resemble the tradition established through Marx and Engels, according to which humans both shape and are shaped by their tools – dialectally; see Frederick Engels, »The Part Played by Labour in the Transition from Ape to Man«, in: *Selected Works, Karl Marx and Frederick Engels* (Volume 2) (Moscow: Foreign Language Publishing House, 1962). This is also the approach developed out of the material structuralism of the French anthropologist Leroi-Gourhan that is continued in the work of Derrida, among others. For anthropologists such as Malinowski, tools were interpreted in the Maussian tradition – as »total social facts.« A slightly different approach was developed by the pioneering feminist Shulamith Firestone, whose enthusiastic technofuturism drew in no small part on the example set by the British socialist biofuturists of the interwar period, such as Haldane, Huxley, and Waddington, see Sarah Franklin, »Revisiting Reprotech: Firestone and the Question of Technology«, in: *Further Adventures of the Dialectic of Sex: Critical Essays on Shulamith Firestone*, ed. by Mandy Merck & Stella Stanford (London: Palgrave, 2010), pp. 29–60. One question motivating this chapter is what it means for a human embryo to become a tool.

7 An interesting example in this context is the argument made by eco-futurist Stewart Brand, founder of the *Whole Earth Catalogue*, who suggested to the Financial Times in an interview about his recent book, *Whole Earth Discipline*, that IVF was a good model for the beneficence of technological engineering solutions applied to the most elementary processes of biology and biochemistry. See Stewart Brand, *Whole Earth Discipline: An Ecopragmatist Manifesto* (London: Viking, 2009); Stewart Brand, »Lunch with the FT«, interviewed by David Honigmann, in: *Financial Times*, 8 January 2010.

widely. What kinds of future imaginaries engender, or are evoked by, the increasing number of technologies through which reproduction is variously assisted and remade?[8]

The IVF Platform

An example of how the history of IVF unfolds into the present is its new interface with stem cell research.[9] Over the course of its development in mammals, the IVF technique gradually evolved from an experimental scientific method into a variety of clinical and agricultural applications.[10] Since its successful translation into human clinical medicine in 1978, IVF has similarly undergone a rapid evolution as a platform for newer techniques such as intracytoplasmic sperm injection (ICSI) and preimplantation genetic diagnosis (PGD). The vast increase in the scale of human IVF now undertaken worldwide, combined with the ease of cryopreservation and storage of fertilized eggs, embryos, and blastocysts, means that IVF has

8 See, for example, Adele Clarke's pioneering work *Disciplining Reproduction*, in which she charts the emergence of reproductive biology and »the problems of sex« in the 20th century. Adele E. Clarke, *Disciplining Reproduction: American Life Sciences and »The Problems of Sex«* (Berkeley: University of California Press, 1998). See also Hannah Landecker, *How Cells Became Technologies* (Cambridge, MA: Harvard University Press, 2006).

9 Sarah Franklin, »The Cyborg Embryo: Our Path to Transbiology«, in: *Theory, Culture and Society* 23 (2006a), 7/8, pp. 167–188; Sarah Franklin, »The IVF-Stem Cell Interface«, in: *International Journal of Surgery* 4 (2006), 2, pp. 86–90.

10 For useful histories of IVF, see John D. Biggers, »In Vitro Fertilization and Embryo Transfer in Historical Perspective«, in: *In Vitro Fertilization and Embryo Transfer*, ed. by Alan O. Trounson & Carl Wood (London: Churchill Livingstone,1984), pp. 3–15; Jack Challoner, *The Baby Makers: The History of Artificial Conception* (London: Macmillan, 1999); Robert G. Edwards, »The Bumpy Road to Human In Vitro Fertilization«, in: *Nature Medicine* 7 (2001), 10, pp. 1091–1094; Simon Fishel & Edward M. Symonds (Eds.), *In Vitro Fertilisation: Past, Present, Future* (Oxford: IRL Press, 1986); or Robin M. Henig, *Pandora's Baby: How the First Test Tube Babies Sparked the Reproductive Revolution* (Boston, Houghton Mifflin, 2004). For useful feminist histories see Clarke, »Disciplining Reproduction«, op. cit. (note 8); Gena Corea, *The Mother Machine: Reproductive Technologies from Artificial Insemination to Artificial Wombs* (New York: Harper & Row, 1985); or Naomi Pfeffer, *The Stork and the Syringe: A Political History of Reproductive Medicine* (Cambridge: Polity, 1993).

become intimately linked with the futures of stem cell research, tissue engineering, and regenerative medicine. In sum, the IVF industry generates what is now called »the embryo supply« or more specifically »the population« of research embryos, the preservation, governance, use, and handling of which has required the development of new forms of biological control and quality control that are deemed necessary for the manufacture of safe, reliable, and ethical human cell-based products.[11] Without IVF, human embryonic stem cell (hES) research would be impossible, and the new epigenetic understandings of basic cellular processes that are central to these fields, such as imprinting, reprogramming, methylation, and dedifferentiation, could not be studied (»in man«) during the crucial early embryonic stages of development when they are most accessible experimentally (*in vitro*). Retaining a lead at the bioknowledge horizons of this high-profile research frontier is a major economic priority of both the UK government and the EU, especially with the US doubly hampered by Right-to-Life and controversies over patenting and intellectual property.[12]

In the UK the strong government push to accelerate hES derivation is evident in a new generation of specialized labs that have been commissioned and built over the past 5 years. They are designed to facilitate the most efficient, economical, and ethically robust use of human research embryos produced in the UK. These new labs embody the goal of enhancing UK hES derivation, banking, and standardization, with a view to establishing a new source of »life stock,« or biolife, that promises, in the neoliberal parlance of successive governments, »substantial health and wealth deliverables« for future Britons and their offspring.

I visited the largest and most state-of-the-art of these new laboratories at Guy's Hospital in London in the autumn of 2008 with three of my research colleagues. Professor Peter Braude, a consultant obstetrician, ge-

11 Sarah Franklin, »Embryonic Economies: The Double Reproductive Value of Stem Cells«, in: *Biosocieties* 1 (2006c), 1, pp. 71–90.

12 For an international perspective on the stem cell debate see Ingrid Geesink, Barbara Prainsack, & Sarah Franklin (Eds.), *Science as Culture Special Issue: Stem Cell Stories 1998–2008* 17 (2008), 1; Barbara Prainsack, Ingrid Geesink & Sarah Franklin (Eds.), *Science as Culture Special Issue: Stem Cell Technologies 1998–2008* 17 (2008), 4; and Herman Gottweis, Brian Salter & Catherine Waldby, *The Global Politics of Human Embryonic Stem Cell Science: Regenerative Medicine in Transition* (London: Palgrave, 2009).

neticist, and head of the lab, led the tour. The timing was ideal because the lab was just beginning the process of decontamination. So we could see everything and wander round freely without wearing bunny suits and masks. Peter's is the largest of seven new UK labs that have been constructed with government funding to bring IVF and human embryonic stem cell derivation physically closer together, so that any spare or clinically useless embryos can go straight into a quality controlled cleanroom laboratory if a couple decides to donate them to research (which approximately 70% of those asked in the UK will be likely to do). The new labs are thus designed to join together a so-called »dirty« surgical room, where eggs are aspirated from women patients undergoing IVF, with a »clean« laboratory that complies with the highest quality standards of sterility. The two rooms are separated by a hatch, or hole in the wall. The eggs go through the hatch to be fertilized, and, if they grow and develop normally, one of them returns through the door to be transferred into the uterus of a woman IVF patient. Other fertilized eggs or embryos can be frozen for future use, donated to other couples for treatment, donated to research, or disposed of, depending on what the IVF patients decide to do with them.

The new labs offer a path forward – in the current idiom of scientific innovation they represent the cutting edge of *biomedical translation*. What the Food and Drug Administration (FDA) denominates as »the critical path« is the path to application (now known as translation) and thus not only a movement »from bench to bedside« but »from bench to market.« The labs manifest this ambition as a bespoke, purpose-built architecture to facilitate more efficient use of the embryo supply by creating a direct interface between IVF clinics (or Assisted Reproductive Technology, ART) and hES derivation, storage, and banking. They establish a new state of ART. At the IVF-stem cell interface is a new form of passaging human gametes and embryos, not only from one dish to another or even from one room to the next, but from a specific clinical context (a patient having treatment in a surgery) to a new biological order of things (quality controlled facilities that can be process-validated for the safe handling of human cell-based products – a.k.a. the future production of clean and certified human cell-based biological products). This form of propagating human cells represents the latest evolution of the IVF platform – broadly speaking it enables IVF to become a source of embryo supply for regenerative medicine.

Embryo Movements

What I realized as I investigated the embryo transfers through the hatch at the IVF-stem cell interface was that this interface is not as new as it seemed. IVF and stem cell research come from the same stable, and the story of their co-culture is a well-established theme in historical accounts by scientists active in these fields.[13] Although novel, the transfer of eggs and embryos through the hole in the wall of the cleanroom is only the latest extension to a chain of embryo transfers that define the origins not only of IVF and stem cell research, but experimental embryology and the study of biological development – especially in the late 20th century, especially in mammals, and especially in the British Isles.[14]

These egg and embryo movements, or transfers, have been a staple technique of reproductive and developmental biology since the late 19th century, and their practical applications in livestock breeding have had enormous consequences for world agriculture as well as zoological conservation (especially in combination with cryopreservation). Indeed, one of the simplest means of tracking the history of IVF is by tracing the extension of these transfers from animals into humans – or indeed by considering IVF itself as a »critical path« of embryological knowledge transfer. In other words, IVF was the translational bridge that enabled ET to make its »human turn« – initially as a means of redressing the burden of human reproductive and developmental deficits, later for stem cell research, and now for regenerative medicine. The ET of »IVF and ET,« which is used to describe the surgical transfer of an embryo into an IVF patient's uterus, belongs to a long lineage of related, or ancestral, embryo transfers extend-

13 Cf. Edwards, »The Bumpy Road«, op. cit. (note 10).

14 Chris Graham, »Mammalian Development in the UK (1950–1995)«, in: *International Journal of Developmental Biology* 44 (2000), pp. 51–55. For an important cultural history of this British interest in »babies in bottles« see Susan M. Squier, *Babies in Bottles: Twentieth-Century Visions of Reproductive Technology* (New Brunswick, NJ: Rutgers University Press, 1994).

ing back at least a century.[15] Today, human embryo transfer belongs to an expanding global diaspora of reproductive trafficking, or »tourism«[16] as well as to networks of international scientific exchanges, commercial transactions for research eggs and embryos, and biobanking.[17]

This global movement of embryos is part of a dialectic of translation through which new knowledges generate new applications, and vice versa. IVF and ET epitomize this process, having an equally robust importance on both sides of the »pure« and »applied« domains of the biological sciences. As I argued in my previous work on cloning, embryo exchanges continue to cement clinical-scientific collaborations in the busily expanding bioscientific present, just as they have done historically by facilitating mutually beneficial veterinary-scientific and agro-scientific partnerships (such as those uniting Britain and Australia in livestock breeding).[18] At work propelling embryos through the doors of the new labs at the IVF-stem cell interface, then, are historically well-established goals of maximizing efficiency through cooperation, promoting economic growth, exchanging scientific knowledge and materials, and generating technological progress as well as »paybacks« to the general public (who funds much of the research). The new labs express the intention to rationalize the thousands of transfers of research embryos all over the UK, to standardize and validate

15 Cf. Keith J. Betteridge, »An Historical Look at Embryo Transfer«, in: *Reproduction and Fertility* 62 (1981), pp. 1–13; Keith J. Betteridge, »A History of Farm Animal Embryo Transfer and Some Associated Techniques«, in: *Animal Production Science* 79 (2003), 3, pp.203–244; or Biggers, »In vitro fertilization and Embryo Transfer«, op. cit. (note 10).

16 See contributions by Sven Bergmann, Marcia Inhorn and Michal Nahman in this volume.

17 This practice, which conjoins modern transportation with culture and cryopreservation methods to enable a complex worldwide trade in human germplasm, extends the long history of livestock egg and embryo transfers, some of which as early as the 1950s were co-sponsored by commercial airlines such as TWA. The airline industry also features prominently in the online video promoting the American Embryo Transfer Association and its goal of »Global Genetic Improvement through Embryo Technology« (www.aeta.org).

18 Franklin, »Dolly Mixtures«, op. cit. (note 5); Sarah Franklin, »Crook Pipettes: Anglo-Australian Exchanges in Embryology«, in: *Journal of the History of Biology*, Special Issue, ed. by Sarah Wilmot, »From Farm to Clinic«, December (2007); Ian Wilmut, Keith Campbell & Colin Tudge, *Second Creation: Dolly and the Age of Biological Control* (London: Headline, 2000).

procedures, to increase biosecurity and ethical oversight, and eventually to remunerate the British population through »health and wealth gains« in the future.

Although the new labs facilitate more proximate transfers of IVF embryos directly into stem cell research, they are also embedded in a larger system of national embryo exchanges reflecting the specialist expertise in different research centers. Thus, in a complex national choreography of embryo movements, Manchester sends its »failed to fertilize« embryos to Edinburgh, while Leeds sends its past-their-shelflife frozen and research-consented embryos to York. London sends others to Cambridge, which also collects up unused local embryos when they are available. It may well be that a distinctively new type of transfer occurs when the human embryo is passed through the hole in the wall, or the hatch, from the »dirty« IVF surgery into the cleanroom, with quality control and graded air.[19] But it was only after several years of studying the future of these transfers, and the expansion of the IVF-stem cell interface through new labs such as the one in London, that I began to realize that embryo transfer is the signature theme, and conduit, of a much longer history.

In other words, the new future-oriented embryo transfer involved in the passage from the dirty surgery into the clean derivation laboratory at the IVF-stem cell interface is the offspring of a complex genealogy of kindred embryo transfers stretching back more than a century to the first, and most famous, transfer of mammalian reproductive cells – that of Walter Heape, who transferred eggs from one rabbit to another in 1890 to determine the influence of uterine foster mothers on the genetic constitution of their offspring.[20] Embryo transfer is both a core idiom and a basic experimental method in the medical, scientific, and agricultural lineages to which contemporary human IVF and its stem cell interface are heir. As

19 See Franklin, »The Cyborg Embryo«, op. cit. (note 9); Franklin, »The IVF-Stem Cell Interface«, op. cit. (note 9); Franklin, »Embryonic Economies«, op. cit. (note 11).

20 For a review of the history of embryo transfer in light of the work of Walter Heape, see Biggers, »In vitro fertilization and Embryo Transfer«, op. cit. (note 10). See also Betteridge, »An Historical Look«, op. cit. (note 15) or Betteridge, »A History of Farm Animal Embryo Transfer«, op. cit. (note 15). For the original procedure, see Walter Heape, »Preliminary Note on the Transplantation and Growth of Mammalian Ova within a Uterine Foster Mother«, in: *Proceedings of the Royal Society* 48 (1891), pp. 457–458.

a consequence, and crucially, embryo transfer is both a way of knowing and an output, a product and an application, a technique and a world-view. What is important about »IVF and Embryo Transfer« is that, like nuclear transfer, it fuses research technique, proof, experimental material, knowledge generation, and application not only with the reproductive process itself (which becomes both a tool and an outcome, or »deliverable«) but with a new, aspirational (sic.) ethos of reproductive control and improvement – whereby the control, the improvement, and the reproductive process »itself« become impossible to separate. This is the fusion which IVF epitomizes.

The IVF Synechdoche

In pursuing the genealogical question of how the biocultural history of IVF is linked to its future, it is important to point out that although this question can be described as understudied, there are notable exceptions. Feminists and anthropologists were among the first to provide empirical and theoretical accounts exploring how we might reckon the forms of cultural change associated with the dawn of the *in vitro* human embryo – itself, of course, a product of improved culture medium.[21] Among the

21 The prescient work of Shulamith Firestone deserves special mention: Shulamith Firestone, *The Dialectic of Sex: The Case for Feminist Revolution* (New York: Bantam, 1970); or see Franklin, »Revisiting Reprotech«, op. cit. (note 6). For early feminist accounts of IVF, see Rita Arditti, Renate Duelli Klein & Shelley Minden (Eds.), *Test-Tube Women: What Future for Motherhood?* (London: Pandora. 1984); Lynda Birke, Susan Himmelweit & G. Vines, *Tomorrow's Child: Reproductive Technologies in the 90s* (London: Virago, 1990); Corea, »The Mother Machine«, op. cit. (note 10); Christine Crowe, »Women Want It: In Vitro Fertilisation and Women's Motivations for Participation«, in: *Women's Studies International Forum* 8 (1985), pp. 547–552; Renate Klein, *Infertility: Women Speak Out About their Experiences of Reproductive Medicine* (London: Pandora, 1989); Lene Koch, »IVF – An Irrational Choice?«, in: *Reproductive and Genetic Engineering* 3 (1990), pp. 225–232; Maria Mies, »›Why Do We Need All This?‹: A Call Against Genetic Engineering and Reproductive Technology«, in: *Women's Studies International Forum* 8 (1985), 6, pp. 553–560; Barbara Katz Rothman, *The Tentative Pregnancy: How Amniocentesis Changes the Experience of Motherhood* (New York: Norton, 1986); Margarete Sandelowski, »Women's Experience of Infertility«, in: *Journal of Nursing Scholarship* (1986); Margarete Sandelowski, »Fault

most prominent scholars to have considered this topic is Marilyn Strathern, who argued in the early 1990s that the most significant legacy of IVF is *a new reproductive model* in which »the natural facts« of sexual reproduction are understood as *engineerable*, *replaceable*, and *intervenable*.[22] Strathern argued this new understanding of conception affected the ability of natural facts to operate as a »grounding function« for other meanings. IVF thus not only altered the facts of life, it altered the way a naturalized model of the facts of life could establish a context, a background, or a »before« for the social. Indeed, the way in which nature provides a model for context is arguably one of the things that has been changed »*after IVF*.«[23]

Especially in the wake of cloning, stem cells, and the human genome project, as we enter the »age of biology« in the wake of what has been called »biology's big bang,« it sometimes seems that the importance of IVF as a new model of biological facts has been overshadowed by the cloning

Lines: Infertility and Imperilled Sisterhood«, in: *Feminist Studies* 16 (1990), 1, pp. 33–51; Margarete Sandelowski »Compelled to Try: the Never-Enough Quality of Reproductive Technology«, in: *Medical Anthropology Quarterly* 5 (1991), 1, pp. 29–47; Margarete Sandelowski, *With Child In Mind: Studies of the Personal Encounter With Infertility* (Philadephia: University of Pennsylvania Press, 1993); Patricia Spallone & Deborah Lynn Steinberg (Eds.), *Made to Order: The Myth of Reproductive and Genetic Progress* (London: Pergamon, 1987); and Michelle Stanworth (Ed.), *Reproductive Technologies: Gender, Motherhood and Medicine* (Cambridge: Polity, 1987). For a summary of feminist monographs on IVF see Sarah Franklin & Maureen McNeil, »Reproductive Futures: Recent Literature and Current Debates on Reproductive Technologies«, in: *Feminist Studies* 14 (1988), 3, pp. 545–561; for later debates see Dion Farquhar, *The Other Machine: Discourse and Reproductive Technologies* (New York: Routledge, 1996). For more recent feminist monographs on IVF, see Gay Becker, *The Elusive Embryo: How Women and Men Approach New Reproductive Technologies* (Berkeley: University of California, 2000); Sarah Franklin, *Embodied Progress: A Cultural Account of Assisted Conception* (London: Routledge, 1997); Debora Spar, *The Baby Business: How Money, Science, and Politics Drive the Commerce of Conception* (Cambridge, MA: Harvard Business School Press, 2006); Charis Thompson, *Making Parents: The Ontological Choreography of Reproductive Technologies* (Cambridge, MA: MIT Press, 2005); and Karen Throsby, *When IVF Fails: Feminism, Infertility and the Negotiation of Normality* (London: Palgrave, 2004).

22 Marilyn Strathern, *After Nature: English Kinship in the Late Twentieth Century* (Cambridge: Cambridge University Press, 1992); Marilyn Strathern, *Reproducing the Future: Anthropology, Kinship and the New Reproductive Technologies* (Manchester: Manchester University Press, 1992).

23 Sarah Franklin, Celia Lury & Jackie Stacey, *Global Nature, Global Culture* (London: Sage, 2000).

of Dolly the sheep (quickly followed by stem cell science, regenerative medicine, and synthetic biology). Five million miracle babies later, however, we might look back on Dolly mania and the stem cell wars as delayed reactions. Why else would the birth of a sheep or a few dishes of skin cells occasion such global diplomatic consternation if not that it confirmed exactly the same sequence inaugurated by IVF, which was developed in sheep as a model for humans? Is it perhaps that cloned sheep and cell lines did not presage a Brave New Biology so much as reveal the significance of *what had already happened in 1978*? Can we not see in the writings of Frances Fukuyama, Bill McKibben, or Jürgen Habermas examples of this oversight in their identification of PGD, the so-called designer-baby technique, developed 12 years after IVF and never practiced on anything like its scale, as the threshold technique auguring a loss of our humanity?[24] Doesn't IVF demonstrate that the most relevant question about technologically assisted futures is not if or when they will make us post- or transhuman, but whether those conditions have already been normalized by the reproductive model of ART, through which offspring are born whose »artificial conception« both embodies and confirms the benefits of scientific progress by incorporating technology into the human germline?[25]

Of course when we speak of »IVF« we run into problems right away, since this term, as many feminists have pointed out, nominates the center of action as the fertilization of an egg in a Petri dish.[26] As the abbreviated name for a lengthy and complex procedure, »IVF« effects both a detachment and a substitution in the process of becoming symbolic shorthand for reproductive biomedicine as a whole. Controversially successful in hu-

24 Cf. Francis Fukuyama, *Our Posthuman Future* (New York: Farrar, Strauss & Giroux, 2002); Bill McKibben, *Enough: Staying Human in an Engineered Age* (London: Macmillan, 2003); or Jürgen Habermas, *The Future of Human Nature* (Cambridge: Polity, 2003).

25 The larger question about technology and human regeneration has been mentioned earlier, and could be seen through the emergence of agriculture to have already become part of the human condition, and thus human biology, much earlier. This is argued, for example, by both Marx and Engels, who describe both agriculture and industrialization as dialectical historical processes that have literally reshaped the human body. See Engels, »The Part Played by Labour«, op. cit. (note 6). In this sense we could argue technology is »already genetic.«

26 E.g. Deborah Steinberg, *Bodies in Glass: Genetics, Eugenics and Embryo Ethics* (Manchester: Manchester University Press, 1997).

mans at the end of the 1970s, IVF came to signify a triumphant coupling of social will to scientific potency in the service of creating new families: in the media, Parliament, and in mainstream public discourse, IVF was defended because of what it *delivered*, in the form not only of healthy take-home babies but as proof of the benefits of modern scientific progress.[27] It could even be argued that IVF was imagined to manifest human biological destiny as a technological solution to the suffering of infertility and genetic disease. The technique »itself« thus became, among other things, the placeholder for an evolving social contract whereby the moral obligation to improve the human condition could be pursued by increasingly »radical« technological means, so long as they were proven safe and subject to appropriate regulation. Increasingly, the proof of this contract's ethical validity – and the basis of its widespread popular acceptance – is found in the lives of children conceived through IVF who would not otherwise have been born.

This is why it is important to consider what »IVF« has come to mean, to stand for, and to symbolize, as both a method and a metaphor for coming into being, for »reproduction,« and for technologically assisted human reproductive futures more generally – and thus for the meaning of »biological control« writ large. If »IVF« is, among other things, an abbreviation for a new conception model in which biology and engineering are united in the name of an improved human future, realized literally at the moment of fertilization in glass, how can we evaluate its significance forty years and five million offspring later? As well as being an abbreviation, a metaphor, a symbol and a model, »IVF« is a synechdoche, a part that stands for the whole – as in boards for stage, sail for ship, or man for human. In sum, it shows us that reproductive control is in many ways the template for what is now known as »biological control.«

But it also tells us a great deal about the biopolitics of such a situation. As many feminists have pointed out, the part that is named, or acronymed, in IVF – *in vitro* fertilization – is technically the part of the procedure that is furthest removed from the woman patient, or couple, undergoing it. Fertilization *in vitro*, which takes place over a period of 24 hours in an incubator, is a notoriously unpleasant hiatus of anxious, passive waiting for IVF patients, who can do nothing but sit by the phone

27 Franklin, »Embodied Conception«, op. cit. (note 20).

while they wait to see how many, if any, eggs have fertilized, and if so how well. Non-fertilization *in vitro* is the statistically more likely outcome of this penultimate stage in a cycle, and such 'non-events' are typically unexplained. The name of the procedure – IVF – is thus partial, and anticipatory, or even optimistic, in referring to a process that occurs only in a minority of cycles. When cycles fail, which they still do roughly 75% more often than they succeed, they are said to have been »abandoned.« A young healthy woman at a top IVF clinic has about a 50–50 chance of succeeding on her first cycle. If her first cycle fails, her chances of ever succeeding drop precipitously, initially by another 25%, and further with each subsequent cycle. The longer she has treatment, the older she is, and since age is a primary determinant of successful IVF, her worsening odds are compounded over time. »Successful IVF« requires much more than successful fertilization *in vitro* – which itself comes relatively late in the sequence of procedures that will only lead to a successful outcome in a minority of cases.

We use »IVF« because it is shorthand, and it is not the only medical technique whose popular moniker is an abbreviation. It is habitual to over-condense technological agency through such shorthand – as in the »IT revolution,« as if IT were the cause when it is a collective noun and an abstraction. Similarly at issue in the »history of IVF« is the common tendency to reify technology as the source of social or historical action – as in the »impact« of this or that new discovery, or the influence of »TV.« Technology »itself« did not bring about the first successful extra-corporeal human conception: the technology, and more importantly the aims and goals that inspired the development of the technology, had to be imagined, desired, funded, legitimated, and tenaciously pursued in order to succeed, and this was done exclusively by *people*. Pressure from patients throughout the 1970s played an important role in the development of successful IVF techniques, as did the ambitions and perseverance of Robert Edwards indexEdwards, RobertindexEdwards, Jeanetteand Patrick Steptoe, their dedicated research team headed by Jean Purdy, the nursing staff of the Oldham Infirmary, various colleagues who provided the team with eggs, equipment, energy, and encouragement, and the many women and couples who agreed to take part in what was until 1978 still an unproven method of overcoming infertility. The momentum building towards the eventual clinical application of IVF was increasingly evident as its success in other mammals became well established from the 1950s onwards (often, ironically, as part of the effort to develop better contraceptives). All of these efforts were fueled by expectations and anticipations that in turn were shaped by cultural values, such as the sense of obligation to alleviate human suffering, and to improve human futures.[28]

IVF as a Means

Although it is problematic to reify »IVF« as a causal agent or as an inevitable outcome of scientific and technological advances, however, it is nonetheless important to address its specificity as a technology, and to chart its genealogy as the offspring of a specific intellectual, political, and experimental culture – for example the British biological pragmatism born out of food shortages, livestock management, family planning, and later the post-war emphasis on energy and radiation. Like the discovery of the structure of DNA, IVF is an offspring of shifting national, economic, and military priorities in the UK in the immediate aftermath of World War II. The IVF story, like that of somatic cell nuclear transfer (a.k.a. Dolly), unfolds at the intersection of agriculture, science, and medicine and within the intertwined histories of developmental biology and genetics, as they in turn are shaped by the socio-political influences of both institutions and individuals.[29]

Without attributing to IVF »itself« an agency or causality, however, it is still important to engage with IVF as a *means*. It does not have to be posited that IVF had inherent properties or potentials in order to claim that its successful development in humans has made other, subsequent technological achievements possible – such as human embryonic stem cell research, for example. In this sense IVF *is itself a kind of transfer*, or »bridge,« enabling

28 Robert G. Edwards & Patrick Steptoe, *A Matter of Life: The Story of a Medical Breakthrough* (London: Hutchinson, 1980).

29 Sarah Wilmot (Ed.), »Between the Farm and the Clinic: Agriculture and Reproductive Technology in the Twentieth Century«, Special Issue, *Studies in History and Philosophy of Science Part C: Studies in History and Philosophy of Biology and Biomedical Science* 38 (2007), 2.

new possibilities for *in vitro* human embryo culture – such as improvements in preimplantation genetic diagnosis (which, although developed in tandem with IVF and stem cells, was not clinically successful until 1990). I would even venture to suggest that if IVF and ART have been somewhat overestimated in terms of their »impact« on society, they have probably also been underestimated in terms of their role in reshaping biomedicine and bioscience. Since the 1980s it is no exaggeration to claim that the rapid worldwide expansion of IVF has provided the experimental ground zero for a whole new chapter of biological exploration into the mechanisms of human reproduction, genetics, regeneration, and development.

The importance of IVF as a means or method is complemented by its importance as a model. What IVF »modeled« was the successful imitation of life – or more specifically »the facts of life« – *in vitro*. Successful fertilization *in vitro* minimally required a viable culture system and reliable surgical means of identifying, removing, and transferring eggs, sperm, and embryos. Numerous obstacles beset the path to successful IVF in mammals before it was first achieved in the rabbit by Min Chueh Chang at the Worcester Institute for Experimental Biology in 1959. The technique was initially pursued in studies using small, prolific, and inexpensive animals whose ova were relatively accessible and plentiful – i.e. rabbits and mice. In livestock animals, such as cows and sheep, access to ova was limited by the inability to induce ovulation as well as the greater expense in acquiring, costs of maintaining, and difficulty of handling larger mammals. Primate *in vitro* culture systems were almost non-existent until well after human IVF had succeeded due to the difficulty of inducing ovulation.

The *in vitro* systems developed for culturing the eggs and embryos of rabbits and mice thus provided the main animal model systems for IVF. The achievement of successful IVF in a wide range of species served as models for its eventual transfer into humans. The ability to achieve fertilization of human ova in culture, by Edwards, Bavister, and Steptoe in 1969,[30] enabled further study of the *in vitro* human embryos for many years before such embryos were transferred into patients. As Robert Edwards
indexEdwards, RobertindexEdwards, Jeanettecommented in a lengthy re-

30 Robert G. Edwards, Barry D. Bavister & Patrick Steptoe, »Early Stages of Fertilization In Vitro of Human Oocytes Matured in Vitro«, in: *Nature* 221 (1969), pp. 632–635.

view article on the ethics of IVF in 1974, the ability to observe human and non-human mammalian embryos *in vitro* (»preimplantation embryos«) confirmed they were reassuringly robust. As he noted of the *in vitro* embryo culture systems of rabbits, mice, sheep, or cows that ultimately performed the role of nearest-to-man models for therapeutic IVF:

»Preimplantation embryos can obviously adapt to the artificial conditions of culture and undergo normal development, a conclusion supported by other forms of evidence showing that early embryos have considerable powers of regulation even after their total disorganization in culture. Embryos of rabbits, mice, sheep, cows and other species have been separated into individual blastomeres and then reaggregated, single cells or groups of cells in an embryo can be destroyed, pieces have been removed from blastocysts and large parts of the embryonic disc destroyed, yet in all these studies there has been literally no increase in malformed fetuses. *The degree of embryonic regulation during these early stages is indeed remarkable.*«[31]

IVF thus involves two different kinds of relationships to animal models. Each animal model involves slightly different embryo culture systems and variations in the procedures for IVF. In this sense IVF comprises a plurality of forms across a range of animal systems in which fertilization can be achieved *in vitro*, but with species-specific variations. Each of these animal systems provides a model for others, in the sense that parts of hamster IVF are »modeled after« rabbit IVF and so forth. A widening comparative range of animal models of IVF enhances the ability to assess the role of crucial factors such as sperm capacitation or culture media, and to detect new factors, such as the significance of maternally or paternally derived centrosomes, genomic imprinting, and Y-chromosome deletions.[32]

On the other hand, IVF also introduces an alternative to animal models by enabling the observation of fertilized eggs *in vitro* up to and beyond the blastocyst stage, and, as Edwards notes, through a range of experimentally induced injuries to both human and non-human embryos that would be impossible to control, replicate, or observe *in vivo*. From this perspective the importance of IVF should be understood as having provided the first »test-tube« human culture systems long before it provided the world's

31 Robert G. Edwards, »The Ethics of In Vitro Fertilisation«, in: *Quarterly Review of Biology* 49 (1974), pp. 3–26, in particular p. 5, emphasis added.

32 These have become more apparent in more recent primate models, see Laura Hewitson, »Primate Models for Assisted Reproductive Technologies«, in: *Reproduction* 128 (2004), pp. 293–299.

first »test-tube« baby. In its first incarnation, IVF was a modeling device that could substitute for »nearest to man« *by being human*. Early IVF, in both animals and humans, in other words, was not only a model but a *tool*. Since the purpose of both animal and »dish« models is to identify potential hazards for humans, they are complementary. The ability to interpret them together requires the kind of merographic logic described by Marilyn Strathern, in which it is not the *parts* of different systems that are themselves precisely analogous (mouse ova, rabbit ova, human ova), but *the logic between the parts* that enables them to be models for each other (which is a partial logic in more than one sense, since they are composed of parts, and are both different and partially alike). What is anthropologically interesting about the composite knowledge of IVF that results from this »logic of the overlap« is that it both separates and combines humans and animals, *in vivo* and *in vitro* processes, and both »technologically assisted« or »artificial« conception with their »natural« counterparts – thus setting up precisely the complex ricochet in analogies that enables merographic thinking to be flexible and plural whilst also loyal to singular logics.[33]

IVF Pragmatism

The scientific and medical line of thought connecting human and animal models, and the moral and legal justifications for protecting the value of IVF as a model system as well as a form of infertility treatment, have been essentially pragmatic over the course of the past century. From the late 19th century onwards, IVF and embryo transfer were seen to offer potential solutions to a wide range of problems in science, medicine, and agriculture, from the reproductive to the developmental and genetic. These pragmatic goals also lay at the heart of the protracted legislative debate in the UK, a century later, which lasted for 12 years after the birth

33 The flexible logic of IVF, through which it can be both natural and technological, miraculous and biological, familial or scientific, exceptional and normal, etc., is itself metonymic with the larger logic of plastic biology, of which, I am suggesting, the logic of IVF is not only a part, but an important precursor. The fusion of the biological with the technological at a cellular level is the constitutive condition of what I am calling biolife.

of Louise Brown (a debate, it is worth remembering, that was less about clinical IVF than embryo research). Although this debate involved considerable deliberation over the need to protect the rights *of* embryos, the HFE Act ultimately protected a collective human right *to* human embryos and specifically to their use *as tools* in the effort to alleviate human suffering.

For example, as the Cabinet Minister for Women, the Right Honourable (Labour) MP from Barking Jo Richardson, argued in the British House of Commons 20 years ago, in December 1988, as part of the debate over the first Human Fertilisation and Embryology Bill:

»It is of course true that the fundamental principles of human IVF were established with the use of animal models, but different animal species – including the human – differ from each other in biochemical and developmental details. That means that however much enormously useful information can be provided by animal models there will ultimately be a point in the research when the human system must be directly examined. That is why it is necessary that we ensure that there is an opportunity for the research to continue.« (HL Hansard, 16 Dec 1988, co 1268)

Based on more than half a century of experimentation with fertilized mammalian embryos *in vitro*, the eventual clinical application of IVF showed that human ova could be removed from the body, cultured in media, fertilized *in vitro*, and transferred to the uterus to produce viable offspring.[34] This not only confirmed a transferability of principles from other animal models to human, but an isomorphism between *in vivo* and *in vitro* conception. Put simply, IVF proved the viability of a substitution of an *in vitro* model for the »real thing,« and the HFEA confirmed the inestimable value of this new tool for human progress.[35]

34 An overcomplicated way to describe this transformation is that it combines material-semiotic reduction and performative substitution: both imitation and reduction enable a model to occupy the place of an original, or, for that matter, *to become a new original* (it is now a tool). As both a name and a technique, IVF performs all of these functions.

35 This addition, or supplement, of technological assistance neither removes nature from the process of conception, nor replaces it by technology: it combines both. What Strathern articulated so clearly was how IVF establishes new roles for biology and technology *based on their interchangeability.* This substitutability is what, in Strathern's view, displaces an understanding of technology as a set of tools *that can be applied*

Marilyn Strathern's predictive argument was that these transformations would generate new understandings – after all, IVF is a reproductive model. And so we arrive back at the IVF-stem cell interface where, again, new models and analogies generate others. In the same way IVF is implicated in the birth of new persons and the culturing of new lives, so too is the means by which it does so productive of new ideas of life and new understandings of embryonic induction and regulation (which can now be artificially assumed and replicated). These new facts of life usher in the next stage of ART – the cleanroom facts of life now adjacent to the IVF surgery at Guy's – which belong to a more fully characterized, quality controlled, and performance-validated successor version of reproductive control. Like previous innovations, the pragmatic argument to improve human futures through the use of new human tools is driven by the most conventional and familiar humanist values, such as the obligation to alleviate human suffering, empathy with the sufferers, and the consequent duty to improve the conditions of human life.

This brings us to the question of whether the IVF-stem cell interface, the hole in the wall for safe embryo passage, reaffirms and extends the pervasive synechdoche through which assistance to human reproduction »stands for« a far more encompassing project of human biological reverse engineering, such as that proposed in the context of tissue engineering and regenerative medicine. To what extent is the hope of IVF and regenerative medicine, stem cells, tissue engineering, etc. the same familiar hope for safe biological passage, biological rescue, or biological repair? And to what extent is IVF a template for these hope technologies? If IVF babies are in a sense the living proof of the ethos of experimental embryology – that you have to interfere to understand and improve the reproductive process – then what is the connection between biology, reproduction and technology these definitions of »life« or »control« imply? Does the »critical path« from IVF lead not only to offspring or stem cells, but to synthetic biology (whose maxim, »in vivo, in vitro, in silico,« rather neatly encapsulates the »next stage« of reverse engineering via computational biology)? The reason to ask »Foucault's question« about IVF is not to exaggerate or overplay its importance by appearing to make it belong to a seismic historical shift in

to biology or nature. *In vitro*, the distinction between embryo, tool, and experiment disappears.

biological or economic terms. In fact, from a Foucauldian perspective the point would be the reverse – that what IVF might help us to understand is how cultural change of the kind in which it can now be seen, 30 years later, to have been »foundationally« implicated *is often very ordinary and mundane at the same time as it may be revolutionary.* Is this not one way in which the very word »revolutionary« has changed – so that it is now more likely to be used for a new MP3 player than for radical social change?

Biological Relativity

The question to be asked, then, is not so much »is IVF good or bad?«; »Where is it leading us?«; »Is it the thin end of the wedge?«; or even »Was Gena Corea right when she said it would all lead to a reproductive brothel (or factory)?« Perhaps, in other words, we should take IVF a bit more seriously as a techno-cultural template for what is meant by »biological control.« More pointedly, the question is whether it is through reproductive biology that we have moved to *the condition of being »biologically relative,«* which is increasingly an »obligatory passage point« for understandings of the human I suggest IVF has helped to produce. I am suggesting that IVF makes explicit the ways in which biological facts *in general* belong to *multiple transferable logics*, which are serially and partially stabilized to perform certain functions or create certain effects in different contexts. This »biological« is what Strathern called »merographic,« in that biological facts belong to multiple contexts, or logics, that can be emphasized, separated, or recombined according to context or situation.

We do not have to argue any of this is new to be interested in how it works.[36] The model for Strathern's concept of »merographic« (which she invented) is kinship – notably the segmentary lineage structure of the Tallensi described by Meyer Fortes, in which individuals alter their status, get help, or resolve conflicts by shifting the emphasis of belonging from the matriline to the patriline, or vice versa. As Fortes notes of the social

36 Indeed, if »the biological« always worked this way (which it arguably does within biology, where facts are seen as highly contingent), the question of how it ever came to represent fixity and unchangeability becomes more important than whether it is so.

utility of what he calls »breaches« or »divided loyalties,« they are crucial to »the solidarity of the unit,« especially when »genealogical boundaries« need to be »adjusted« through »mediation«:

»From the point of view of the total social structure the most important function of extra-clan kinship is to make a number of breaches for the individual in the rigid genealogical boundary of the maximal lineage and clan. It creates bonds of amity and loyalty for him with members of other clans, irrespective of the corporate, political relations that may prevail between clans and other clans. The individual is not confined within the boundaries of his clan for social purposes. He has not only channels of communication with other clans but sources of material aid and moral support outside his own clan....As we saw in the case of uterine kin, it meant that people could move about the country with some security...in spite of the tendency to be on terms of latent hostility [with other clans]. [Similarly], disputes between members of different clans can be adjusted through the mediation of common kinsmen without setting in motion the organs of corporate political life.«[37]

Fortes argued these »partial connections« provided both the socio-spatial »room« and the practical means for individual adjustment of fixed, inherited systems of ascribed identity. Merographic reasoning describes how divergent logics can be electively mobilized against shifting backgrounds to enable otherwise intractable conventions or truths to be »adjusted.«

Borrowing from kinship theory to make the suggestion that assisted conception similarly enables a logic of »adjustable« genealogy to become more explicit is only to repeat the argument from the many well-known ethnographic studies of ART,[38] which have confirmed a point Marilyn Strathern herself had argued decades earlier in numerous pioneering studies of English kinship (in which she showed, among other things, how the allegedly »unbreakable« bond of blood descent, or genealogy, was cross-cut by other, equally powerful, idioms of belonging). What I am suggesting here is that this logic can be doubly extended by IVF, which not only literally introduces new possibilities of »genealogical transfer« but a whole host

37 Meyer Fortes, *The web of kinship among the Tallensi: the second part of an analysis of the social structure of a Trans-Volta tribe* (Oxford: Oxford University Press 1969).

38 E.g. Marcia Inhorn, *Quest for Conception: Gender, Infertility, and Egyptian Medical Traditions* (Philadelphia: University of Pennsylvania Press, 1994); Thompson, »Making Parents«, op. cit. (note 20); Charis Cussins, »Ontological Choreography: Agency through Objectification in Infertility Clinics«, in: *Social Studies of Science* 26 (1996), 3, pp. 575–610.

of associative or symbolic transfers as well. Hence, again, IVF's »unremarkableness« could be read along these lines to suggest that its normalization through naturalization (it is just like nature) requires a logic of transferability (in vivo – in vitro – in vivo) that »travels back« as an analogy to make of »human reproductive biology« itself a kind of »hole in the wall« or a »passaging« technology.[39]

The »Logic of IVF«

This »genealogical transfer« model of IVF can be given a more concrete, albeit unfamiliar, kinship context by charting the actual and figurative »biological relatives« of the newly socially interfaced *in vitro* human embryo and its contested connections to a plural social world. The animated debate over the contested meanings of the »intervenable« human embryo is a good place to look for endless examples of »merographic« social and political processes, and it is also a high-profile social arena to which we have ample empirical access. The stem cell debates in the US are a good example, and 2008 was also an eventful year in the UK, during which the 30th anniversary of the birth of Louise Brown coincided with the unamended passage of a new Human Fertilisation and Embryology Bill. In conspicuous contrast to the US, the UK has long hosted the most highly regulated but scientifically permissive climate for human embryo research anywhere in the world. Embryo research, including human embryonic stem cell derivation, enjoys strong support from all of the major political parties and the general public, as does the production of cloned human embryos for research and human-animal cybrid embryos. Indeed, this area of research is something of a jewel in the crown as far as UK bioscience and biomedicine are concerned.

In order to consider briefly how the »logic of IVF« has evolved in the UK over the past 30 years, it is thus useful to revisit the most recent round of embryo debates in the UK, many of which were centered on the ques-

39 Incidentally, this is another way to describe the de- and re-naturalizing processes described by Rabinow as biosociality, in which nature is modeled on »culture« – a phrase with a convenient second meaning in the context of IVF. Paul Rabinow, *Essays on the Anthropology of Reason* (Princeton: Princeton University Press, 1996).

tion of deliberately creating so-called cybrid, or human-cow, embryos for basic scientific research into the »ground state« of cellular renewal. By so doing it is possible to reflect on some of the more abstract arguments developed so far in the context of more specific empirical examples.[40] Arguably, these debates can be interpreted as evidence of the increasing influence (at least in the UK) of what I am calling the »logic« of being »after IVF.«

In the autumn of 2008, not long after I had visited the stem cell lab described above, I attended one of the major demonstrations outside Parliament in support of, and against, the new Human Fertilisation and Embryology Bill at a key point during its passage through Parliament. It was a beautiful sunny day and it is a short bike ride from my office at the LSE down the Embankment to Old Palace Yard, where I arrived just after 1 pm. In the announcement of the 12 May 2008 pro-embryo research demo, »Show Your Support,« organized by the office of (Liberal) MP Evan Harris, it was suggested that:

»In recent months there has been intensive lobbying of MPs, particularly from groups who are opposed to embryo research to continue in the UK, including embryonic stem cell science and the animal-human hybrid work. MPs may not have heard quite so clearly from those who strongly support the proposals in the Bill, and know that it is vitally important that the legislation is not watered down.«

It went on:

»A YouGov poll in August 2005 showed that 77% of people accept embryo research for life-threatening diseases. But for far too long, the most prominent shows of feeling on this issue have come from those who wish to impede carefully regulated embryo research and important and ethical clinical interventions like preimplantation genetic diagnosis.«

The announcement concluded that on 12 May 2008, just before the start of the Bill's second reading in the House of Commons, »hundreds of patient groups would join with scientists, doctors and other supporters to represent the breadth and depth of support for the Bill, and in particular to confirm support for the government proposal that embryo research

40 Although the following examples are taken from public debate, similar data can be drawn from both patient interviews and lab observations.

should continue in the UK, and should include animal-human hybrid work as well as embryonic stem cell science.«

In fact, on the day there were fewer than a dozen patients and representatives of patient groups available to comment to the media – most of whom had left by the time I arrived. The only scientists present were some members of leading stem cell scientist Stephen Minger's lab, who joined the small demo – without their white coats. The fear that the pro-embryo research lobby would be swamped by the pro-life rally also scheduled the same afternoon just before the start of the second reading at 2 pm proved groundless, as it too was poorly attended and lack-lustre. The weather was perhaps too glorious to support a mood of indignation.

Riding back to my office to watch the second reading live on Parliament TV, I reflected on what a different situation it had been in the late spring of 1990, when the first Human Fertilisation and Embryology Bill was passed. At that time, not so long after a private member's bill by Conservative MP Enoch Powell had attempted to ban embryo research entirely, the question of how Parliament would vote on the amendment to allow embryo research was far from certain. The pro-life lobby was much larger and better organized. In a dramatic show of opposition to abortion, they had showered the chambers of Parliament with postcards of aborted fetuses.

However, the reduced size and fervor of the demonstrations for and against embryo research were not the only measure of the difference between 1990 and 2008. Looking back, we can see that although some forms of reproductive technology, such as cloning, human-animal hybrids, and stem cells, still engender controversy, the logic of IVF has been sedimented into a naturalized trajectory of intervention in the name of improvement, in which technological manipulation of human embryos is not only a viable alternative to »natural« reproduction, but human embryo experimentation is *a necessary path* to the continued improvement of human health. If severe, debilitating, and destructive conditions can be alleviated, they should be, and if *in vitro* methods are available they are preferable to using animals or human subjects. In a sense, the connection between IVF and fertility – or even conception – has been superceded (as it was preceded) by a more general isomorphism between improvements to human life and the ability to culture human life »in glass.« This is the »biological relation« IVF establishes as a »model system« and as a path. Thus, the contemporary condition that is variously described as being after nature, posthuman, or biologically relative, is, in an important sense, that which is epitomized by being *after IVF.*

To underscore this hypothesis, it is worth noting the somewhat surprising scale of IVF's popularity – in spite of its many failings, high cost, and known and unknown risks when used for fertility treatment or preimplantation genetic diagnosis. Contrary to most expectations at the time of its initial success, and indeed throughout the 1980s, IVF has become a popular and widespread technology worldwide, with success rates that are more or less comparable to those of normal conception. Although accurate records are not maintained, it is estimated that approximately five million IVF babies have been born worldwide from this technique. In Israel and Denmark, IVF is responsible for as much as four percent of the annual birth rate. The leading IVF center in China last year completed 5000 cycles of IVF. More than 10 000 women underwent IVF in the UK in 2005.

The recent debate in the UK suggests the cultural shift over the past 30 years is not only a process through which the axiomatic status of natural facts has been displaced, but one in which newly partial, and often technologically assisted, understandings of these »facts« are used »merographically« – much as Haraway similarly described through her figure of the cyborg.[41] We might say that IVF has made biology newly relative in the process of making new biological relatives. Importantly, the new plastic, recombinant »transbiology« born of the cyborg embryo is today in constant use to propagate new biological entities, such as cultured transgenic stem cell colonies, human-animal cybrids, clones, chimeras, and – most recently – induced pluripotent embryoid bodies (iPS cells – made in Japan and named for the iPhone).[42]

41 Donna Haraway, »A Manifesto for Cyborgs: Science, Technology, and Socialist-Feminism in the Late Twentieth Century«, in: *Socialist Review* 80 (1985), pp. 65–108.

42 A telling feature of the worldwide debate over the post-IVF technologies of cloning and stem cell cultivation is the explicitness with which the biological mechanisms of development have been fused with the helping hands of science – as is often seen in short clips of footage from the micromanipulators used in both IVF and research labs that are now common on the evening news, in Hollywood films, and in advertising. The fact that we can *see* the *in vitro* human embryo being biopsied or transferred

Post IVF, and especially three decades post IVF, the fact that the »built« embryo has become a naturalized construct is very much what was predicted from within social science. The comparative lack of contemporary public opposition to stem cell research in the UK could be read as confirming this pattern (as might recent events in the US). Very much in contrast to the debate that took place in Parliament throughout the 1980s concerning embryo research, the high-profile UK debate in 2008 concerning human-animal hybrids, or cybrids, relegated the Catholic church right-to-life position to the »extreme« fringe of public debate. Cardinal Keith O'Brien's strident 2008 Easter sermon condemning the revised Human Fertilisation and Embryology Bill was widely perceived to damage the reputation of Catholicism in the UK (where, despite former Prime Minister Tony Blair's thinly concealed leanings toward the Papacy, it has never been well-liked). »It is difficult to imagine,« O'Brien claimed, »a single piece of legislation which, more comprehensively, attacks the sanctity and dignity of human life than this particular Bill«:

»What I am speaking of is the process whereby scientists create an embryo containing a mixture of animal and human genetic material. If I were preaching this homily in France, Germany, Italy, Canada, or Australia I would be commending the government for rightly banning such grotesque procedures. However here in Great Britain I am forced to condemn our government for not only permitting but encouraging such hideous practices.…This Bill represents a monstrous attack on human rights, human dignity and human life… One might say that in our country we are about to have a public government endorsement of experiments of Frankenstein proportion. May God indeed help us to be Missionary at this present time and to hand on the saving message of Jesus Christ in a world which does not seem prepared to receive it.«[43]

has intensified the intimacy of our encounter with its direct manipulation – not least because the spectators occupy the same »hands on« viewpoint as the manipulator. In front page coverage of famous human blastocysts, such as the cloned embryos from Newcastle announced two years ago created through somatic cell nuclear transfer, we participate in a form of witnessing in which the spectacle of »biological control« of human life *in vitro* is not unlike the experience of viewing the earth as seen from outer space. These are recontextualizing, literally re-grounding, forms of visual engagement that now connect basic laboratory science with mainstream popular culture.

43 Keith O'Brien, »Easter Sunday Homily«, 23 March 2008. Online publication http://news.bbc.co.uk/1/hi/scotland/7308883.stm [last accessed: 5.10.2010].

Among those challenging this view was the prominent geneticist Mary Seller, also a Christian, whose commentary on cybrids published in *The Tablet* cited the teachings of Jesus Christ as a motivation not only to heal the sick but to marvel at the splendor of God's creation.

»God certainly intends healing of the sick. Jesus always healed when he encountered a person in need: he never passed one by. Indeed he often flouted authority to do so: he healed on the Sabbath, he touched untouchables, and vociferous criticism did not stop him. Furthermore, he gave power and authority to his disciples to go out on the highways and byways to do likewise. If today we are able to heal anyone through our new scientific endeavors, it is an expression of our discipleship, and can also be construed as another way in which we legitimately ›play God.‹«[44] Seller's pragmatic interpretation of Christ's teaching closely follows the mainstream UK position of support for science based on a sense of moral duty to explore new avenues for the relief of human suffering. In her view, God's intentions are consistent with instrumental intervention, including scientific experimentation. She evokes a tradition of active, mobile evangelism – flouting the state's authority to take to the road, »the highways and byways,« with tools to heal the sick. Scientific experimentation, in this view, is no less than a form of discipleship.

In their press release prepared to accompany the debate in Parliament on human-animal hybrid embryos, the Genetic Interest Group representing patient groups in favor of the new legislation took a similar view – describing the human *in vitro* embryo as »a vital tool to advance the progress of research into the potential of embryonic stem cells,« and thus as »a potentially vital avenue for research which could greatly increase our understanding of serious medical conditions such as Parkinson's, motor neurone disease, Alzheimer's disease and cystic fibrosis.«[45] Such a statement strongly reinforces the initial UK government position set in place by the debate over Warnock – that some embryo research should be permitted in the effort to provide relief from human suffering – whilst also

44 Mary Seller, »Slipping on the Slippery Slope of Progress«, in: The Tablet (5 April 2008), http://www.thetablet.co.uk/article/11258 [last accessed: 9.10.2010].

45 GIG, »Human Admixed Embryos«, 2008. The Genetic Interest Group (GIG) whose leaflet on *Human Admixed Embryos* is referred to here has changed its name, as of May 2010, to the Genetic Alliance UK. The pamphlet can be accessed at: http://www.geneticalliance.org.uk/policy_archive_2008.htm.

confirming, as does passage of the new legislation unamended, that this position has stood the test of time. As the (lack of) cybrid debate reveals, support for this view has, if anything, been strengthened to the extent that the value of the *in vitro* human embryo culture system as both a tool and a way has come to occupy the moral high ground.

We might, on reflection, suggest that the IVF embryo, having been technologically admixed, *was already hybridized*, so that further mixtures might differ in content, but not in form. The progress-driven analogy that procreation can be assisted, and that nature and technology can be productively fused or mixed, could be said to have *returned* in such a manner that *this is what human reproductive biology has come to signify*, as is made explicit in the GIG analogy between a human embryo *and a tool.* Similarly, the Genetic Interest Group refers to human embryonic stem cell research as »a vital avenue...that may ultimately lead to new treatments and cures.« Here, then, is the social genealogy of the *in vitro* human embryo – it has been literalized as a tool of progress, not so much canceling as morphing its status as an embodiment of shared reproductive substance to become a helping hand to future generations, and thus a »way forward« for humankind.

Conclusion

Although today considered largely unremarkable, and now a widespread medical procedure that has proven globally very popular, what I have tried to suggest in this chapter is that IVF is for this very reason implicated in, and indicative of, a wider shift in how human reproductive biology is understood – socially, scientifically, and technologically. In the post-IVF context, a new backdrop of re-engineerable human biology has been normalized. IVF is thus not only an instance, but a model of a wider process – as we would expect a reproductive model to be. It is implicated in a new model of biology comprised of movable and recombinant parts – a biology we can denominate as transbiology. And it is also a grounding idiom for a new definition of life. This is not so much life »itself« – as some kind of singular entity linked through shared descent, as Foucault or Darwin argued – as biolife, an array of disparate lives that are inseparably bound up with technological »assistance.« Although IVF may affect a limited number of people directly, I have suggested that its significance as a model of new biological relations, as a template of both transbiology and biolife, as an *experimental tool,* and as a translational path together comprise its under-recognized and overlooked »thick genealogical« legacies. IVF thus introduces new models of biological relationships among parts as well as wholes, and of the use of parts to make new wholes – or indeed new parts. These models simultaneously operate as means of reproduction, substitutability (between *in vivo* and *in vitro* models), and intervenability (via the *in vitro* window, hatch, or »hole in the wall«), through which alterations can be made that »travel back« to change the »ground state« of human biology, or biological renewal (which is increasingly synonymous with »biological control«).

Enlisting assistance from the *in vitro* embryo and its indigenous idioms of genealogical and embryo transfer to map the cultural legacy of IVF leads, then, to some other speculations.

1. The legacy of IVF in terms of the extent to which human biology has become more »intervenable« in general has probably been underestimated. While attention is paid to stem cells, PGD, and cloning, it is in fact IVF that should be seen as a historical turning point for the basic analogy between the *in vivo* and the *in vitro* human.
2. This would mean that possibly much of what we imagine to be in the future concerning issues such as designer biology, posthumanism, etc., is already behind us.
3. In turn this would suggest the characterization of new biological futures is wrongly imagined to be unfamiliar. It might instead be most legible where it extends the familiar – for example kinship models.
4. If so, then the huge global expansion of IVF and its new role as a conduit, or passage, to stem cell research should alert us to some important aspects of its legacy that differ significantly from the version of posthuman futures depicted by mainstream cultural commentators such as Lee Silver, Frances Fukuyama, Bill McKibben or Jürgen Habermas. Far from an unfamiliar posthuman future, the history of IVF suggests that the ethos of scientific helping hands being extended into the mechanisms of biological reproduction is already well established. In fact,

what IVF suggests is the successful »transfer« of experimental embryology into human reproduction as the model for its next »passage« into human regeneration.

5. The British case also suggests that a high degree of regulation and open debate has increased public confidence in the ethical basis for a view of human *in vitro* embryos as »special« because they have »special« instrumental value, whereas the reverse situation characterizes the United States (little or no regulation has privatized much research and decreased public confidence in more radical avenues of experimentation).
6. From the point of view of kinship, and in particular of shared reproductive substance, this means the embryo (as shared human reproductive and also regenerative substance) now still ethically »codes« for conduct, except the conduct of »biological relationality« is the obligation to use the embryo as a *tool* of medical innovation. Such an argument would have consequences in the debates about, for example, biosociality or biological citizenship.

A key oversight may be the importance of the *in vitro* embryo culture systems that were established for many mammals prior to humans, and in humans for more than a decade prior to the birth of Louise Brown. Linked to this is the interpretation I am foregrounding here, of IVF *as a model that instantiates a recombinant imaginary based on transfers*. It is perhaps worth pointing out that in the very idea of a conception model is the suggestion of analogy, for the simple reason that a model relies upon comparison, and thus on movement between one domain of meaning and another. If, following this train of thought, the flow of genealogy was previously imagined to follow the lines of shared reproductive substance along the template of biogenetic inheritance (»lines of descent«), then perhaps what has truly been altered is the content of this lineage. IVF »models« the flow of knowledge as progress, and progress as linear and cumulative. IVF babies are, in a sense, a fusing of this knowledge with reproductive substance – or the embodiment of this knowledge as genealogy. In this case, perhaps it is *the movement between instrumental knowledge and genealogy* that the embryo now increasingly embodies. The global research population of *in vitro* human embryos in culture, which can be used for research into human regeneration, now comprise »a vital avenue« to future life, thus confirming an instrumentalized biological relationship that remains highly ethically charged and filled with a sense of urgent obligation.

This would mean that the IVF embryo is indeed the embodiment and representative of a human genealogical frontier – *but not one that is in front of us*. Like other frontiers, it is already behind us, part of us, and its conditions have already become heritable and genealogical (just like Frederick Jackson Turner's version of the manifest destiny that »made« the American character – which was the labor forged in the »crucible« of the frontier). If so, then this is a point at which we might venture to be predictive, for this would mean biogenetic substance can still be understood as »coding« for conduct in the sense of conveying a sense of moral imperative, duty, obligation and reciprocity. And so we might understand what the sense of »specialness,« preciousness, or awe still attached to the human embryo as »one of us« or as a »biological relative« is: it is unique as a »tool« because it extends our connections and attachments to each other, and this, increasingly, appears as a first-order obligation. If so, this would be the most powerful biocultural legacy of IVF – that it has refashioned the relationship between substance and code for conduct not only by making the substance the object of conduct, but conduct (e.g. scientific research) the origin of substance (e.g. replacement parts, artificial gametes, cultured hES lines, biobanking, etc.). It is also where we might understand the power of IVF as a technology of »genealogical transfer,« because being »after IVF« has changed what »genealogical« and »biological« are, can do, and mean.

Localizing In Vitro Fertilization: The Cultural Work of Encounters with Medical Technologies

Legacies and Linkages: Episodes in the Establishment of New Reproductive Technologies in Contemporary Sri Lanka

Bob Simpson

Introduction

At the IVF as Global Form conference, Sarah Franklin began with a striking and thought-provoking assertion. Whilst attentions are invariably drawn to high-profile technological developments in stem cell research, PGD, and cloning, the rapid rise and diffusion of IVF has played a far more consequential role in transforming the way people think about developments in genetics and reproduction. More specifically, with its appeal to the plight of those who are involuntarily childless and the sympathies and passions that this stirs, IVF has ushered in wide and surprising levels of acceptance of new forms of intervention in reproductive processes, as well as novel forms of substitution and artificiality. Echoing an earlier prediction made by Paul Rabinow in relation to the new genetics, the power to re-shape society is such because developments of this kind »will be embedded throughout the social fabric at the micro-level.«[1] A major contribution of anthropologists in understanding this process in the context of IVF has been the move beyond IVF's development and use in Euro-American and Anglophone societies, and into its global diffusion and incorporation into other modernities.[2] In these studies, detailed, situated, and comparative accounts of how IVF operates in different set-

1 Paul Rabinow, »Artificiality and Enlightenment. From Sociobiology to Biosociality«, in: *Essays on the Anthropology of Reason* (Princeton: Princeton University Press, 1996), pp. 99–103.

2 Marcia Inhorn & Frank Van Balen (Eds.), *Infertility around the Globe: New Thinking on Childlessness, Gender, and Reproductive Technologies* (Berkeley and London: University of California Press, 2002). Also see Marcia Inhorn, *Reproductive Disruptions: Gender Technology and Biopolitics in the New Millennium* (Oxford: Berghahn, 2007) for an overview and comprehensive bibliography; and Faye Ginsberg & Rayna Rapp (Eds.),

tings have highlighted the capacity of IVF to alter conceptions of identity and relationality within distinctive »national« IVF cultures. The emphasis in these studies is on the ways in which technologies do not simply and passively »transfer« but are shaped by the cultural, social, political, and economic circumstances that prevail in the contexts in which they are brought into use.[3] Yet, as this volume amply demonstrates, »national« IVF cultures are also part of IVF as »global form.« Indeed, familiar reference points such as national territories, sovereignties, and states, are passed over and through as the reach and availability of IVF continue to expand and encompass provision in different countries.[4]

Appadurai's notions of transnationality and translocality take us part of the way in attempting to understand the flows of technology, knowledge, personnel, and money that underpin the global spread of IVF.[5] However, despite attempts to think beyond the nation, flows largely remain dependent upon distinct models of nationhood and sovereignty in order to be made visible. As Appadurai himself also points out in later works, these flows also bring disjunctures, »problems that manifest themselves in intensely local forms but have contexts that are anything but local.«[6] While these disjunctive flows bring acute problems for equality, well-being, and governance, Appadurai's assessment is not entirely pessimistic. He also sees in these spaces the possibility of re-capturing a place for the imagination in social life. In this sense, the imagination operates both at the level of the agents who are responsible for creating, engineering, and manipu-

---

Conceiving the New World Order: The Global Politics of Reproduction (Berkeley and London: University of California Press, 1995).

3 For recent examples, see: Monica Bonnacorso-Rothe, *Conceiving Kinship: Heterosexual, Lesbian and Gay Procreation, Family and Relatedness in Southern Europe* (Oxford: Berghahn, 2008); Aditya Bharadwaj, »Introduction«, in: *Culture, Medicine and Psychiatry* (special edition *Sacred Conceptions: Religion in the Global Practice of IVF,* 2006); Sarah Gibbon & Carlos Novas (Eds.), *Genetics, Biosociality and the Social Sciences: Making Biologies and Identities* (London: Routledge, 2007).

4 For example, the IVF worldwide directory and website boasted 2995 clinics worldwide after only three months of registration. http://www.ivf-worldwide.com/ [last accessed: 16.10.2009].

5 Arjun Appadurai, *Modernity at Large* (Minnesota: University of Minnesota Press, 1996).

6 Arjun Appadurai, *Globalisation* (Durham and London: Duke University Press, 2001), p. 6.

lating flows, as well as at the level of how we, as social scientists, might conceptualize these emergent spaces. The anthropological challenge then, continues to provide accounts of how the global-local binary might be not only contextualised but transcended altogether.[7] The work of Ong and Collier has provided an important contribution in this regard.[8] Drawing their inspiration from Deleuze and Guattari, they develop the notion of global assemblages as a methodologically workable and locally specifiable approach to understanding the international reach and effects of a variety of globally transferable forms such as technologies, policies, protocols, and guidelines. In so doing they draw our attention to the »minor histories that address themselves to the ›big‹ questions of globalizations« rather than grand structural transformations.[9] Examples brought together by Ong and Collier include HIV prevention, ideas of citizenship, banking, and the regulation of food production.[10] All of these cases reveal the ways that ideas and practices travel and embed in a wide variety of locales. Key to the mobility and applicability of these forms in diverse contexts are the ways in which their scalability renders them fluid and adaptable. Rather like Latour's immutable mobiles, they bring change without themselves being changed.[11] In this essay I consider IVF as such an assemblage in which regulatory guidelines, training, conferences, technology transfer, and the spaces in which the business of IVF is daily transacted reveal ideas and practices in motion. These are the places where the work of rendering IVF a global form is carried out and the power of the assemblage begins to transgress other readings of reproduction, gender, and parenthood.

7 For an example from political geography, see Neil Brenner, »Globalisation as Reterritorialisation: The Re-scaling of Urban Governance in the European Union«, in: *Urban Studies* 36 (1999), 3, pp. 431–451.

8 Aihwa Ong & Stephen J. Collier (Eds.), *Global Assemblages: Technology, Politics and Ethics as Global Problems* (Oxford: Blackwell Publishing, 2005).

9 Ibid., p.15.

10 For example, see essays in Ong & Collier, *Global Assemblages,* op. cit. (note 8) by Vinh-Kim Nguyen, »Anti-retroviral Globalism, Biopolitics and Therapeutic Citizenship«, pp. 124–144; Nikolas Rose & Carlos Novas, »Biological Citizenship«, pp. 439–463; Douglas Holmes & George Marcus, »Cultures of Expertise and the Management of Globalisation: Toward the Re-functioning of Ethnography«, pp. 235–252; Elizabeth C. Dunn, »Standards and Person-making in East Central Europe«, pp. 173–193.

11 Bruno Latour, *Science in Action* (Cambridge, Massachusetts: Harvard University Press, 1987), p. 227.

My own attempt to understand the formation, transformation, and impact of these activities is assisted by further reflection on the notions of de-territorialization and re-territorialization as they have figured in the works of Deleuze and Guattari.[12] It begins ethnographically, with reflections on what it is to study the unruly assemblages of people, knowledge, and objects that globalization represents. Drawing on fieldwork carried out in Sri Lanka into the reception of new reproductive and genetic technologies, I go on to document various moments in the development of IVF in Sri Lanka as a publicly visible form. These are points at which the assemblage unfolds, stimulating movements, connections and novel combinations of existing ideas and practices. These, in a Deleuzian sense, are the »cutting edges« of the assemblage; the points where creative potential is most apparent. At these points, new technologies and the expertise that goes with them bring a creative engagement with alternative codes, classifications, and values. In the process of de-territorialization, local practices are re-aligned and made to articulate with the global, IVF assemblage. However, as in Deleuze and Guattari's original conceptualization, de-territorialization and re-territorialization are not oppositional processes but dynamically linked; they are inextricably bound within any given social field. Just as there is the possibility of an assemblage cutting through local forms and bringing standardization to otherwise diverse elements, there is also the possibility of these emergent forms being reclaimed and becoming »something that ›has-the-value‹ of home.«[13] Re-territorialization can be seen in the re-casting of rhetorics of linkage and acceptance, as acts of assertion, challenge and resistance to universalizing

12 Gilles Deleuze & Felix Guattari, *A Thousand Plateaus* (Minnesota: University of Minnesota Press, 1987). The work of Deleuze and Guattari has had limited use in the context of ethnography and in the spirit of their original work my own foray is tentative and experimental. For other forays, see Lisa Malkii, »National Geographic: The Rooting of Peoples and the Territorialization of National Identity among Scholars and Refugees«, in: *Cultural Anthropology* 7 (1992), 1, pp. 24–44; also Rachel Douglas-Jones & Salla Sariola, »Rhizome Yourself: Experiencing Deleuze and Guattari from Theory to Practice«, in: *Rhizomes* 19 (2009), http://www.rhizomes.net/issue19/sariola.html [last accessed: 16.10.2009].

13 Deleuze & Guattari, *A Thousand Plateaus*, op. cit. (note 12), p. 360.

forms of science, economy, and morality. Re-territorialization seeks to counter »the reduction of all to the same.«[14]

The backdrop of this account is Sri Lanka, a multi-ethnic and multi-religious society made up of some 20 million people. In recent times the country has become widely known for the ethnic strife and bloodshed arising from a bitter secessionist struggle between the government of Sri Lanka and the Liberation Tigers for Tamil Eelam [LTTE], who were fighting to establish an independent state in the north of the island. The insurgency was brought to a bloody and decisive end in the early months of 2009, when LTTE forces were routed in the north. The island has also suffered considerable turbulence and instability as a result of insurgency attempts in the 1970s and 1980s inspired by movements combining leftist and nationalist politics and eager to dismantle and displace the island's neo-colonial political and economic heritage. IVF and the reproductive potential that this ensemble of clinical practices and procedures opens up first appeared in this complex social and political landscape in the late 1990s and I have been following its development over that period.[15] This work entailed interviews with key stakeholders (doctors, clinicians, lawyers, and interested parties and representatives from religious communities) who, in a context of weak regulation and limited public awareness, were involved with both the formulation of regulatory responses as well as attempts more generally to shape public responses to the variety of new technologies which were making their appearance. I also carried out participant observation in meetings, at conferences, and in various clinical settings in order to understand the forms that local engagement with these technologies was taking. In what follows I hope to set out the way that some of these processes have unfolded, as Sri Lanka has become part of the global IVF assemblage: a mosaic of institutional forms and clinical practices in which the business of making ethical, legal, and social sense

14 Michael M.J. Fischer, *Emergent Forms of Life and the Anthropological Voice* (Durham and London: Duke University Press, 2003), p.3.

15 The research on which this article is based was carried out as part of a wider exploration of the reception of new reproductive and genetic technologies in Sri Lanka. This research was funded by the Wellcome Trust in the form of a fellowship under the Medicine in Society Program (Biomedical Ethics GR067110AIA) for the year 2002–03. This work was preceded by a pilot study carried out in the summer of 2000 funded by the Nuffield Foundation (Social Science Small Grants Scheme).

is an ongoing and unfinished project. This paper focuses on the role of various experts as key agents in this process. These are the people not only responsible for attracting new developments, but also for keeping them in place, moving them forward, and shaping the moral and regulatory frameworks crucial to the local meaning and impact of the new technologies.[16] In the section that follows I juxtapose two very different accounts of this process; one from the perspective of the »official« story of IVF, and the other from my own field notes.

Legacies and Linkages: Sri Lanka's »first« IVF Baby

In 2008 a newspaper report appeared celebrating a decade of activity in Sri Lanka's premier reproductive clinic, the Vindana Reproductive Health Centre [Sunday Times of Sri Lanka – May 4th 2008]. The article reported that:

»In a cosy home many miles from Colombo, while a family prepares to celebrate the sixth birthday of a little girl on July 1 with a »small party,« in Colombo on Friday, a young mother experiences the joy of childbirth.
What is the link between the bubbly nearly-six girl and Friday's newborn … both are inextricably linked to Vindana, which helps »mimic nature«. The six-year-old is Vindana's very first baby and the newborn the 101st. Both of them and all the others in between have been born through the process called in vitro fertilization or in lay terms known as »test tube« babies.
A fine record within six years, and though Vindana has the atmosphere of a family gathering in its waiting room than that of a clinic and the walls are plastered with photographs of smiling babies, some alone and two together, this Reproductive Health Centre has passed many milestones, including many firsts in the country, since its inception in 1998.«

The account replicates a familiar narrative and draws on widely used metaphors of progress and advance in the field of assisted reproduction. It

16 Dominic Boyer, »Thinking through the Anthropology of Experts«, in: *Anthropology in Action* 15 (2008), pp. 38–46. Also cf. Adriana Petryna, *When Experiments Travel: Clinical Trials and the Global Search for Human Subjects* (Princeton: Princeton University Press, 2009) for an account of the role of local experts in the reception of and responses to clinical trial activity.

tells of »milestones« and »journeys« and later on casts the clinicians in the role of »helping hands« who are able to »mimic nature« in circumstances where it is in some way found to be deficient. The article moves on to speak of the bold steps that were involved in creating the »first« IVF child, and what the public can now glimpse in the pages of a newspaper as an exemplary and profound normality in the form of a six-year-old girl, unaware of her extraordinary origins. The focus in the article is on the products of IVF (the much-wanted babies) and the sociality that is created through the collective efforts of all to achieve successful conception and birth. These sentiments are hinted at in the evocation of the deep empathy between couples with a shared predicament who find themselves in the clinic's waiting room. Essentially, what we are given in this newspaper story and the many others that appeared like it, is a narrative, perhaps even one that has taken on canonical proportions, that moves from desperation to fulfillment in the form of a child born through the bold endeavors of committed and dedicated doctors willing to engage with progress and its challenges.

Beneath this account, however, is a complex history of engagements and episodes; these are the »cutting edges« which make for uncertainty and unpredictability in the way that the narrative will unfold. The newspaper captures one, widely acknowledged, endpoint but there could have been a multiplicity of others. To illustrate this point I would like to contrast this account with something that I wrote in my field notes while in the thick of fieldwork in July 2002. This was a period in which there was much activity in the development of IVF and a growing public awareness of it as a locally available reproductive option:

»… an item appears in several Sri Lankan English newspapers showing a photograph of a »miracle« baby. The baby is the first to be born on Sri Lankan soil as a result of IVF carried out by an all-Sri Lankan team of specialists. On seeing the photograph of the said miracle baby, a woman writes to the medical problems page of a newspaper expressing concerns that the child's picture should have been displayed in this way and asking what would happen to the child in future. The letter is passed on by the doctor who edits the page to a member of the Sri Lanka Medical Council Ethics Committee. He is moved by the woman's anxieties and prompted to voice wider concerns within the medical community about the lack of regulation of these technologies. He produces a paper in which he proposes guidelines based on Australian frameworks for regulation. A Tamil doctor, on seeing the image in the newspaper, is disgruntled that his team of Tamil and UK specialists produced an IVF child in Sri Lanka long before the »Sri Lankan« team but received little acclaim. A Sinhala daily goes on to point out that the child born was a Sinhala Buddhist child and that it was not a gift from God but the work of a clever team of doctors from »our country.« An imam in a local mosque gives a sermon in which he refers to the first IVF baby: »sperm and eggs come from God and there is nothing miraculous in mixing them together. Only God can do miracles.« A pub quiz team in a bar in Colombo make light of their ethnic hybridity by calling their team›IVF-mix-up. ‹« This account was written as I attempted to capture and make sense of the linkages set in train as the »miracle baby« newspaper item appeared to ricochet around various domains – public, legal, religious, and social – in the weeks following its publication. It hints at the extent of the connections that might be followed once immersed in the networks of connection, association, and coincidence that make up ethnographic fieldwork. Unlike the myth of origin outlined above, it also reveals the non-linear paths which might lead to some stories becoming fixed and part of a common currency of ideas about and attitudes towards IVF; what might at one point have been thought of as contingent and open to variation, over time becomes an obvious and inevitable aspect of local response.

In grasping the significance of this observation about being »in the field « the idea of the assemblage as a rhizomatic form is helpful; it foregrounds the notions of connectivity, multi-dimensionality, variation, expansion, and capture which seemed to be going on around me as I wrote my field notes.[17] Of particular interest in this paper is the way the concept invites reflection on the interplay between de-territorialization and re-territorialization in the way that scientific, institutional, and bureaucratic forms are replicated in different settings across the globe. In these processes, the work of de-territorialization is apparent in the way local forms are drawn into wider networks and hierarchies. Thus, establishing IVF in Sri Lanka entails the development of, and commitment to, trans-national connections and collaborations (economic, professional, supervisory,

17 Deleuze and Guattari, *A Thousand Plateaus*, op. cit. (note 12).

regulatory, personal etc.). These linkages are key to establishing authority, authenticity, and legitimacy in the transfer of novel clinical techniques, their ethical oversight, and commercial exploitation. The movement back and forth of persons, information, drugs, and equipment results in a creative de-territorialization whereby the delivery of IVF treatment in Colombo is actively made to look the same as IVF delivery anywhere else in the world. But hierarchy is also complemented by independence, that is, the establishment at the local level of autonomous and self-sufficient versions of these forms. Here we might identify the quest for an appropriate ethics, locally sensitive regulations, and the creation of distinctive markets and publics. In these activities are found imaginative attempts to re-territorialize the assemblage such that IVF in Sri Lanka is not merely a replication of clinical practices and their governance as found elsewhere, but also an attempt to frame IVF such that it carries traces of beliefs and values that will resonate with local users and providers alike. Before considering this process further, it will be helpful to locate them within some broader discourses about infertility and reproduction in Sri Lanka.

IVF in Sri Lanka

Producing offspring in Sri Lanka satisfies deep-rooted expectations on the part of partners, extended families, and women themselves that they should become mothers in the early years of marriage. Frustration of this desire is one of the major catastrophes of personal and family life. In a society in which there are few social spaces for a childless couple to occupy comfortably, absence of children and the frustration of social reproduction that this entails is a cause of deep anguish and social stigma. Against this backdrop, IVF has been propagated as a technology with immediate and powerful appeal: it offers relief to couples facing the most desperate of social circumstances and does so with the authority of advanced technological interventions fresh from Europe, North America, or Singapore. However, while awareness of the promise of these technologies has reached many, they are not available through the National Health Service and the numbers that can afford the treatments privately are currently very small.[18] IVF remains an expensive service that can only be accessed in the private sector.

Nonetheless, it has been recognized that there is a significant market for IVF in Sri Lanka. Prior to 1998, those wealthy enough to afford IVF would travel to India, Singapore, or Europe for treatment. Some enterprising doctors realized that providing these services locally would save considerably on travel costs and, even though drug costs would remain more or less constant, the costs of labor and services at local rates would ensure that further savings could be made. Indeed, some clinics even began to generate inward-coming health tourism with expatriates returning to Sri Lanka for treatment in surroundings that, some doctors claimed, were more attuned to cultural sensitivities than northern European clinics, as well as being considerably cheaper. Other markets were identified in India, Singapore, and the Maldives. However, one of the more important markets was, and continues to be, found among the burgeoning numbers of urban dual-earner professional couples in Sri Lanka. Such couples find themselves with heavy financial commitments in the early years of marriage and opt to delay childbearing until careers have been established and there is greater financial stability. Meeting one set of desires thus means disaggregating and sublimating others, and later childbearing often means that reproductive problems are exacerbated. For these and other reasons, couples are finding their way onto the waiting lists of the capital's private infertility clinics in increasing numbers.

The development of these clinics requires a good deal of investment of time, money, and clinical expertise from local doctors and entrepreneurs. These developments also relied heavily on collaborations with overseas providers in the early stages. Initially, these collaborations took the form of »getting down« specialists such as embryologists from the UK, Europe, and Singapore to complement local teams. As more local specialists have been trained, the evidence of foreign practitioners has reduced, although the collaborations around the transfers of expertise in clinical techniques,

18 The five major private clinics offering IVF in Sri Lanka are located in Colombo. Smaller clinics exist in Kandy and Kurunegala. There have been attempts to initiate IVF in government hospitals, but these have proved unsuccessful due to the cost to the NHS, the high laboratory standards needed for successful IVF, and the difficulty of attracting sufficient numbers of trained personnel.

technological capability, and organizational support are still common. The profile of local doctors involved in these collaborations is high. They are seen to be bringing important technologies to Sri Lanka for the benefit of people who might not otherwise be able to afford the costs of overseas travel. Moreover, where Buddhists are concerned, these are doctors carrying out highly meritorious acts in that they are doing »service« (sevaya) and relieving suffering. Doctors undertaking IVF also gain high status by virtue of the fact that they are working to assist reproduction against a backdrop in which, in recent decades, violence and the threat of national disintegration have never been far from people's thoughts. In these circumstances, pro-natalist ideologies have come to the fore and new reproductive technologies become a powerful symbol of the ability to overcome reproductive crisis.[19] Finally, the development of new reproductive technologies has a wider symbolic significance in terms of national development. The ability to participate in global scientific advance is in itself a powerful statement of the nation's development credentials and a source of great kudos for the doctors who are seen to accomplish this.

However, behind the headlines proclaiming bold advance, concerns were voiced from various quarters about the headlong rush into areas of reproductive medicine that unsettled accepted moralities. Underlying the celebration of reproductive technologies and the demand that this stimulates, there were expressions of disquiet about how the country, or more specifically the medical and legal professions, were responding or rather failing to respond to this and other biomedical revolutions.[20] Anxieties about the inadequacy of regulation in relation to the new reproductive technologies were first triggered by doctors concerned about the possible transmission of HIV/AIDS due to lack of screening in relation to sperm donation. Attempts to address this problem soon revealed the extent to which a range of other transactions in sperm, eggs, and embryos were

19 Bob Simpson, »Localising a Brave New World: New Reproductive Technologies and the Politics of Fertility in Contemporary Sri Lanka«, in: *Reproductive Agency, Medicine and the State*, ed. by Maya Unnithan-Kumar (Oxford: Berghahn, 2004), pp. 43–58.

20 For example, in March 2000 Professor Rohan Jayasekera, Sri Lanka's leading human geneticist gave a public lecture entitled »Genethics in Sri Lanka: The Slumbering Sentinels.« In it he provided an overview of the range of ethical, legal, and social challenges resulting from the island's engagement with new reproductive and genetic technologies and highlighted the failure of the professions to address these issues.

already being practiced without ethical or regulatory oversight. Indeed, foreign teams were rumored to operate freely in the island, providing a range of reproductive services using local clinics as their platform. Concerns were expressed that such teams might be practicing in ways that fell below the ethical standards of their countries of origin. One major source of anxiety lay in the possibility that IVF might be taking place using gametes that had originated from outside of a married couple who had consented to treatment. The consequences of unregulated transactions in gametes was seen by some practitioners in this field as a threat to the stability of marriage and the family; lack of clarity about the relationship between donors, genetic material, and its recipients would be likely to cause offense to Buddhists, Catholics, and Muslims alike. A second major concern was that large sums of money were being handed over for treatments that were poorly targeted and implemented and therefore prone to failure. National bodies such as the National Science Foundation, National Science and Technology Commission, and Sri Lanka Medical Council Ethics Committee all debated these issues and pressed for tighter regulation. The need was expressed for clearer guidelines that would inform the actions of those engaging in this burgeoning field, with the desire that these guidelines would, in due course, be given »teeth« in the form of an underpinning legislation that would establish an »authority« to license and monitor all centers carrying out IVF, gamete donation, and storage. Models from the UK [Human Fertilisation and Embryology Act 1990 and Australia [Infertility (medical procedure) Act 1982] were regularly invoked as models worthy of replication. Such a framework was seen by many practitioners as crucial in building defenses against external agents using Sri Lanka to carry out activities that were not acceptable elsewhere, as well as preventing local practitioners from operating, intentionally or unintentionally, in ways that might offend local sensitivities and, more importantly, cause people harm. The fact that other countries had already »been down this road« was a self-evident justification for using regulatory templates from elsewhere and, moreover, for adopting key elements of their deliberations as major building blocks of a local response.

Part of the study undertaken in 2002–03 concerned the attempts to create such regulatory defenses. The activities I focused on were those of expert working groups and their various efforts to prepare guidelines which would, in due course be underpinned by acts of parliament similar to those in place in the UK and elsewhere.[21] Undoubtedly, there will at some point emerge an official »story« of regulation of the new technologies in Sri Lanka; it will be linear and show how different expert groups begat guidelines which begat laws. However, almost ten years on, there is some guidance but no regulation. The development of the assemblage continues to be strategically fluid, made up of many minor instances of connection and capture.

In the sections that follow, I describe three brief episodes that took place during my fieldwork in 2002–03. I have characterized these as »cutting edges« as they represent points at which the global assemblage of IVF was brought decisively into connection with local networks of medical professionals and their publics. In these encounters, the negotiation of IVF as a kind of duplex can be glimpsed, that is, an ensemble of practices that is both emergent from, and therefore a part of, the global IVF assemblage, yet is distinct and autonomous within it.

»Cutting Edges«: IVF as De-Territorialization and Re-Territorialization

Whilst in the field in 2003, considerable excitement was generated among those interested in the treatment of infertility in Sri Lanka by a visit from Dr. Simon Fishel, an embryologist and the director of the Nottingham-based CARE network of fertility clinics. As well as being director of a network of clinics in the UK, Fishel has been involved with an extensive network of international collaborations which has brought technical expertise and advice to emerging fertility services in many different countries. These collaborations have included Sri Lanka and the Vindana clinic

21 The National Science and Technology Commission produced its report, *New Genetics and Assisted Reproductive Technologies in Sri Lanka: A Draft National Policy on Biomedical Ethics* in 2003. As a direct recommendation of this report the *Sri Lanka Medical Council's Assisted Reproductive Technologies: Code of Practice* was published in 2005. Here proposals were made for an Act of Parliament to regulate ARTs. On a visit in 2008, I was informed that the Act had been partially drafted but was not yet ready for submission.

referred to at the beginning of this paper. This association was marked by a high profile visit in March 2003, to sign a memorandum of agreement and participate in a series of consultations, lectures and meetings in which he would share his considerable experience and offer advice to various groups of stakeholders as to how they should proceed with the challenge of embracing technological advance within suitable ethical and regulatory frameworks.

At the time, a picture appeared in the Ceylon Daily News showing Dr. Fishel lighting a traditional brass oil lamp. This is an auspicious act that marks occasions of importance. It not only signifies welcome but demonstrates good-will and shared purpose at the beginning of a joint venture (such as a marriage); it thus locates the commercial act of signing an agreement within a broader cultural etiquette. In the picture, the act is overseen by Dr. P.R. Anthonis, a medical luminary in Sri Lanka and a former chancellor of the University of Colombo, and Dr. Athula Kahandaliyanage, at that time director of Health Services. The caption reads: »The Vindana Reproductive Health Centre signed an agreement with CARE UK …[ ]… to facilitate the introduction of latest international technology on test tube baby birth to the in vitro fertility programme in Sri Lanka.«

For the Vindana team, the collaboration with Dr. Fishel and the CARE Network offered the opportunity to work with what the director described as a »good« group, that is, a group containing professionals who are recognized, experienced, and with a reputation for working outside the UK. The implicit contrast here was with the ad hoc arrangements with itinerant clinicians of the kind who had worked elsewhere in Sri Lanka and with little by way of accountability in the longer-term. The »good« collaboration would include training, technical support, help with quality assurance oversight and advice on some of the more challenging cases that assisted reproduction generates. The collaboration was widely trailed in the media and served as a powerful statement of linkage and legitimation for local audiences regarding the clinic's present and future work in assisted reproduction. The three »cutting edges« I wish to draw attention to are as follows:

1. Pioneering Genealogies: The birth of Louise Brown in 1978 was an event of profound significance in the development of IVF. It was a notable first for Edwards and Steptoe as well as members of their team. Dr. Fishel was part of the original team, and this is noted as one of the many »firsts« in which members of the CARE's UK team have been involved with.[22] A prominent feature of the news reporting of the visit to Sri Lanka was the attention paid to this direct linkage with the birth of Louise Brown, the »first« IVF child; a critical point of connection that Dr. Fishel brought into the Sri Lankan setting. Dr. Fishel was a »pioneer,« and it seemed entirely appropriate that the collaboration was with local »pioneers.« The rhetorical import of this event was thus not only in terms of the clinical practice and organizational procedures that the collaboration would bring – the replication of »good practice« – but also in terms of the canonical narratives that surround the relief of the »desperate« needs which those who are involuntarily childless carry with them. As Vindana Centre had had the first all-Sri Lankan team to produce an IVF baby back in July 2002, the linkage with Dr. Fishel and CARE established a genealogical link of sorts back to Louise Brown. However, the claim to be »first« also sent out a number of other important messages. First, it made a powerful statement to the outside world about technological competence and independence: the relationship with CARE could be entered into without the need to draw directly on their practical expertise to perform IVF, as this had already been established in 2002. The relationship was cast by the director of the center as one between collaborators looking to future developments and not merely as one between a patron and a client. The team had thus succeeded in staking their claim in progress and modernity. Second, it signaled to local audiences the achievement of Sri Lankan scientists. This achievement was widely reported in the press with the essence of its newsworthiness being the achievement of technological self-sufficiency in this most vital of interventions. The Sinhala press was also keen to point out that this was a »Sinhala Buddhist« child that was born to a group of doctors who were an »all-Sri Lankan« team.[23] This was not just any old connection but one that could be made to carry a significant political load once placed in the turbulent ethno-politics in which the island is currently gripped. This loading becomes all the more significant when it is noted that the first IVF child born on Sri Lankan soil was actually born

22 See http://www.carefertilityweb.co.uk/aboutus/firsts.shtml for the CARE segment of the genealogy.

23 Divayina newspaper, 26th Septemper 2002.

in November 1999 to a Tamil couple from Batticaloa (The Sunday Times of Sri Lanka 14th November 1999). Crucially, the team that achieved this birth contained UK specialists and was led by a Tamil doctor. Although the director of the Vindana team was always keen, both in public and in private, to point out that they were not the first team to deliver an IVF baby in Sri Lanka, the earlier birth has been largely superseded by their achievements. The Vindana team members are now widely acknowledged as the ones who were the first to render global IVF as Sri Lankan IVF.

2. Regulation and the State: The visit by Dr. Fishel was also intended to operate as another kind of »cutting edge« in the development of IVF as a local practice. As already stated, regulation of the new technologies is not very strong in Sri Lanka. This problem is further compounded by the fact that the communities of interest that have formed around IVF in Sri Lanka as in other places are relatively small, with the result that regulators and practitioners are often the same people wearing different hats. Thus, managing the desire to regulate and control the activities of clinics alongside concerns about interference and unhelpful bureaucratization is a process that takes on a curious circularity. In one sense, this is the replication of a tension familiar in the UK and other settings where mixed medical economies operate involving professional, public, and commercial interests.[24] At several points in meetings and talks to various audiences, Dr. Fishel returned to his own experience of the relationship between private clinics and the HFEA in the UK. Along with a number of other high profile directors of UK private clinics, Dr. Fishel's relationship with the HFEA has been a somewhat turbulent one in which the potential of new reproductive technologies had been, in his view, needlessly restrained by an over-cautious regulatory machinery .Essentially, in his view clinicians know best and should be left to self-regulate with minimum interference.[25] In keeping with this pioneering spirit, the view he advocated was that clinicians should be allowed to address their patients'

24 Martin H. Johnson & Kerry Petersen, »Public interest or public meddling? Towards an objective framework for the regulation of assisted reproduction technologies«, in: *Human Reproduction* 23 (2008), 3, pp. 716–728.

25 At the time of his visit, Fishel was engaged in an attempt to get HFEA approval for the creation of a »savior sibling« for Zain Hashmi, a child with Thalassaemia. A special license was granted for this procedure in the House of Lords after being refused by the HFEA. More recently (May 20th 2008), the House of Commons voted to endorse

needs without having to request permission at every turn for licenses from an intermediary authority. It is taken as part of the inexorable progress of the biosciences that what is greeted with concern and scepticism today will be commonplace tomorrow. In a country like Sri Lanka, in which there is considerable antipathy towards bureaucracy as the primary source of a more general inertia and indifference, such comments had an immediate appeal, albeit a rather different one than originally intended by Dr. Fishel. Specifically, it offered support to a strategy of keeping regulation at arm's length vis-à-vis the practitioner community. They also invited a contrast to be made between the entrepreneurial and scientific success of the private sector clinic and the weakness of the state to act in areas such as the new reproductive technologies. The effect was to add to a familiar dynamic in Sri Lankan society, namely the appearance of governance which masks a state of considerable openness and flexibility. Under these circumstances, the space that opens up between the intention to act and its realization in the form of different kinds of engagement with the new technologies is considerable. As one clinician put it, ethical and regulatory issues are likely to remain, a matter of »common sense« and individual »self-discipline« of a kind that doctors from all parts of the world might assume that they share. In this view, beyond ensuring that practitioners have the right qualifications, that laboratories are properly equipped and licensed, and that protocols and procedures are in place to meet patient needs and protect their rights, then there is little that the state or anyone else should be called on to do when it comes to the conduct of IVF. This is indeed the way that it has remained until the present. Clinics are required to be registered with the Sri Lanka Medical Council as the interim authority identified in its Code of Practice on Assisted Reproductive Technologies produced in 2005. However, the prospect of regulation remains a long way off, given that the push from practitioners is not strong as they regulate themselves to a large extent. Also, such legislation is unlikely to be a state priority as the country enters into what is effectively a period of post-war reconstruction. Under the cover of anticipated policy and regulation, many novel techniques and practices can slip into place with little by way of scrutiny or oversight.

---

revisions to the Human Fertilisation and Embryology Bill which would allow for the creation of »savior siblings« in cases where there was a serious illness.

3. Meanings of the Embryo: While on his visit, Dr. Fishel gave a public lecture to the Medico-Legal Society of Sri Lanka entitled »Ethico-legal Issues in Assisted Reproduction: International Experience« (Colombo, 19th March 2003). The meeting was opened with a welcome from no less a personage than Sarath Silva, the Chief Justice of Sri Lanka. In his opening remarks, the Chief Justice began by referring to a question put to a Buddhist priest (by whom, it wasn't clear): Are the techniques in question »compatible« with Buddhism? The priest's response was positive and the Chief Justice explained why. In Buddhism, he opined, there is a basic distinction made between physical processes of the body and those of the mind. Developing this somewhat Cartesian view, he went on to explain that artificial reproductive technologies posed no problem for Buddhists because they only dealt with the physical aspect of reproduction and not the mental or spiritual aspects. By the latter, he was referring to a key point of differentiation in a Buddhist understanding of the early stages of conception, namely the arrival of consciousness (vinnāna) that is believed to enter into the physical configuration of cells which forms in the womb at conception. The vinnāna that falls or descends into the womb is believed to be released at the death of another being and, whether instantaneously or following a period of disconnection, it passes on into another incarnation. This emphasis on the role of the vinnāna in reproduction not only served to dismiss a swathe of ethical concerns, but also aligned Buddhism with these new and challenging technologies. The Chief Justice went on to use a Buddhist reading of conception to explain the failure rate of approximately two thirds of all attempts at IVF. Quite simply, these were instances where the all-important vinnāna had failed to make its appearance.[26] As a prelude to a lecture on the global promise and challenges of assisted reproductive technologies, the Chief Justice had provided an open door. There was no conflict between the island's predominant religious tradition and the IVF revolution that Dr. Fishel was there to promote and extend.[27] In-

26 In textual accounts, the *vinnāna* is but one of the five constituents or *skandha* necessary for a living being to come into existence, the others being material form (*rūpa*), sensation (*vedanā*), perceptions (*sannā*), and mental formations (*samkhāra*). In the Pāli canon there is repeated emphasis on the fact that the conjunction of all five groups is necessary for the constitution of a living being.

27 For a more extended version of this argument, see Bob Simpson, »We Have always Been Modern: Buddhism, Science and the New Genetic and Reproductive Technolo-

deed, a Buddhist rendition of the ethics of reproductive technology could contribute its own universalizing discourses to the development of IVF as global form.

Conclusion

In this essay I have offered what might be thought of, following Deleuze and Guattari, as a slice into the rhizome; a brief ethnographic insight into the conjunction of power, reproduction, and bureaucracy as articulated by experts and professionals operating in an elite sector of medicine in contemporary Sri Lanka. The account reveals that in becoming part of the global IVF assemblage, there would appear to be a submission, often eager and willing on the part of local doctors and clinicians, to its commercial, technological, and ideological potential. As I have argued, the assemblage is powerfully expansive and de-territorializing in its effects. Through a replication of a genealogy of practice, the clinic takes on familiarity in terms of its treatments, the way they are presented, and the justifications that are used for the forms that these take. Similarly, the construction of governance in the form of guidelines and regulations also falls into readily discernible patterns modeled on those from other parts of the world. In short, IVF in Sri Lanka is made to look like IVF anywhere else. To participate in the making of the assemblage in its local forms is therefore to be demonstrably part of the bigger projects that IVF betokens: progress, modernity, and the future. However, what I also hope to have thrown light on is the way that those who work hard to replicate these forms are also at the forefront of rhetorical attempts to differentiate, that is, to render the delivery of services compatible with the expectations of local publics, whether made up of consumers of the technologies, potential ones or audiences who are at some remove. The work carried out in this regard involves imagination and creativity in rendering IVF »culturally appropriate« or, more accurately, culturally appropriated and therefore bounded, autonomous, and distinct. There is, in short, the possibility of

gies in Sri Lanka«, in: special edition of *Culture and Religion* (ed. by Yulia Egorova) 10 (2009), 2, pp.137–158.

perspectives on emergent biotechnologies that can be taken as definitively Sri Lankan. The assemblage thus always appears duplex; both the same as in other parts of the world yet different; imposed from without while owned from within; contrived and artificial yet somehow inevitable and natural. The challenge for the ethnographer wishing to capture these aspects of IVF as a global form, is not to render these oppositions as polar and somehow fixed but to convey their connection and relative mutability; their propensity to de-territorialization and re-territorialization. In the interplay of parts and wholes, it is the task of the ethnographer to look beneath the apparent smoothness of the narratives describing the arrival of IVF and at the partial connections that belie these homogenous representations.[28] Such connections link the anthropological account with the history of elisions, omissions, and condensations in which processes once messy and contingent become tidy and linear in their routine presentation and performance. Furthermore, in the work of converting commerce, creativity, and contingency into »the legacy of IVF« – reducing all to the same – there is not an endpoint; there are always questions of how to engage with its present and future possibilities for substitution, artificiality, and exchange. The legacy in all its rhetorical and naturalizing force has to be created at every turn, and the ethnographic challenge is to capture the systematicity in this process without losing site of its unruly, serendipitous, and contingent aspects.

28 Marilyn Strathern, *Partial Connections* (Savage, Maryland: Rowman & Littlefield Publishers, 1991).

Practitioners as Interface Agents between the Local and the Global: The Localization of IVF in Turkey[1]

Zeynep B. Gürtin

One of the most striking aspects of assisted reproductive technologies (ARTs) has been their rapid globalization. However, as highlighted by a growing body of ethnographic research, ARTs have been subject to diverse contextual interpretations in different locations. The practice of ARTs is subject not only to scientific developments, but also to intricate negotiations between these and local concerns, possibilities, and morals. While the processes of localization can have a variety of drives and drivers (including regulators or patient support groups, see Polat in this volume), this paper focuses specifically on the role of in vitro fertilization (IVF) practitioners. Examining the ways in which practitioners interact at both the global and the local levels of IVF practice, and the ways in which they enable communication and connection between these (separate and sometimes incompatible) spheres, I conceptualize their role as *interface agents* who transform universal scientific knowledge about assisted reproduction into culturally expedient applications for their patients.

Based on ethnographic work between 2005 and 2009 and in-depth interviews with 28 senior practitioners, I take Turkey as my case-study and

1 Subsequent to the writing of this paper in July 2009, substantial changes were made to the regulation of assisted reproduction in Turkey. Interestingly, the core changes pertain directly to the examples discussed in this chapter: the new statute, introduced in March 2010, prohibits reproductive travel and its facilitation for the purposes of gamete donation, and compels single embryo transfer for all women undergoing their first cycle of IVF with a maximum of two embryos on subsequent cycles. These recent changes are currently facing strong opposition from various groups, including a patient support organization, professional organizations and practitioners, and many individual patients. The current debates and their resolution, one way or another, will likely have a profound impact on how IVF is practiced in Turkey. This paper must therefore be read as describing a particular period of IVF practice in Turkey, which will already be history by the time it is published.

explore the material and discursive practices by which Turkish IVF practitioners moderate, modify, and mold IVF practice. Taking account of and accountable to both global and local sensibilities, demands, and preoccupations, practitioners must find the right balance in ART practice. Moreover, they are not only required to define the parameters of practice in their own clinics and more broadly in their nation, they must also represent and justify these decisions to the scrutiny of various constituencies and audiences. There may be myriad means to achieve these ends, but I focus on two in this paper: *negotiating trans/nationalism* and *designating sameness and difference*. The former is illustrated with reference to the choreography of ART treatments involving donor gametes, and the latter with an analysis of discourses surrounding embryo transfer numbers. Both of these cases demonstrate the multiple obligations practitioners have at both the global and the local level (to the scientific community, to national regulators, to their patients) and the complex and intricate ways in which they need to work in order to successfully localize a global techno-science.

Global assemblages?

During the past three decades, IVF and its descendants have led to the »miracle« birth of millions of »test-tube babies« around the world. These treatments have transformed the global (in)fertility landscape and have profoundly altered the reproductive trajectories of countless involuntarily childless individuals. Although often marked and marred by resource and access inequalities, which further stratify reproduction[2] both between and within populations, ARTs continue to expand their appeal, reaching from Europe and the United States to Asia, South America, and the Middle East. However, this global spread has been far from homogenizing in its effects: rather than a series of replicas, ART practice around the world is characterized by great diversity engendered through processes of indigenization and context-specific application.

2 Faye D. Ginsburg & Rayna Rapp (Eds.), *Conceiving the New World Order: The Global Politics of Reproduction* (Berkeley, University of California Press, 1995).

To better understand the diversity of ART practice it is important to bear in mind that these technologies are not transferred into »cultural voids.« Indeed, as medical anthropologist Marcia Inhorn explains, »local considerations, be they cultural, social, economic, or political, shape and sometimes curtail the way these Western-generated technologies are both offered to and received by non-Western subjects.«[3] As ARTs are introduced to or practiced in specific contexts, they become subject to various »arenas of constraint« with different structural, ideological, and practical obstacles and apprehensions serving to limit access, define prohibitions, and delineate parameters for their application.[4] Indeed, these constraints and opportunities define the character of ARTs in each of their different incarnations, with a possibility of endless variations. The resulting heterogeneity has been, and continues to be, the subject of a growing body of social science literature, illustrating through rich and vivid ethnographies the multiplicity of ways in which ARTs are localized and tailored to specific populations.[5]

Moreover, these detailed and diverse ethnographies, with the aid of theoretical perspectives that emphasize the co-constitutive relationships of societies and technologies,[6] increasingly negate a unidirectional model of technology transfer. It is not (any longer?) a case of exporting ARTs »from the West to the rest,« but rather a range of dynamic and pluridirectional exchanges between multiple contexts that dis-locate and re-locate these technologies and practices. Local parameters for ART application serve not only to translate scientific knowledge and practice, but also to generate improvements and innovations. A clear example of this may be

3 Marcia C. Inhorn, »The ›Local‹ Confronts the ›Global‹: Infertile Bodies and New Reproductive Technologies in Egypt«, in: *Infertility Around the Globe: New Thinking on Childlessness, Gender, and Reproductive Technologies*, ed. by Marcia C. Inhorn & Frank van Balen (Berkeley: University of California Press, 2002), p. 265.

4 Marcia C. Inhorn, »Global Infertility and the Globalization of New Reproductive Technologies: Illustrations from Egypt«, in: *Social Science and Medicine* 56 (2003), pp. 1837–1851; Marcia C. Inhorn, *Local Babies, Global Science: Gender, Religion, and In Vitro Fertilization in Egypt* (New York: Routledge, 2003).

5 For a review of this literature, see Marcia C. Inhorn & Daphna Birenbaum-Carmeli, »Assisted Reproductive Technologies and Culture Change«, in: *Annual Review of Anthropology* 37 (2008), pp. 177–196.

6 E.g. Aihwa Ong & Stephen J. Collier (Eds.), *Global Assemblages: Technology, Politics, and Ethics as Anthropological Problems* (Oxford: Blackwell Publishing, 2005).

seen in Italy, where practitioners invested in the development and improvement of oocyte cryopreservation following the prohibition of embryo storage in 2004.[7] These developments demonstrate the interactional processes that facilitate the (at times unexpected) pluridirectional movements of techno-science, and also exemplify the potential for »arenas of constraint« to simultaneously act as catalysts for ingenuity and development. When global technology is localized, local permutations contribute back to the body of global knowledge and science, the total sum of which is continually available to processes of dis-location and re-location. It thus becomes increasingly difficult, or meaningless, to speak of some nations as the ones that generate and distribute and others as the ones that receive and replicate these technologies, or to put it another way, to speak of center and periphery models.

In addition to these technological dispersals, pluridirectional ART pathways increasingly admit the disjunctive flows, to use Appadurai's terminology, of experts and patients, material, processes and protocols, pharmaceuticals, debates, and gametes from one location to one or more others. Indeed, as inter-national disparities between techno-scientific or financial resources, mismatch, for example, the availability of biological material or the social desirability of the conditions of practice, the global ART landscape becomes typified by variable and incommensurate stratifications, where surplus in one area may accompany deficit in another. These stratifications push and pull both need and demand in different directions in a bustling hypermarket. One result of this is the growing phenomenon of »reproductive tourism,« whereby men and women seek fertility treatments across national borders for a variety of reasons, from avoiding local restrictions to accessing scarce resources. Via geographical mobility and economic capital, these »fertility tourists or global consumers«[8] can trade their unfavorable »home« conditions (including prohibitions, waiting lists, high costs, or a range of other factors) for more favorable offers from other jurisdictions. Whether these

7 Guila Scaravelli et al., »Analysis of oocyte cryopreservation in assisted reproduction: the Italian National Register data from 2005 to 2007«, in: *Reproductive BioMedicine Online* 21 (2010), pp. 496–500.

8 Lorraine Cully & Nicky Hudson, »Fertility Tourists or Global Consumers? A Sociological Agenda for Exploring Cross-Border Reproductive Travel«, in: *The International Journal of Interdisciplinary Social Sciences* 4 (2010), 10, pp. 1833–1882.

practices are framed as »reproductive tourism« or »reproductive exile«[9] makes little difference to their allusion to a global fertility market that makes it increasingly difficult to contain ARTs within national borders.

On the one hand, then, it is possible to theorize the spread of ARTs as an exemplary illustration of a strikingly new interactive system, in which deterritorialized technological know-how, money, persons, commodities, images, and even ideologies »are involved in ceaselessly chasing each other around the world.«[10] Yet, on the other, ethnographic accounts repeatedly describe processes of localization by which transported ARTs are translated and, sometimes laboriously, made appropriate, acceptable, and meaningful for local populations. One means of reconciling these reflections may be to bring under the analytical gaze of social science not the de- or re-contextualization of techno-science, but its concomitant capacity for both, as proposed by Ong and Collier (2005).[11] It is, they argue, in *assemblages* – »the actual and specific articulation of a global form«[12] – that we find the animated details of practice and can begin to tease out interactions. However, in defining global forms by their »distinctive capacity for decontextualisation and recontextualisation, abstractability and movement, across diverse social and cultural situations,«[13] it is possible to overstate their fluidity and thus to inadvertently eclipse the very *work* often necessary to enable their travel. Taking this potential blind-spot as a starting point and IVF practitioners as its focus, this paper articulates the work that interweaves the local with the global, with specific reference to the Turkish example.

9 Marcia C. Inhorn & Pasquale Patrizio, »Rethinking Reproductive ›Tourism‹ as Reproductive ›Exile‹«, in: *Fertility and Sterility* 92 (2009) 3, pp. 904–906.

10 Arjun Appadurai, *Modernity at Large: Cultural Dimensions of Globalization* (Minneapolis: University of Minnesota Press, 1996), p. 38.

11 Stephen Collier & Aihwa Ong, »Global Assemblages, Anthropological Problems«, in: *Global Assemblages: Technology, Politics, and Ethics as Anthropological Problems*, ed. by Aihwa Ong & Stephen Collier (Oxford: Blackwell Publishing, 2005).

12 Stephen Collier, »Global Assemblages«, in: *Theory, Culture and Society* 23 (2006), pp. 399–401, in particular p. 400.

13 Collier & Ong, »Global Assemblages«, op. cit. (note 11), p. 11.

Practitioners as Interface Agents

»Interface (*noun*)
1. A surface lying between two portions of matter
or space, and forming their common boundary.
2. A means or place of interaction between two systems, organizations, etc.; a
meeting-point or common ground between two parties, systems, or disciplines.
Interface (*verb*)
1. To connect (scientific equipment) *with* or *to*
so as to make possible joint operation.
2. To come into interaction *with*.«
Oxford English Dictionary

When talking about senior IVF practitioners, I am referring to key actors who not only see patients on a daily basis, but often also make important resource allocation and pricing decisions as directors of IVF clinics, sit on national committees debating regulation, make television appearances and engage in public education, regularly attend conferences and contribute to scientific publications, and partake in international discussions regarding the present and the future of assisted reproduction. As members of both global scientific networks and local communities or cultures, these practitioners are intermediaries that facilitate both the transnational abstraction and successful national application of ART practice. In order to succeed, they need to represent, mediate, and interpret across contexts, as well as at times to produce exact replications. As the connection between the local and the global, practitioners are required to translate between these two spheres and to balance competing demands at transnational and national levels. It is primarily through their mediation that the concerns or commodities of one collective can become audible, legible, and functional forms for the other, and thus they also play a central role in generating representations. Moreover, practitioners are key to the abstraction, dispersal, and/or re-assembly of techno-scientific knowledge, protocols, and patients, commonly acting as vectors that define the distance and direction in which these travel. I therefore propose conceiving of practitioners as *interface agents.*

The concept of *interface agents* encapsulates the role of practitioners between the local and the global, and directing ethnographic attention to the work they do provides empirical grounding by which abstract connections can be made manifest through concrete, contextualised examples. Although IVF practitioners have various material, collective, and discursive means of intersecting the local and the global, in this paper I wish to discuss two in particular: *negotiating trans/nationalism* and *designating sameness and difference.* Negotiating trans/nationalism involves enabling or disabling transnational demands, identities, and connections by selectively breaching or bolstering a variety of national boundaries and borders. It is the process of judgment and prioritization by which some avenues for transnational exchange are opened and widened, while others are constrained and narrowed. Designating sameness and difference refers to acts of representation and comparison by which practitioners explain and justify why ARTs are practiced as they are in a particular context (with implicit or explicit comparisons to alternatives), and from where (the local or the global) they derive constituent aspects of their character. The total sum of practitioners' actions – including which technologies to offer, to whom and in what manner, and how to represent, explain, and justify these decisions to internal and external audiences – is central to developing the national character of ARTs in any particular location. This national assemblage then will necessarily take account not only of global scientific developments, standards, and decisions, but also of what people want, need, or find morally appropriate at the local level.

A methodological focus on practitioners and their practices can thus be used to interrogate the assemblage of ARTs from a particular angle. Analyzing my ethnographic research in Turkey from this angle has the advantage that my informants' (i.e. practitioners') reflexive accounts are made audible and their intricate work of assembling highlighted. Practitioners themselves define certain constituent parts as »local« and others as »global« through flexible boundary-practices and designations of sameness and difference. Moreover, their reflexive constructions or accounts are fundamentally malleable and inherently relational – a means of impression management[14] – where IVF in Turkey, for example, may be portrayed differently to different audiences. The (context-specific) allocation or amplification of certain characteristics as definitive of or integral to IVF practice in Turkey foretells much about the perceived priorities or prej-

14 Erving Goffman, *The Presentation of Self in Everyday Life* (London: Penguin Books, 1959, 1990 reprint).

udices of the audience, as well as of the priorities of the presenter. The layered image that emerges shows a global assemblage that is continuously re-assembled through the individual and collective efforts of practitioners, with the result being a unique and localized version of ART practice.

IVF in Turkey

> »Sure some technologies may take a long time to come to our country, but our desire for *tüp bebek* technology in this country is very high. [...] So these technologies – I mean it is related to the need, it is about supply and demand – so, as you see, these technologies quickly reach our country.«
>
> Senior IVF practitioner, Turkey[15]

IVF technology – or *tüp bebek* (literally tube-baby) as both its process and products are ubiquitously known – has become one of the most arresting hallmarks of contemporary Turkish society. Ever-present in popular media coverage, from celebrity endorsements on daytime television shows specializing in conversation targeted at housewives (*sohbet programları*) to cutting-edge news items on the front pages of broadsheets, *tüp bebek* stories regularly pique the national interest. Illustrated by the common motifs of happy families created after long personal struggles and the successes of diligent Turkish doctors, *tüp bebek* is a source of palpable national pride and valorized as a cutting-edge product of modern medicine.

Since 2005, the Turkish IVF industry has undergone rapid growth and development. Although the prevalence and popularity of reproductive technologies are commonly attributed to their cultural aptitude (as illustrated by the quote that opens this section), marked increases in demand with their concomitant opportunities for market expansion are undoubtedly also associated, in this context, with the advent of funded treatment cycles. Introduced by the state and social security institutions during 2005 and 2006, funding for two cycles of IVF, redeemable against treatment in

15 Quote taken from an interview with the senior IVF-practitioner of a public hospital in Istanbul, February 2005. Interview conducted by Asiye Kaya, as part of the »Reproducing Kinship« project, Department of European Ethnology, Humboldt University at Berlin.

state institutions or available as part-payment for treatment in private clinics, is available to all eligible Turkish couples.[16] The significant widening of participation in assisted reproduction facilitated by these provisions can be inferred from the rises in clinic numbers and annual treatment cycles. According to Prof. Bülent Tıraş, the President of TSRM at the time, the number of treatment cycles in Turkey doubled from approximately 20 000 in 2005 to 40 000 in 2007[17], and during the same period the number of IVF clinics increased by almost 50%, from 66 to 91, with private clinics accounting for *all* of this increase[18]. Turkey's total IVF expenditure in 2007 was reported to be in excess of 300 million dollars, which according to national newspapers ranked Turkey as »The World's 7th Biggest IVF Market« (behind Israel, France, Spain, England, US, and Germany).[19] The records of the Ministry of Health, which is responsible for the licensing and registration of ART practices, state that there are currently 118 fertility clinics operating in Turkey, with a dense concentration in the larger cities of Istanbul, Ankara, and Izmir, but increasingly also in the country's furthest corners, from Trabzon on the Black Sea coast to Diyarbakır in the East.

The spread of IVF across Turkey communicates as much about the disintegration of cultural obstacles as it does about the traversing of geographical distance. The locally welcomed establishment and successful operation of IVF clinics in the most conservative, traditional, and religious areas of the country is a testament to the broadening social acceptability and desirability of high-tech fertility treatments. The increased social acceptability of IVF in Turkey can, at least in part, be attributed to the synchrony between moral, religious, and civic laws, which confine the

16 Eligibility criteria include marriage duration of a minimum of three years, an absence of any living children, and limits the woman's age to between 23 and 39 years.

17 *Hürriyet*, 31 January 2008.

18 These figures have been obtained from the archives of the Ministry of Health. Most recent data are available through their website at http://www.saglik.gov.tr.

19 This »finding« was announced by Ilknur Karakulak of Er-Kim Pharmaceuticals, one of the four companies distributing IVF drugs in Turkey, and also disseminated by representatives of the Turkish Society of Reproductive Medicine (TSRM) and The Turkish Society for Obstetrics and Gynecology (TJOD), appearing in the briefs of several news agencies, e.g. HaberTurk, 31 January 2008; NetHaber, 31 January 2008; Hürriyet, 31 January 2008. These figures were subsequently widely incorporated as background information in news coverage of Turkish IVF.

use of fertility treatments to heterosexual married couples using their own gametes. Third-party reproductive assistance (e.g. donor sperm, eggs, or embryos, or the use of surrogacy), a culturally problematic proposition prohibited by the local religion of Islam,[20] is also prohibited according to Turkey's ART regulation.[21] Confining IVF within strict parameters, so it can only be used to aid the medically impeded reproduction of married couples, designates it as simulacrum for traditional procreation. This pivotal emphasis on the marital unit (both practically indispensable and legally central) and their presumed medical need was often presented to me, by both patients and experts, as a self-evident justification for the moral absolution, and indeed virtue, of IVF treatment.

ARTs in Turkey, then, are perceived as a much needed »cure« for the tragedy of involuntary childlessness and have wide appeal for an emphatically pro-natalist population. Offered by a wide spectrum of institutions, from state hospitals to state-of-the-art private clinics, which cater to different socio-economic demographics, IVF is increasingly available to and sought after by broader sections of the population. Indeed, Prof. Bülent Tıraş, the President of the Turkish Society for Obstetrics and Gynecology, estimated that demand would only be met if at least 150 000 IVF cycles were undertaken per year.[22] The expansion of ARTs has been facilitated through the interplay of moral arbitration, geographical accessibility, the provision of funding, and, perhaps most crucially, the growing familiarity and promotion afforded by sustained, enthusiastic, and populist

20 The majority of Turkish Muslims (70–80%) belong to the Sunni branch of Islam. For an exegesis of Islamic attitudes and rulings regarding ARTs, including the differences between Sunni and Shi'a stances with regards to donor gametes, see Morgan Clarke, »Islam, Kinship and New Reproductive Technology«, in: *Anthropology Today* 22 (2006), pp. 17–22; Marcia C. Inhorn, »Making Muslim Babies: IVF and Gamete Donation in Sunni versus Shi'a Islam«, in: *Culture, Medicine and Psychiatry* 30 (2006), pp. 427–450; Marcia C. Inhorn, »Islam, IVF and Everyday Life in the Middle East: The Making of Sunni versus Shi'ite Test-Tube Babies«, in: *Anthropology of the Middle East* 1 (2006), 1, pp. 42–50.

21 The Ministry of Health introduced the »Statute for Centers for In Vitro Fertilization and Embryo Transfer« on 21 August 1987 (Official Gazette no. 19551). It was superseded on 19 November 1996 by the »Statute Concerning Assisted Reproduction Treatment Centers« (Official Gazette no. 22822), which has received several updates, with the latest on 8 July 2008 (Official Gazette no. 25869). The Ministry of Health provides an archive of Official Gazettes through its website, http://www.saglik.gov.tr.

22 Hürriyet, 31 January 2008.

media coverage. Through their involvement in techno-scientific as well as regulatory and commercial networks and via prolific media appearances, senior practitioners have been key architects of IVF in Turkey, arbitrating techno-scientific possibilities and developments with social and cultural expedience.

Negotiating Trans/Nationalism

> »A global culture, in whatever form, appears culturally fragmented, historically shallow and affectively neutral, by comparison with the emotive, easily intelligible and vibrant national cultures with which the vast majority of human beings have become familiar.«
> Anthony D. Smith[23]

Most, if not all, senior IVF practitioners in Turkey consider themselves to be part of a global ART community. Their membership is secured through the completion of training or internship placements in prestigious clinics, usually in the UK, Germany, or the United States, and is kept active through participation in international conferences, avid consumption of and contribution to the latest publications in leading journals, and personal communications with colleagues from other locations. Some senior practitioners can even trace their affiliation to particularly esteemed lineages: one pointed out to me a framed photograph of himself with Robert Edwards
indexEdwards, RobertindexEdwards, Jeanettein his office with the jovial remark, »Look, here is the man who made the earliest *tüp bebek*, with the man who is making the latest!« These biographical details of direct expertise inheritance, displayed in various, and variously targeted, formats in offices, CVs, or clinic websites, are professional-cum-personal assets with considerable value in a country that fetishizes Western techno-science. However, aside from their individual importance these transnational connections and collaborations in sum are credited with keeping the IVF

23 Anthony D. Smith, »Nations in Decline? The Erosion and Persistence of Modern National Identities«, in: *Nationalism in a Global Era: The Persistence of Nations*, ed. by Mitchell Young, Eric Zuelow & Andreas Sturm (London: Routledge, 2007), p. 18.

sector in Turkey up-to-date and apace with global (read: Western) developments.

Yet alongside an emphasis of the importance of transnational connections for scientific development, the very same practitioners also emphasize that being »a good doctor« is only possible if you understand your patients' concerns and respond to them with intimate contextual resonance. It is not their elite training but their tacit local knowledge that enables them to empathize with their patients and thus to treat them in the most suitable manner. Practitioners tailor their communication and the delivery of treatments to their heterogeneous patients, gaining trust and giving care in ways that sometimes resemble pseudo-kinship relations. Shared local understandings – referenced by my informants simply as »our culture (*bizim kültürümüz*)« or »our character (*bizim karakterimiz*),« where »our« denoted »Turkish« – are conferred as particularly essential to the practice of assisted reproduction.

Many practitioners explained to me that an appreciation of cultural taboos, and the extent to which infertility could be »a personal, emotional, and family catastrophe in Turkey,« necessitated that it must be approached »not mechanically, but receptively« by the medical profession. Practitioners saw it as their job to be mindful not just of the physical, but also of the psychological, familial, and social welfare of their patients. It was a sensitivity to situated values, preoccupations, and considerations – to Turkish culture or character – that enabled practitioners to exercise sound judgment in regulatory discussions and professional arbitration, to appropriately engage in »public enlightenment« through a »media-medicine nexus«[24] when promoting not just their own clinics but often ART in general, and to establish practices and protocols agreeable and attractive to Turkish men and women. In short, while transnational links enabled the development of expedient scientific knowledge, it was only through the filter of local know-how that this was converted into culturally prudent practice.

24 Aditya Bharadwaj, »Conception Politics: Medical Egos, Media Spotlights, and the Contest over Test-Tube First in India«, in: *Interpreting Infertility: Childlessness, Gender and Reproductive Technologies in Global Perspective*, ed. by Marcia Inhorn & Frank van Balen (Berkeley: UCLA Press, 2002).

It is possible to conceptualize these practitioners, with their diffuse transnational links and nationally rooted cultural sensibilities, as *interface agents* occupying a third space within which they are both Turkish and »world-citizens.« They embody both »objective« scientific knowledge and »subjective« local know-how, and are required to navigate their identities in order to successfully translate the vernacular of one into an intelligible form for the other. However, their role comprises not just interpretation, but also advocacy and gate-keeping practices. Through their actions, comportment, and information, be it in international conferences or national media coverage, in the form of »data« made available for international comparisons or expert advice for patients, they variously personify and project IVF as it is practiced in Turkey to national and international constituencies, who then make judgments based on these representations. The authority of practitioners may be variously experienced as connoting »Turkish perspectives« or »medical expertise« based on the relational vantage point of their audience, but will nevertheless lead to judgments regarding how IVF in Turkey is/should be practiced.

In addition, through professional, political, and commercial connections, practitioners act as gatekeepers. They have the ability to help or hinder the flow of protocols, materials, debates, discussions, professionals, patients, as well as information between national and transnational spaces. Whilst it may not be impossible to bypass these practitioners, for example through recourse to foreign news websites or reproductive travel without referral, the practitioners nevertheless occupy a central position as interface agents, commonly mediating meaning, access, and mobility through designations of inclusion and exclusion. This means that practitioners are required to engage in a variety of material, collective, and discursive practices of boundary management in their attempts to define the context-appropriate application of a global techno-science. Accordingly, as a sector they are accountable for the very character of IVF in Turkey, and must therefore be able to justify themselves and their efforts to frame and police its parameters to various internal and external constituents. Hence practitioners must not only designate the boundaries of national ART practice, but also engage collectively in impression management.[25] As one senior practitioner reminded his colleagues at a national

25 Goffman, »The Presentation of Self«, op. cit. (note 14).

ART symposium in December 2008, »We are watching each other, but we must not forget that everyone else is watching us too, by which I mean the patients, the Ministry [of Health], and abroad. [...] We need to project a positive image of ourselves both nationally and internationally.«

My ethnographic observations of practitioners' efforts at reflexive boundary-practices[26] suggest that, with regards to IVF in Turkey, there is a pluralization of boundaries and boundary-making efforts[27] rather than their negation.[28] However, the bolstering or breaking of boundaries are not necessarily mutually exclusive practices: the same actions may have mixed consequences, upholding some boundaries while simultaneously impeaching others, or they may render boundaries permeable to differing degrees. Moreover, the discriminatory porosity of boundaries can serve as a primary stratifying factor: the facilitation of greater mobility and access for some conversely signals frustrating immobility and restraint for others.[29] This remains true for a range of material and immaterial national boundaries and borders. Thus, whilst »[pushing] aside the blinders of methodological nationalism« it is important not to become dazed by emerging transnational connections and to fail to appreciate the continuing significance of (some) national boundaries for at least some groups or individuals.[30] Without even entering a discussion of the state's waxing and waning powers, it is possible to interrogate the continued iconic potency of nations and their rhetorical purchase through self-definition, myth and memory making, territorialization, public culture, and law-making

26 I follow Shields's definition of boundaries as material or virtual (immaterial) semiotic entities that are used to mark edges and borders, and employ his terminology of »boundary-practices.« See Rob Shields, »Boundary-Thinking in Theories of the Present: The Virtuality of Reflexive Modernization«, in: *European Journal of Social Theory* 9 (2006), 2, pp. 223–237.

27 Ulrich Beck, Wolfgang Bonß & Christoph Lau, »The Theory of Reflexive Modernization: Problematic, Hypotheses and Research Programme«, in: *Theory, Culture & Society* 20 (2003) 2, pp. 1–35.

28 Appadurai, »Modernity at Large«, op. cit. (note 10).

29 Zygmunt Bauman, *Globalization: The Human Consequences* (Cambridge: Polity Press, 1998).

30 Andreas Wimmer & Nina Glick Schiller, »Methodological Nationalism and Beyond: Nation-State Building, Migration and the Social Sciences«, in: *Global Networks* 2 (2002), 4, pp. 301–334, in particular p. 326.

practices.[31] It is this rhetorical engagement with national identity, and not an assessment of state power, that is thrown into relief as practitioners negotiate trans/nationalism and partake in boundary practices, as I go on to discuss with references to the choreography of ARTs involving donor gametes.

Managing Donor-Gamete Treatments

As I have already mentioned, IVF in Turkey is practiced within strict marital parameters. This means that ARTs involving donor eggs or donor sperm are legally prohibited and therefore not nationally available. The prohibition of donation is often neutralized – by regulators, religious authorities, and »lay« people – with the »common-sense« claim that there is no demand for donation. Various actors represent Turkey and Turkish men and women, through the territorialization of certain attitudes and behaviors, as against and averse to the use of donor gametes in fertility treatment. The stigma and immorality of extra-marital procreation, the desire of men and women to raise »their own« children, and the apparent absence of demands from invested individuals are all advanced as support for the view that donation is antithetical to local morals and local culture. The argument is that Turkish people would not resort to donation and would not accept it even if it was offered. While this is undoubtedly a true reflection of the views of many Turkish men and women, it is not exactly a complete picture.

Despite strong cultural taboos, which undoubtedly do exist, there are nevertheless many opinions regarding the use of donor gametes in assisted reproduction. For example, a study of general public opinion in Turkey found that only 15% of those asked showed »complete objection« to egg donation.[32] Moreover, according to a survey of Turkish female ART pa-

31 Smith, »Nations in Decline?«, op. cit. (note 23).

32 Mete Isikoglu et al., »Public Opinion Regarding Oocyte Donation in Turkey: First Data from a Secular Population among the Islamic World«, in: *Human Reproduction* 21 (2006), 1, pp. 318–323.

tients, 23.3% would accept egg donation, 15.1% would accept surrogacy, and 3.4% would accept sperm donation if it was required.[33]

Almost all clinicians have come across some Turkish couples who, having failed to conceive a child through »standard« IVF, are willing (albeit sometimes with reluctance and apprehension) to try ART treatments involving donor gametes. This was interpreted to me by one practitioner as evidence that »the desire for a child is stronger than morals, or religious beliefs, or cultural conventions.« Yet perhaps there is also a social paradox, since it seems to be precisely the same cultural values – to have one's own children within marriage – that simultaneously stigmatize using donor gametes *and* drive some childless couples to covertly resort to such ART treatments as their final option. So strong is the normative mandate for reproduction, and individuals' desires to conform to these social expectations, that for some it is better to have a child that is conceived by the use of donor egg or donor sperm, and to keep this stigmatized conception a closely guarded secret, than to remain involuntarily childless.

I was told many anecdotes by different practitioners who had faced requests for covert solutions to intractable infertility from the most »unexpected« or »conservative« patients driven (as I was told) by utter desperation. One clinician, for example, recounted how a policeman »who by his profession ought to be dedicated to upholding the law!« pleaded for some »solution (*çare*)« to his azoospermia, promising that it would remain just between him and the doctor. Another told me of his observation that the »covered« (i.e. more religious) sectors of the population were more willing to consider donor gametes, and explained this apparent contradiction by suggesting that it was because in these families it was »even more essential to have children.« Practitioners explained how these irremediable requests proved frustrating for both patients, who were sentenced to remain childless, and for clinics, which could not help these men and women in their quests for conception. This was given as the background context to what eventually became a more or less sector-wide circumventive solution to the problem of how to deal with these patients.

In response to patient requests for a solution to intractable infertility, some Turkish IVF clinics have been operating trans-border donor

33 Baris Baykal et al., »Opinions of Infertile Turkish Women on Gamete Donation and Gestational Surrogacy«, in: *Fertility and Sterility* 89 (2008), pp. 817–822.

treatment programs. These successful programs involve directing Turkish patients wishing or willing to use donor eggs or donor sperm to (Northern) Cyprus, where the treatments are legally available. Patients begin their IVF treatment cycle in Turkey, undergo the usual ovulation induction or preparatory protocols under the observation of their doctors, and are then referred to particular clinics in Cyprus, where eggs are collected (either from the patient or a donor), fertilized with sperm (from the husband or a donor), and embryos transferred to the patient, usually all within three days. In many cases, home clinics in Turkey are developing intimate economic, professional, and commercial connections with destination clinics in Cyprus, some even referring to them as »our Cypriot branches (*Kıbrıs'ta ki şubemiz*).« This circumventive solution has two key elements. Firstly, from the perspective of clinics and practitioners, the nationally illegal aspects of treatment (i.e. the use of donor eggs or donor sperm) are designated to spaces outside national jurisdiction, and therefore not subject to Turkish regulation. And second, from the perspective of patients, the trip to Cyprus is short enough to be explained as a holiday or disguised altogether, meaning that the donor procedure can be effectively hidden even from intimate others.

The supra-legal choreography of transnational donation – incorporating the movement of finances, expertise, gametes, patients, treatment cycles, and even clinic brands in and out of national borders – is dependent on the professional regulation and personal discretion of practitioners. The practitioners thus function as gatekeepers between patients and donor treatments. They make not only medical decisions regarding which patients require such treatments, but also exercise judgments regarding which patients have the appropriate attitudes (i.e. suitable moral framework), financial resources, and emotional temperament to accept such treatments. Practitioners do not talk about the possibility of donor sperm or donor eggs with every patient, but make careful decisions on whether this is an appropriate subject to raise with a particular couple. As the senior nurse responsible for coordinating the donor program of one large clinic told me, in doing this doctors use their »acumen (*sezgi*)«: »When you have been doing this job for many years, it takes just one look to understand whether you should mention this to a particular couple.«[34]

In the absence of specific legislation applicable to traveling patients, some practitioners also feel responsible for considering the social consequences of these treatments, and some who offer transnational donation apply personally defined limits to its practice. One practitioner, for example, stated that he is happy to refer couples to Cyprus for donor egg treatment, but only if the woman is not »too old.« He explained that he sees ARTs involving donor eggs as an appropriate treatment option for premature ovarian failure or for infertility in reproductively aged women, but that he feels uncomfortable about its use to help older post-menopausal women to conceive. According to him, using the technology to make middle-aged mothers amounts to an »unnatural exaggeration« of maternity which is not the role of medicine. However, rather than looking simply at the age of the woman, he bases his decision on whether or not to refer a couple to Cyprus on a range of factors, including »the woman's general health, looks, and social condition.« He is thus exercising limits, as he sees appropriate, on who is suitable and who is considered »too old« to be a mother in order to guard not just the medical and personal welfare of individuals, but also to guard the proper social and moral parameters of ART practice.

The choreographies of transnational donation can be conceptualized as simultaneously breaching and bolstering different boundaries and borders. Legal boundaries – or prohibitions – regarding the use of donor gametes are successfully transgressed by using the donor gamete itself outside national borders (although the product, if there is one, will no doubt

34 There is an interesting incongruence to be explained between accounts (such as this one) of practitioners easily and accurately assessing with which patients to broach the topic of donation, and accounts of practitioners' surprise at requests for third-party solutions from »unexpected« patients (as discussed earlier). Most practitioners expect only the most »modern« patients (by which they refer to educated, secular, Westernized individuals) to be »open« to donation. Thus, when faced with alternative examples of »traditional,« »conservative,« and »religious« patients asking for such treatments, they feel compelled to explain what they see as an inherent »contradiction« with reference to cultural paradoxes. For a further discussion of this point, see Zeynep B. Gürtin »Assisted Reproduction in Secular Turkey: Regulation, Rhetoric, and the Role of Religion« in: *Islam and the Biotechnologies of Human Life,* ed. by Marcia Inhorn & Soraya Tremayne (forthcoming).

return to the nation). However, at the same time the secrecy and discretion with which donation is pursued enables the practice to be rendered essentially invisible, keeping moral boundaries intact and perpetuating the impression that donor gametes are not used or accepted by Turkish couples. Moreover, the judgments made by practitioners regarding who is offered donation occur within flexibly-bounded frameworks that police the social impact of these treatments according to what they believe »Turkey is ready to handle.« In making these judgments, practitioners are required to effectively negotiate trans/nationalism and act as boundary-arbiters.

Demarcating Sameness and Difference

> »[T]he central feature of global culture today is the politics of the mutual effort of sameness and difference to cannibalize one another and thereby proclaim their successful hijacking of the twin Enlightenment ideas of the triumphantly universal and the resiliently particular.«
> Arjun Appadurai[35]

In the interviews I conducted with practitioners, I was always struck by their reflexive assessments, in which they characterized certain aspects of IVF in Turkey as »the same *(aynı)*« and others as »different *(farklı)*« in various comparisons. Often, interestingly, they did not specify a direct object of comparison for this sameness and difference, but simply referred to »outside *(dışarıda)*« or »abroad *(yurt dışında)*.« Although, of course, IVF outside Turkey is as varied as the number of locations in which it is practiced, this unspecified other connoted a Western or European location that symbolized the epitome of modern medicine. Sometimes, it was impossible to situate the comparator location, and at other times it was clearly an amalgam of practices from different European jurisdictions, always serving more the rhetorical purpose of comparison between Turkey and »global standards« than to provide specific information. In turn, in the uses of my informants »global standards« or »world standards« referred only West-ward, and to best practices rather than to averages. There was

35 Appadurai, »Modernity at Large«, op. cit. (note 10), p. 43.

no interest in comparing Turkey with developing nations or Middle Eastern countries, although perhaps this was partly a function of what they imagined I (as a social scientist living in England) would be familiar with. So it was against imagined (and sometimes imaginary) Western locations as others that IVF in Turkey, either as practiced in particular clinics or as the national ART sector, was judged, compared, and represented by practitioners, and assessed depending on the case to be superior, matching, or inferior.

Accounts from practitioners displayed both consistency and some variation regarding the representation and assessment of IVF practice in Turkey. While the discourse on »sameness« was quite dependable, different practitioners noted and pinpointed various aspects as »different,« attributed differing levels of importance to these differences, and appealed to various explanatory factors as the causes of the differences. Although it was acknowledged that there might be considerable variation between IVF clinics in Turkey, as demonstrated by the quote from the senior practitioner below, it was usually »best practice« that was subjected to transnational comparisons.

»Here, in Turkey, there are over one hundred [IVF] centers. Of course we cannot assume that all of these are the same quality. But, there are clinics that are excellent, that immediately follow scientific developments and activities, that engage in stringent quality control measures – and here, Turkish IVF standards are truly world-class.«

Most accounts, as the one above, began with »science (*bilim*)« as the first component of comparison. This was usually assessed to be »exactly the same in Turkey as anywhere in the world!« because, as discussed previously, transnational links were seen to enable the global communication of a scientific community, de-territorializing universal techno-scientific knowledge and facilitating its replication in various global locations. Turkish practitioners' ability to access »the latest information (*bilgi*)« simultaneously with their European or American counterparts, for example via online subscriptions to the leading journals, kept them up-to-date with this global knowledge and ensured that the global ART community practiced according to »the same« cutting-edge scientific developments. Thus, the science that informed and directed IVF practice in Turkey was characterized by its sameness, and the similarities between clinics in Turkey and elsewhere (e.g. regarding methods for oocyte retrieval, the medium used for the storage of gametes and embryos, laboratory conditions, etc.) were seen as replications of this supra-cultural global science.

The display of direct international connections and collaborations through the establishment of clinical franchises and clinics' applications for ISO standards can be seen as efforts to support, strengthen, and verify these claims to sameness in Turkish IVF practice. Thus, for example, Bahçeci Clinic, Turkey's largest private IVF center, provides prominently on its website not only a direct comparison for its impressive success rates – »While average success rates in America for 2006 were 38%, ours are 48%« – but also the assurance that its quality is confirmed by JCI accreditation and ISO standards[36]. However, within Turkey, the appeal of these systems of assessment or measurement reside less in their transcontextual meaning as »immutable mobiles«[37] and more in their contextual interpretation as signifiers of prestige, seen to authenticate claims of »global standards« within qualifying clinics. Likewise, despite rhetoric the success and attraction of clinical franchises, for example with eminent American clinics, to Turkish patients depends less on exactly replicating what happens in the equivalent clinic in the US, and more on an ability to balance sameness with difference. While it may be desirable to replicate certain aspects (for example, treatment protocols leading to high success rates or tried and tested equipment), it is more important to modify others with sensitivity to local desires, values, and expectations (for example, the decor, the interaction between the doctor and his patients, or the clinic's opening hours). It is, thus, not quite an exact »aura of German or American locality«[38] that is transmitted by these franchises, but rather an impression that is locally recognized as connoting a desirably »world-standard« practice.

36 The International Organization for Standardization (ISO) and Joint Commission International (JCI) are both standard setting bodies. The former is an international organization setting quality standards in a wide variety of industrial and commercial areas, and the latter is a predominantly United States based body which operates voluntary accreditation programs in healthcare settings. A clinic's ability to meet these standards can guarantee a certain level of quality and enable international comparisons.

37 Bruno Latour, *Science in Action. How to Follow Scientists and Engineers through Society* (Milton Keynes: Open University Press, 1987).

38 Stefan Beck, »Transnational Lab-Benches: Transforming Experience«, in: this volume.

However, the equivalence accorded to the scientific practice of IVF by Turkish practitioners also necessitated an explanation of why there were nevertheless differences to be found. The differences that could be observed between IVF practice in Turkey and IVF »outside« – for example in the preference for the use of intracytoplasmic sperm injection (ICSI) over IVF, the increased occurrence of multiple pregnancies, or the behavior of doctors or patients – were sometimes judged to be »worse« and sometimes judged to be »better.« In some respects IVF in Turkey was considered superior, in others it had not yet become as good as it should be, but in either case differences were attributed to a variety of territorialized characteristics. The three central (sometimes over-lapping or co-constitutive) characteristics referenced by practitioners were national character and culture (with or without the inclusion of Islam), differences in regulatory structures, and socio-economic conditions.

For example, during my observations in Turkish IVF clinics it was very striking to note the frequency and intimacy of patient-clinician interactions. In addition to medical care, most practitioners made concerted efforts to attend to the emotional welfare of their patients and their families, often forming pseudo-kinship relations in which they acted like benevolent uncles. Many practitioners, dealing with a diverse range of patients, perceptibly varied their choice of words and general demeanor to facilitate a »dialog« and to enable better communication with each and every type of patient. Even the most senior practitioners provided their patients with their mobile telephone numbers and accepted that calls from patients at all times of day and night (sometimes for very minor reasons) were a central and routine feature of their occupation. In this aspect, summarized as greater »personalization,« Turkish doctors reflexively recognized themselves as »different« to their Western or European colleagues. They explained this through an appeal to national character – »Turkish people are generally warm-blooded and always value a human connection« – and assessed this difference to have a beneficial impact on their patients and on their practice. In this respect, then, different was judged to be »better.« As one practitioner put it, »Which German or English patient would not prefer to have such easy access to their doctor?« These appeals to national culture were easily understandable explanations because they drew on readily recognizable identifiers and assumptions regarding Turkey and Turkish people.

Designations of sameness and difference are also used as an internationally effective marketing tool. While franchises or ISO standards are designed to provide security, reliability, and assurance through the promise of familiarity for international patients, it is only the coupling of this similarity with different regulatory, financial, or personal conditions that makes them attractive and desirable for foreign patients. Appeals to internationally resonant stereotypes or images of »Turkishness« can become a valuable shorthand in the lucrative and competitive global market of reproductive travel. Building on Turkey's already existing reputation as a tourist destination (comprising elements of hospitality, affordability, relaxation, etc.), Jinemed clinic in Istanbul, for example, promotes itself and more generally IVF treatment in Turkey to »reproductive tourists.« Through its website, www.ivfturkey.com, dedicated to attracting and communicating with foreign patients, Jinemed advertises »world-class treatment, personalized service« in its Turkish IVF clinic, where »excellent healthcare meets low cost and leisure.«

These appeals to sameness and difference are not evident propositions, but impression management by the »over-communication of some facts and the under-communication of others.«[39] By comparing the practice of IVF in Turkey against practices that takes place »abroad,« and in selectively explaining sameness through transnationalism or difference through a variety of territorializations (of culture, regulation, or socio-economic conditions), these designations also function as discursive boundary-making practices. Moreover, in addition to framing and description, both sameness and difference can be used to justify why IVF is practiced as it is and from where it derives its national character, as I discuss with reference to embryo transfer numbers.

39 Goffman, »The Presentation of Self«, op. cit. (note 14), p. 136.

Explaining Embryo Transfer Numbers

In recent years, with the growing recognition of the risks and complications of multiple gestations in ART practice, both the European Society for Human Reproduction and Embryology (ESHRE)[40] and the American Society for Reproductive Medicine (ASRM)[41] have advised reducing the number of embryos transferred in an IVF cycle, and have recommended single embryo transfer (SET) for younger patients with a favorable prognosis. Thus, the general worldwide trend since 2001, as documented in the IFFS Surveillance 04 and subsequently 07, has been a decrease from three or four embryos to one or two embryos transferred per cycle, with double embryo transfer (DET) becoming established practice in many locations.[42] Moreover, the Nordic countries increasingly favor the use of SET, and since 2004 it has become compulsory in Belgium to transfer only one embryo to women under 36 years of age during their first two funded treatment cycles.[43] Turkish legislation allows practitioners to implant up to three embryos after IVF treatment, with a possibility for more in individual cases, subject to professional judgment and documentation. This regulation is more relaxed than the DET norm in several countries (including Australia, Denmark, Israel, Norway, New Zealand, and the United Kingdom), and the three maximum in many others (including Argentina, the Czech Republic, Italy, Germany, Latvia, Slovenia, and Spain). However, it is worth noting that, in addition to Turkey, there remain a number of countries that allow the transfer of more than three embryos, usually to older women or those who have experienced failed cycles. These includes Greece, Hong Kong, Hungary, Croatia, India, Japan, Singapore and the United States).[44]

40 The ESHRE Task Force on Ethics and Law, »Ethical issues related to multiple pregnancies in medically assisted procreation«, in: *Human Reproduction* 18 (2003), 9, pp. 1976–1979.

41 The Practice Committee for the American Society for Reproductive Medicine and the Practice Committee of the Society of Assisted Reproductive Technology, »Guidelines on number of embryos to be transferred«, in: *Fertility and Sterility* 92 (2009), pp. 1518–1519.

42 Howard W. Jones, Jean Cohen, Ian Cooke & Roger Kempers, »IFFS Surveillance 07«, in: *Fertility and Sterility* 87 (2007), 4, Supplement 1, pp. S1-S67.

43 Jones et al., »IFFS Surveillance 07«, op. cit. (note 42).

44 Loc. cit.

Although there are considerable differences between different countries with regards to average embryo transfer numbers, whether multifetal pregnancy reduction (MFPR) is practiced, and the incidence of multiple births following ART treatment, according to the World Collaborative Report 2002, there is an overall twin delivery rate of 25.7% and triplet rate of 2.5% following conventional IVF and ICSI cycles.[45] These numbers, although lower than in previous years, are still high enough to merit concern regarding increased risks in multiple gestations, and the primary reason for reducing the numbers of embryos transferred in IVF is to lower the chance of multiple conception. Multiple gestations are associated with a range of increased risks for pregnant women and their offspring and require greater monitoring by health professionals. Obstetric complications include pre-eclampsia, preterm labor, and intrauterine growth retardation. Neonatal complications include prematurity, low birth weight, and congenital malformations.[46] The percentage of prematurity (<37 weeks) increases from 13.5% for singleton IVF babies to 61.3% for twins and 94.2% for triplets,[47] and rates of perinatal mortality are 5–6 times higher among twins than among singletons.[48] In addition to concerns for the health of the individuals directly involved, multiple pregnancies and births can also raise apprehensions for the economy of the health system and engender debates regarding resource allocation.

In Turkey, discussions regarding embryo transfer numbers and risks of multiple pregnancies became particularly vociferous following the death, in August 2008, of 49 babies at Zekai Tahir Burak Maternity Hospital's neonatal intensive care unit, which received extensive media attention. Although this event was not directly related to ART practice, its shocking nature led to a scrutiny of not only the hospital's practices, but more generally of premature births, multiple pregnancies, and the role of ARTs in both of the aforementioned. Following this episode, Prof. Timur Gürgan, the President of the Reproductive Medicine Association (ÜTD) of Turkey, told me that multiple pregnancies had become »a big headache«

45 Jacques de Mouzon et al., »World Collaborative Report on Assisted Reproductive Technology, 2002«, in: *Human Reproduction* 24 (2009), 9, pp. 2310–2320.

46 Johan Hazekamp et al., »Avoiding Multiple Pregnancies in ART: Consideration of New Strategies«, in: *Human Reproduction* 15 (2000), 6, pp. 1217–1219.

47 de Mouzon et al., »World Collaborative Report«, op. cit. (note 45).

48 Hazekamp et al., »Avoiding Multiple Pregnancies«, op. cit. (note 46).

for the IVF sector, and the ÜTD, with the collaboration of the Ministry of Health, convened a number of professional meetings with renowned international representatives from ESHRE and ASRM to discuss national approaches and to promote lower embryo transfer numbers. As can be deduced from these meetings, Turkish IVF practitioners are indeed engaged in the same scientific and medical discussions as their international colleagues, and are keeping up-to-date with global debates and developments.

However, despite the evidence of increased risk that makes multiple pregnancies and higher embryo transfer numbers medically inadvisable, multiples – especially twins – remain highly desirable for many infertile men and women.[49] Especially in pronatalist cultures, like Turkey, with a strong procreation mandate and low voluntary incidence of single-child families, it is easy to understand why patients might consider twins the optimum result of fertility treatment. Among involuntarily childless Turkish couples, who may have limited financial, emotional, or physical resources and who wish to complete their families as soon as possible, twins are usually seen as a »blessing (*bereket*),« akin to what one father-to-be of IVF twins jokingly termed »a buy-one-get-one-free deal (*birini alana diğeri bedava*).« Indeed, many practitioners I interviewed articulated their empathy for the desperate desires of the men and women who consulted them and the pressure or »obligation« they felt to achieve conceptions. Accountable to both the global scientific community and their patients, practitioners sometimes felt torn as they attempted to balance global scientific data and the advice of the international scientific community to lower embryo transfer numbers with the local demands of their resource-poor patients who strongly desired multiple children. As one practitioner in a state hospital explained:

»When the man in front of you has sold his livestock to come for treatment, and this is his last chance to become a father, and he says to you, ›Please Doctor, make us pregnant,‹ you feel a certain pressure to deliver, to maximize his chances. It is not easy to tell him with a clear conscience (*vicdan rahatlığı*) that you are going

49 Tim J. Child, Anna Maria Henderson & Seang Lin Tan, »The Desire for Multiple Pregnancy in Male and Female Infertility Patients«, in: *Human Reproduction* 19 (2004), 3, pp. 558–561.

to transfer only two embryos, because that is what is internationally regarded as best practice.«

The pressure to balance success rates with risks was not unique to this practitioner, and formed perhaps one of the most persistent collective pressures for the profession. Indeed, according to a survey conducted by the Turkish Society of Reproductive Medicine (TSRM) in 2008, 86% of Turkish practitioners would choose to transfer either two or three good-quality embryos to a patient under the age of 35, and almost none would consider SET even under optimal conditions. Practitioners judged this »difference« between their practices and (what they considered to be) practice in »European clinics« as attributable not to scientific differences but to differences in regulatory and more importantly in economic and cultural conditions. As Dr. Bülent Urman, the President of the TSRM, explained in an interview with *Tüp Bebek* Magazine, Turkish practitioners chose higher embryo transfer numbers despite their awareness of the international moves towards SET because of the specific local conditions under which they practiced:

»There is another very important difference between us and Europe; in most European countries IVF is funded up to the fifth or sixth cycle, and in some of them there is limitless funding available. Hence, there,practitioners can easily (*rahatlıkla*) reduce embryo transfer numbers to one, but when you do that, you also reduce your chances of success. For this reason, if you ask me, at the moment one is not a sensible (*makul*) number for Turkey.«

According to Urman, it is the pressure to make patients into parents within two cycles of funding or within their limited financial resources that leads Turkish practitioners to prefer higher embryo transfer numbers than their European counterparts, and makes SET currently an unsuitable option. In actual fact, the funding of IVF in »most European countries« is not as generous as this quote might suggest, with only six countries (Belgium, France, Greece, Israel, Slovenia, and Sweden) offering complete coverage as part of their national health plan.[50] The two cycles of funding in Turkey compares rather well with many European jurisdictions. Nevertheless, the rhetoric, as demonstrated above, explains and justifies differences in practice with reference primarily to economic conditions, despite the existence

50 Jones et al., »IFFS Surveillance 07«, op. cit. (note 42).

of the same scientific and medical knowledge. In turn, this difference is judged by practitioners to have both positive and negative implications, leading on the one hand to higher success rates, while increasing multiple pregnancies on the other.

Thus, the material and discursive practices of Turkish practitioners regarding embryo transfer numbers provide an illustration by which differences in behavior or outcome are designated to regulatory, socio-economic, and cultural factors, while maintaining claims to the sameness of techno-science. These balancing acts are also indicative of the necessity for situated cultural knowledge in the re-territorialization of de-territorialized »generic« scientific practice.

Conclusion

This paper makes the claim that IVF practitioners function as interface agents between the local and the global. Taking Turkey as a case study, with reference to ethnographic fieldwork between 2005 and 2009 and in-depth interviews with senior practitioners, I examine the work practitioners do to connect the global and local spheres, to balance competing demands at the national and international level, and ultimately to transform a global techno-science into culturally expedient practices. I have argued that through their efforts at translation, mediation, and representation – illustrated here through the processes of negotiating trans/nationalism and designating sameness and difference – practitioners effectively engender particular ways of practicing IVF in specific locations. Although the details discussed here are context specific, regarding for example the choreography of transnational gamete donation or the preference for higher embryo transfer numbers, there may be general applicability and use for a model that situates practitioners at its core and seeks to examine how their material, collective, and discursive practices as interface agents contribute to localizing ART practice. It may be that practitioners' abilities as interface agents or their efficacy at localizing global medical practices will be highly variable, depending on, for example, the extent to which medical professionals are respected and trusted, the degree to which the general population is medically or scientifically literate, and the amount of convergence between the messages from medicine and the popular media. It is possible that in some situations practitioners may be more peripheral to the processes of localization, and that alternative agents such as patient-support organizations, the media, or pharmaceutical companies may serve a more central function. If this were so, it may tell us something interesting about the vacillating role of practitioners in different social contexts, as well as about the variation in processes of localizing global technologies.

If what defines global forms are their »distinctive capacity for decontextualisation and recontextualisation, abstractability and movement«[51] and their assemblage through reflexive arbitration, critical reflection, debate, and contest,[52] then this ethnographic engagement with IVF in Turkey can perhaps be read as the interrogation of an assemblage from a vantage point that emphasizes not the fluidity of transnational movements, but the effort or work necessitated both to facilitate travel and to exercise containment, and hence to conjure local incarnations.

Acknowledgments

This research was undertaken as part of an ESRC PhD studentship at the Centre for Family Research, University of Cambridge. I am thankful to the organizers and participants of the *IVF as Global Form* workshop, following which this chapter was developed. Thanks also to Alex Broadbent, Charlotte Faircloth, Susanna Graham, and Emilia Sanabria who read and provided useful comments on earlier versions. Finally, and most importantly, I would like to express my sincere gratitude to the practitioners who generously gave of their time and their opinions.

51 Ong & Collier, »Global Assemblages, Anthropological Problems«, op. cit. (note 6), p. 11.

52 Collier, »Global Assemblages«, op. cit. (note 12).

Making Connections: Reflecting on Trains, Kinship, and Information Technology

Maren Klotz

When reviewing the field notes of a recent interview trip through southwestern Germany to interview families-by-donation, i.e. families who had used donor sperm to conceive, the notes turn out to be full of stories on making train connections. Full of stories on train connections – and full of stories on sat navs, buses, Google maps, and railway stations. Evidently, the more obvious topics feature as well: The notes reflect on interview dynamics, short episodes of participating in family life, establishing rapport, and my own feelings of entering into so many different »familial worlds« during the trip. But they are steeped with episodes like the following:

»The bus to the train station the next morning is late. I miss the first connecting train, which means I have worryingly little time left to change platforms at Bonn main station. Nevertheless, I make it to the platform in time and notice that there is a previous late train still showing on the departure board. People on the platform seem to be confused. Then an announcement, right when the train is supposed to pull in, that there has been a change in platforms. People hurry up the stairs to get to the other platform. The train pulls in late with compartments not in the order announced. In the middle of the ride the train breaks sharply: people gasp, luggage pieces fall. There are no announcements about the incident and the train continues its journey. I miss my connecting train. When I finally make it to the hotel, I have to hurriedly drop of my stuff and grab my mini–disc recorder and note pad to make it to the interview in time.«

In her gripping analysis of different modes of relationality, Marilyn Strathern claims that making connections, if conceived in relational terms and less mundanely than simply as train connections, is at the heart of the anthropological project, and with this at the heart of kinship (studies) and essentially, as she argues, at the heart of social life – of »the grand project of making society.«[1] »Anthropology uses relations to explore relations,«[2] she contends. We, the contributors to this volume, take part in such forms of relationality, when we try to explore the entanglements, modifications, and consequences of the spread of reproductive technologies around the globe. Finally, Strathern wisely observes that »uncovering connections and making connections can both have the force of a moral imperative.«[3] This is something we can experience in the activities of our interview partners and in our own attempts to establish research relationships. Stretching the metaphor of *making connections* I am drawn back into my field diary and its notes on the necessity and, particularly, on the difficulties of making transport connections in order to set up meaningful face to face relationships with my interview partners:

»My train to the next town was late and as I left the small rural station built of reddish stone I noted that the building was up for sale. It was already dark outside when I walked to the bus station to finally get to my interview partners' house. I had found the bus schedule online and had a printed out version with me. The bus was late and then drove right past me, despite me standing visibly in front of the stop. A woman noticed my waving, but did not deem it necessary to alert the driver. [...] When I ended up taking a taxi, the driver couldn't find my interview partners' newly built house, because it was not in his sat nav. Finally, there was one landmark in the directions I was given he recognized: A newly built shopping center.«

When starting to code the actual interviews with families-by-donation conducted on the trip, they also seem to be full of other modes of »connection making.« Particularly, it is modes of transnational IT-based kinship connections in a broader sense that strike me as worth exploring further for this volume. John Law argues that when analyzing empirical material, concentrating on and working with specific metaphors is about »the need to find or make a pattern against an endless background of noise.«[4] In this article I shall use the metaphor of *making connections* – in transport, infrastructure, and between people – or the failure to make certain connections, as apparent in the quote above, to reflect on doing, *and researching*,

1 Marilyn Strathern, *Kinship, Law and the Unexpected: Relatives Are Always a Surprise* (Cambridge, UK: Cambridge University Press, 2005).

2 Strathern, »Kinship, Law and the Unexpected«, op. cit. (note 1), p. 7.

3 Ibid., p. 11.

4 John Law, *After Method: Mess in Social Science Research* (London: Routledge, 2004).

kinship-by-donation in times of increased globalization. In keeping with the transnational theme of this book, I shall reflexively juxtapose empirical materials on (mostly) transnational IT-based connection making endeavors of my German informants with my own endeavors as a researcher to make different modes of connections to physically and personally reach my interview partners. I shall start off with contextualizing and historicizing the metaphors of making connections and networking some further. I shall then introduce two ethnographic vignettes from my own research and go on to conceptualize and discuss the transnational kinship practices apparent in these vignettes. I will make light of these specific modes of making connections, firstly, with regard to what I call a specific contemporary *convergence* between telecommunication or IT-based networks and kinship which potentially leads to an *informational* »uncontainability« of kinship information. Secondly, I shall interpret them as part of a wider cultural pattern, which has recently been coined »the imperative to connect.« Finally, this article is drawn to a close by using my associative juxtaposition of my own transport connections with the IT-provided kinship connections of my interview partners as a »mechanism« against the potential »autolimitlessness«[5] of network and connection metaphors. i.e. as a strategy to generate new questions on what is being dis-connected or »cut« within the kinship practices described.

5 Marilyn Strathern, »Cutting the Network«, in: *Journal of the Royal Anthropological Institute* 2 (1996), 3, p. 522.

The Ubiquitous Network

»The trip had required quite a lot of e–mailing back and forth with my interviewees and I mainly used the Internet to organize all the details. Most families were not actually living in the bigger south-western cities they had named, but in rather small towns as far as 30 km away from the next town I could place on a map of West Germany. Google maps helped me to locate them and find accommodation near them. The website of Deutsche Bahn was pretty good in telling me which rural bus line to take out of the larger cities in order to get to my families. So here I am, sitting in the train, prepared with printed out schedules, Google maps, seat reservation, and five train tickets.«

Making connections, networking – *the* network – seemingly come across as key metaphors in a globalized world to describe current social and cultural phenomena, ranging from the upsurge of social networking sites on the web, to ubiquitous career advice and grassroots political activism and extending into social science research with the rise of actor network theory and social network theory.[6] As pivotal as another network – the World Wide Web – seems to be for these phenomena and also, to some extent, for my interview partners' transnational activities, as I will also argue later in this paper, Laura Otis still reminds us that the rise of the metaphor of the network and an concomitant alignment »of bodies and technologies,«[7] as it is evident in early comparisons between telegraph nets and nervous systems or contemporary comparisons of the brain with a computer, can be traced back to the 19th century. Although arguing from a more historical perspective than Strathern, she also stresses the relational character of »the network,« which does more than simply join up bounded units:

»Then, as now, sending electronic messages challenged the traditional notion of a bounded, delimited individual. As part of a network, one is defined through

6 Also see Riles and Knox, Savage & Harvey. Riles describes the Network as a reflexive social form both effectual in her informants' (NGO activists) activities and her activities as a social scientist. Annelise Riles, *The Network Inside Out* (Ann Arbor, Michigan: University of Michigan Press, 2001). Knox et al. focus on the history of »network thinking« and associated theoretical and methodological challenges in the social sciences. Hannah Knox, Mike Savage & Penny Harvey, »Social Networks and the Study of Relations: Networks as Method, Metaphor and Form«, in: *Economy and Society* 35 (2006), 1, pp. 113–140.

7 Laura Otis, *Networking: Communicating with Bodies and Machines in the Nineteenth Century* (Ann Arbor, Michigan: University of Michigan Press, 2001), p. 10.

one's connections to others, with an identity that is better represented by a vector diagram than by a bounded cell.«[8]

If it weren't clear that Otis is talking about particular kinds of communication systems, she might just as well be talking about kinship. It is as part of a genealogical network that Euro-American personhood constitutes itself, as Marilyn Strathern asserts: »Kinspersons who find things out about their ancestry acquire identity by that very discovery. [...] Euro-Americans cannot ignore these connections. The information forms (›constitutes‹) what they know about themselves.«[9] Kinship in its »Western version« is at least partly based on the body, on the sharing and passing on of bodily substances, as for instance contemporary kinship studies' founding father David Schneider would argue.[10] It is the traditional idiom then, if one follows Strathern, within which people in the Western world can perceive of connections between physical bodies as such, rather than viewing the connection as lying outside the body of the bounded individual, for instance within a communicative act.[11]

But what if the physical body becomes connected to the communicative network?

»The tendency to see a communications device as a continuation of one's own nervous system developed in the nineteenth century, not in the twentieth. As early as the 1870s, self-conscious telegraphers felt themselves merging with their networks, describing the transmission of signals from their brains, through their fingers, onto their keys, and then on down the line,«[12]

8 Otis, »Networking«, op. cit. (note 7), p. 10.

9 Marilyn Strathern, »Refusing Information«, in: *Property, Substance, and Effect: Anthropological Essays on Persons and Things* (London: Athlone Press, 1999), pp. 64–88, in particular p. 68.

10 David M. Schneider, *American Kinship: A Cultural Account* (Englewood Cliffs: Prentice–Hall, 1968).

11 Strathern, »Kinship, Law and the Unexpected«, op. cit. (note 1), p. 26. Knox et al. also point out that anthropological engagements with networks are in fact to be seen as »re-articulations of an ongoing concern with forms of social relatedness. [...] The use of the term ›network‹ as a separate field of interest hides the fact that anthropologists have long been concerned with questions of connections between people, most clearly demonstrated by the central disciplinary tenets of kinship and exchange...« Knox, Savage & Harvey, »Social Networks«, op. cit. (note 6), p. 115.

12 Otis, »Networking«, op. cit. (note 7), p. 10.

reminds us Otis. This raises ontological questions about our co-implication in technologies as well as questions about persons' individual perceptions of when they merge, or don't merge, with communicative systems; it also brings to mind Donna Haraway's notion of the cyborg. However, I would like to follow a slightly different lead in this paper. If the network as an idea, practice, and technological artifact is not as one might think a phenomenon of the 20th century, but, as Otis argues, of the 19th century, just as much as kinship evidently is not a contemporary phenomenon, a particular alignment of bodies and technologies, to use Otis phrasing, might be *very* 21st century. I see this particular alignment – or *convergence* – in an abundance of present-day kinship practices, which I shall discuss in more detail with regard to my own ethnographic vignettes later: Internet-based half-sibling and donor searches by families-by-donation are part of my core research interests, but convergence figures just as much in new IT-based genealogical research (which sometimes concurrently involves DNA sequencing), for instance, or in Internet-based selection and acquisition of reproductive services and substances (such as ordering donor sperm online). These practices are often transnational in the sense that they breach or connect nationally limited regulatory or physical spaces. Before turning to the discussion and interpretation of this conjunction, I want to present two ethnographic vignettes from my own research.

Ethnographic Vignette One: Single Mother by Choice Maria Lieb

Maria Lieb[13] has been repeatedly interviewed and contacted for my research, the longest conversation between us so far taking place over breakfast in a quiet café conveniently located for both of us. Lieb works as a highly successful scientist and identifies herself as a so-called Single Mother by Choice, i.e. as a single women who decided to become a

13 All names and some further potentially identifying information have been changed in accordance with my interviewees' wishes. This also applies to the Schneider family in the second ethnographic vignette.

mother through sperm donation.[14] Since access for single women to donor insemination (DI) in Germany is very restricted (it basically depends on a doctor's willingness to act against the professional code of the Federal Chamber of Physicians), she decided to travel to the United States to conceive. Lieb had tried relationships with women and men, but when, in her late thirties, she was single and finally found herself in a less stressful job situation and with the strong wish for a child, she decided to try motherhood without a partner. During a longer business trip to the States she more or less spontaneously decided to contact a feminist midwife collective for advice on sperm donation and, with their help, ended up coming back to Germany pregnant with her daughter Julia after just one single insemination.

Lieb chose her donor mainly for his height to balance out her petiteness, she laughingly admits. She also chose him for his academic background and because he was a so-called yes-donor (i.e. a donor who agreed to be contacted once »his« child would reach the age of 18). She has made considerable adjustments to her and her daughter's life in reaction to Julia's genitor being American. This was one of the major reasons for Maria Lieb, for instance, to enroll Julia in a bilingual German and English school. She thinks it a pity, as she tells me during the interview in the café, that Julia cannot contact the donor before coming of age at 18.

Lieb's job enables her to spend substantial time abroad and she recently lived in Ireland with her daughter Julia for half a year. She says she would have preferred going to the States to give Julia the opportunity to experience life there and potentially meet some of her half-siblings. She found those half-siblings through an American website, and she also found out that the donor might have breached sperm bank policies and donated at several clinics:

Maria Lieb (ML): »I have found out through this American donor registry website that Julia has about 30 half siblings; I hope the father will still want to meet her, now, that there are so many others. [...] But at least she is the oldest. [...] I am wondering whether he really is who he claims he is. I mean, I researched this

14 The term Single Mothers by Choice goes back to a book by Jane Mattes, who was also the founder of a self-help organization which goes by the same name: Jane Mattes, *Single Mothers by Choice: A Guidebook for Single Women Who Are Considering or Have Chosen Motherhood* (New York: Times Books, 1994).

project at the University of California he claimed to be working at through the Internet, and it actually exists. But I am not really sure everything he reported to the sperm bank is true. How could they check? I mean, I also found out that he is donating to different banks, and that is kind of against the official policy of these sperm banks. Why would he do that if he is doing ok financially? Maybe he wants to spread his genes… .«

When asked how she found out about this and how the website works in general, she explains to me that the discovery of the »wayward donations« of the donor came about through shared detective work within the websites profiles.

ML: »This website is run by a family-by-donation. You pay a fee and then you can register with the individual number of your donor and the sperm bank you used. That's how you find others who went to the same bank. And then people do research and compare profiles of donors and so on. And that's how we found out he donated at other banks, too. He just put very similar information there. So we have this kind of social network of all the people who believe they used the same donor. So, they don't work with DNA tests.«

She tells me how fascinating it is to compare photographs within this social network and look for resemblances between the children. But there is also information exchanged that worries her: For example, she is concerned about the fact that several of the children in the network have a neurological disorder. Her daughter has already finished elementary school and shows no signs of the condition – which, given the usual course of the disease, she should have if she were affected. Nevertheless, since the disorder is sometimes assumed to have a hereditary component, Maria Lieb is not happy with this discovery and I get the impression she watches her daughter carefully for any signs of this particular disease.

Ethnographic Vignette Two: The Schneider DI Family

Nadine and Marc Schneider live in a newly built house at the outskirts of a metropolitan area in south-western Germany. Nadine used to work as a part-time physician's assistant before she quit her job, partly due to the physical and emotional difficulties she experienced during failed attempts to conceive via ICSI. After recovery, she went back to school to obtain her university entrance degree, which she only received when she was already well into pregnancy with their son Phillip. Phillip has been conceived using donor sperm.

Nadine's husband Marc has an advanced technical job and travels a lot, both nationally and internationally. His low sperm count is due to a childhood medical condition. It has left the couple, who only met and got married in their mid to late thirties, childless in their first year of marriage. After consulting with a clinic they first decided to try ICSI, which they both describe as an extremely invasive and unpleasant experience. The following insemination in comparison to them seemed like »a walk in the park.« After three failed attempts of ICSI they began to think of other options and started gathering information on DI and adoption. For this they mainly used the Internet, as Nadine explains to me in the interview: »We found everything on the net. It's simply *the* medium today, where you can find *all* information.« They got in touch and met with a group of other affected families whom they found through the website of a social worker specializing in counseling families-by-donation. It has been the experience of meeting these other persons – some still childless, some pregnant with their first DI child, some with several older children – combined with the realization of the long waiting periods in adoption as well as the desire to have an at least »half« genetically related child that made them decide in favor of DI.

The Internet and its multiple facilities for very specific and individual (national and transnational) search endeavors and communication have played a decisive role in how they became the family they are today and how they manage their family stories or narratives. It was through the Internet that they chose their sperm donor and ordered the sperm to be delivered from Denmark to a German clinic. Marc Schneider has compiled a vast library of international self-help literature on DI he has found through Internet searches. He is now one of the administrators and programmers of a self-help and networking Internet platform on DI.

It was the availability of certain kinds of information that made the Schneiders turn down their local clinics' donor supply with its highly limited donor information and opt for the large, internationally operating sperm bank Cryos in Denmark instead. Cryos prides itself to be the biggest operating sperm bank network and is organized through a franchise system, which has led to branches being opened in the United States and India. Their sperm is sold and delivered to countries all over the world. In the evening, sitting at their dining table, the Schneiders describe their process of choosing a donor to me during a taped conversation:

Marc Schneider (MS): »I mean, at the end of the day I want to know – I mean, it was important to Nadine as well – that the donor is not an asshole – excuse my language. I want to know whether he is likable.«
Nadine Schneider (NS): »Whether I would find him likable, should I meet him.«

But although the information was more comprehensive than what their clinic provided on its local donors, Cryos' German donor supply list did not convey to them that certain »feel« for the donor's character either. However, what they did like was the way in which Cryos' US website provided information on the donors, and eventually they realized that all of the Danish donors listed there also had to be listed on their more limited German list.

MS: Cryos operates on the American market as well and there you can download much more comprehensive donor profiles. They do not have photographs, but a seven to nine pages paper where…«
NS: »…questions can be answered in an open non-standardized way.«
MS: »Exactly, the donor can answer and the answer is left unchanged. They do not change or schematize it. They give all sorts of additional information. Genetic diseases in the family, how old did the granddads and grandmothers get. What is his favorite animal?«

During the conversation I am more and more baffled about the mass of information they could obtain this way. I tell them that I am quite fascinated. They keep adding more information they gathered through the American donor list: Languages spoken, travel and food interests, eating habits, important life events.

NS: »I had the feeling that I actually got a small impression of him, whether I would like him, through how he answered the questions.«
MS: »It is often not so important what they say but how they say it…«
NS: »How they phrase it.«

Before they started to closely examine donor profiles, they put a filter in place to make sure they would only find donors who matched Marc

Schneider's height and ethnicity and eye color. They decided in favor of a medical student they found sympatico, although he did not match Marc Schneider's hair color. Wanting to avoid the much higher cost of ordering sperm through Cryos USA, they instead set out to make their own match between the German and the American donor list.

NS: »In the German list the donors have numbers, in the American one they have pseudonyms. We needed to find a match using the basic parameters such as height, hair color, eye color, profession, and that fit, it was not hard. [...] We are sure that's him, it has to be him.«

I ask for more details about the process and the sperm delivery to the German clinic. Marc Schneider walks me through the details, obviously enjoying how simple the process was and how clever they were to find their donor on both lists. With a glint in his eyes and a laugh afterwards he adds: »I ordered via fax, paid by credit card and everything basically went as if ordering from Amazon.«

In opposition to many European countries – such as the UK and (although far less clearly regulated) Germany – Denmark has *not* made sperm donation non-anonymous by law. Although Cryos is now offering some possibilities to receive sperm from so-called yes-donors, i.e. donors willing to be contacted by potential offspring, using Cryos at the time for the Schneiders meant that the procedure was fully anonymous. The clinic has in fact informed them that they have destroyed all identifying records on the donor, but Marc Schneider doubts that this indeed is the case: »They say they have destroyed his ›real‹ data because he is not in the active donor stock anymore, but we doubt that they've really done that.« He reflects on the fairly new German regulation, according to which identifying data now has to be stored and potentially made available. This law came in force just after the Schneiders used Cryos. Marc says that they have stored the donors profile electronically and as a paper file, so Phillip could later look at it; and he adds that he seriously doubts the security of the donor's anonymity, should their son ever be earnestly interested in tracking him down:

MS: »So I think, to trace someone nowadays would not be so hard; there was some information in the profile, for instance...And he put down what he studies and when he will finish. So, what I am saying is, I think we actually have enough information to potentially find him.«

I add laughingly: »And Denmark is not so big after all.«
NS: »Not at all, exactly. And how many universities do they have where you can study medicine?«
MS: »It will come down to a fairly small group of people, should Phillip ever go after it.«

Horizontal, Reproductive, plus Wayward Connections

I have chosen to present the two ethnographic vignettes, because part of the story conveyed in them is that they feature three kinship practices which I view as characteristic examples of the contemporary phenomenon of a conjunction of kinship-related and telecommunications-related modes of »connection making« that I discussed before. I shall call them horizontal connections, i.e. the practice of searching for, finding, and communicating with half-siblings as apparent in Maria Lieb's case; reproductive connections, i.e. practices of organizing reproductive processes via online services as apparent in the Schneider case; and wayward connections, i.e. slightly subversive research processes which circumvent the officially intended use of data or establish new, potentially unwanted connections as apparent in both the Lieb and the Schneider case. I have also chosen to focus on these three practices, because they all display modes of transnational connection making.

The practice of seeking out half-siblings through parents of donor offspring or through the children themselves is a very recent and under-researched phenomenon,[15] only made possible on this large scale, I suspect, by the capacity of the Internet to network large amounts of people, with large amounts of data, and bridging large physical distances. It is a practice that highly depends on which data about the donor is available to families-by-donation. The US website Maria Lieb used to

15 But see Tabitha Freeman et al., »Gamete Donation: Parents' Experiences of Searching for their Child's Donor Siblings and Donor«, in: *Human Reproduction* 24 (2009), 3, pp. 505–516. And also Vasanti Jadva et al., »Experiences of Offspring Searching for and Contacting Their Donor Siblings and Donor«, in: *Reproductive BioMedicine Online* 20 (2010), 4, pp. 523–532.

seek out her daughter's half-siblings, the Donor Sibling Registry (DSR)[16], exists since 2000 and, while mainly catering to families who used US clinics, is operating worldwide and has over 10000 members.[17] It was set up by the mother of a DI-conceived son, as Maria Lieb explained, and to access it one needs to pay a membership fee.

The »horizontal connecting« between families-by-donation who used US sperm banks is made fairly easy, because all US donors get assigned a unique number by which half-siblings can find each other. Horizontal connecting is also starting to be a common practice in the UK, for instance, where the regulatory body, the Human Fertilisation and Embryology Authority (HFEA), has opened up a sibling registry in April 2010.[18] While this is a centrally regulated and not a grass-roots initiative, it was only set up because there was a rising demand for such a service. UK parents' and children's individual practices to try to seek out donor offspring included trying to network via donor codes which are, however, composed and assigned differently by individual clinics. There was a worry in the governmental authority that these networking endeavors would lead to false matches or unintended identification of donors. (Clinics had made HFEA aware, for instance, that donors might also know their patient codes and, unaware of »horizontal connecting,« might have used their code somewhere on the Internet, e.g. as part of an e-mail address or a pseudonym, where it could be googled).[19] There is also a voluntary contact register in operation in the UK since 2003, which tries to link donors, offspring, and siblings using DNA tests and which was set up by concerned groups with the help of a government grant.[20] However, possibly because of the more complicated, less web 2.0 like process of having to send in DNA swaps,

16 www.donorsiblingregistry.com [last accessed: 12.8.2009].

17 Freeman et al., »Gamete Donation«, op. cit. (note 15).

18 See, for instance, HFEA Press Release 6.4.2010 »HFEA to help donor-conceived siblings contact each other« www.hfea.gov.uk/5838.html [last accessed: 12.8.2009].

19 Information given to me in an interview with HFEA policy managers (27.05.2010). This was not, as one might think, an overcautious worry, but only came to the authority's attention after at least one comparable incident was reported to them by a fertility clinic.

20 www.ukdonorlink.org.uk [last accessed: 12.8.2009].

which take a long time to get analyzed at this particular service, it has not been as highly used as its US equivalent.[21]

Horizontal connecting in Germany at present only seems possible if the donation has a transnational link, as in Maria Lieb's case or in the case of the Schneiders – who did get hold of the donor's US ID code. Otherwise, a register using DNA testing like the UK contact register would have to be set up privately or by the government. Sperm banks in Germany operate very idiosyncratically, without much networking between the different, fairly small banks.[22] They are also not centrally regulated by a body comparable to HFEA, nor do they have to assign ID numbers that could be used for networking.[23]

The second identified kinship practice, the phenomenon of making reproductive connections via online services, as apparent in the Schneiders' use of Cryos, is evidently part of the broader development of all sorts of economic and social activities being organized via the Internet nowadays. The privatization of much of the reproductive technology sector (DI in Germany, for instance, is not covered by the public health insurance) makes a sleek and customer-oriented web interface necessary. It is not surprising that international corporations market and sell reproductive substances around the globe making use of the World Wide Web. However, similar to the wayward connections described below, there is also a subversive element to this second practice in that it helps to circumvent national regulations or just national conventions regarding the use of reproductive technologies and thereby to avoid either some of their per-

21 Freeman et al make note of the expansive tendencies of the US-based service in opposition to the small numbers at the UK contact register. See Freeman et al., »Gamete Donation«, op. cit. (note 15), p. 506.

22 This was also confirmed to me during an interview with the manager of a large German sperm bank (10.7.2009).

23 Sperm donor anonymity in Germany has only recently come under its first regulatory attention with the so-called Tissue Law (Gewebegesetz 2007), a modification of German national law, incorporating the EU Tissue and Cells Directive (2004). This de facto has lead to a removal of anonymity while there are no detailed guidelines in place yet on what that actually means on the »shop floor.« For further discussion e.g. see Michi Knecht's and Maren Klotz's joint contribution in this volume or Maren Klotz, »Samenspende: Lost in Translation«, in: *Gen-ethischer Informationsdienst* 190 (2008). Sperm donation in the UK is highly regulated and non-anonymous since 2004; the practices in the US differ and are mainly driven by consumer demand.

ceived disadvantages, like the Schneiders did, or, more importantly, some of their social or sexual biases. Lesbian couples, for instance, who have had or still have trouble accessing official reproductive services in their European home countries, rely on the subversive potential of the net to find sperm donors.[24] This brings me to the third kinship phenomenon apparent in the ethnographic vignettes, the phenomenon of making what I call »wayward« kinship connections. (Evidently, what I have termed horizontal and reproductive connections, might also be wayward connections; all these three mainly IT-based phenomena cannot be neatly separated, but are deeply entwined with one another and open to a variety of interpretations). The phenomenon of making »wayward« kinship connections via IT infrastructures is not only apparent in the Schneiders' certainty that it would be fairly easy to find their supposedly anonymous Danish donor, in Maria Lieb's detective work on the potential donation practices of »her« donor, and in the parsimonious matching of US and German donor lists by the Schneiders, it is also evident in HFEA's felt need to »channel« parents' unregulated networking activities into its official registry, i.e. into officially monitored realms of sociality. I would like to argue that these activities of making wayward connections and, to some extent, also the related phenomena of making horizontal and reproductive connections all point to a wider social tendency of increasing *informational* »uncontainability« of kinship. (By this I do not mean to argue that kinship *in general* – whatever this might be – has evolved from something contained to something uncontainable within so-called Western societies. Rather I am specifically referring to kinship *knowledge* and its official regulation.) In my view this tendency, which I will explore in greater detail below, holds fairly unexplored implications for national arrangements to regulate anonymity and data protection within the reproductive technology sector and beyond.

24 See, for instance, BBC News, »Buying Sperm over the Internet«, (2004), http://news.bbc.co.uk/1/hi/health/3423419.stm [last accessed: 24.9.2010].

An »Explosion« of Connections

I would tentatively put forward that what I call the *informational* uncontainability of kinship is rooted in the afore-discussed conjunction of kinship connection-making and telecommunicative connection-making. It would take far more historical and theoretical clarification and research than I can present here to formulate a clear-cut argument on this point, so I shall have to content myself with putting forward a rough sketch, the very first beginnings of an argument. Where kinship, in its Euro-American 21st century genomic guise, and information technology meet, there seems to be an »explosion« of connections, many of which are not in line with nationally or institutionally (nor traditionally) intended modes of making connections in the realm of kinship and data protection in a more general sense. Let me present two further examples of wayward connections, which epitomize the proclaimed contemporary »uncontainability« of kinship knowledge. In a case recently reported in The New Scientist,[25] a US teenager conceived through supposedly anonymous sperm donation used an »ancestry testing service« operating via the Internet to ultimately find his sperm donor father: The ancestry website asks men to send in DNA swaps to have the non-coding regions of their Y-chromosome analyzed and crosschecked with their database, the background to this being that, due to the patrilineal heredity of both last names (as a historical practice) and y chromosomes, there are many correlations between last names and specific base sequences on the male chromosome. The teenager's specific sequence did in fact correlate with a rare last name. Combining this last name with some of the supposedly non-identifying information about his donor, e.g. year of birth and of college graduation, enabled him to eventually trace his genitor. A second example is the recent closure of several public access online DNA databases in the US and Britain after scientists demonstrated their ability to mine specific genetic profiles of individual patients from data that were thought to be just pooled statistical data and not individual-level genotype data.[26] These public access databases are part

25 Alison Motluk, »Anonymous Sperm Donor Traced on Internet«, in: *The New Scientist* 2524 (2005), p. 6.

26 Nils Homer et al., »Resolving Individuals Contributing Trace Amounts of DNA to Highly Complex Mixtures Using High–Density SNP Genotyping Microarrays«,

of research programs seeking to identify and further analyze associations between specific genetic variants and diseases. Given the high cost and the time involved in having the genome of thousands and thousands of individuals mapped, and given the fact that »genotype data is transferable and can be combined with data from other studies, there is a considerable effort to make experimental data publicly available.«[27] Where these data were thought to only show summary statistics, a lengthy application procedure to access the data or specific data protection measures for the individuals who had taken part in the study seemed to be unnecessary. However, if her or his genetic profile is known to the person seeking to identify them, it has now become possible to determine whether a specific individual took part in the study. This is not only problematic because the persons participating in these studies have been guaranteed full anonymity and genetic profiles of individuals might (at least theoretically) be available through other domains, such as biobanks, criminal intelligence DNA databases or Internet-based projects and services such as the Personal Genome Project or 23andme.[28] It is also highly sensitive as the genetic sequences under study relate to disease susceptibilities or specific response patterns to pathogens, drugs, or other agents, i.e. they may contain exceptionally sensitive information which individuals' might have an interest to shield from particular institutions, such as insurance companies.

The perceived link between specific modes of kinship connection making and telecommunicative connection making, in my view, is provided by three entangled historical and material semiotic tendencies: A shared paradigmatic history (1) and resulting »co-evolution« (2), cumulating in something like an interoperability (i.e. the ability of two systems to interlink and work together), mutual constitution, or *convergence* (3) in Bowker's and Star's[29] sense: Both, IT technologies, which enable network-

in: *PLoS Genetics* 4 (2008), 8, pp. 1–9 (e1000167). See also NatureNews, »DNA Databases Shut after Identities Compromised«, in: *Nature* 455 (2008), p. 13. (I am thankful to my colleague Jörg Niewöhner for bringing these incidents to my attention).

27 Homer et al., »Resolving Individuals«, op. cit. (note 26), p. 9.

28 For further information see www.personalgenomes.org or www.23andme.com.

29 Susan Leigh Star, Geoffrey C. Bowker & Laura J. Neumann, »Transparency at Different Levels of Scale: Convergence between Information Artifacts and So-

ing, data storage, and data mining endeavors, and the genetic/genomic research, which informs Western views of what genetic relatedness »is«[30] and underpins current genetic technologies, are rooted in the so-called Information Discourse of the 50s.[31] In other words, kinship information is easily »connectable« to digital communicative networks, because in its contemporary »Western version« it is itself framed in discrete and not in continuous terms. Not only do IT technologies (which have co-evolved with the discipline of molecular biology, cumulating in the subdiscipline of bioinformatics) play an essential part in gene sequencing and thereby making quickly available what is called the »genetic code,« also the resulting 4 base code in its repetitive simplicity particularly lends itself to further computer processing of, say, search and comparison via bioinformatic programs such as BLAST. Imagine, in contrast, ways of obtaining kinship information that rely on information that needs to be »measured and judged« within certain standardized margins rather than on the discrete ATGC code. Such as apparent in, for instance, the evaluation practices of plants in early Mendelian breeding experiments, or in the historical physiognomic categorizations of individual human physical features, or, more blatantly, in non-Western ways of thinking and acting upon kinship knowledge that do not make use of genetics. The resulting »connectivity« between kinship and digital information technologies is difficult to grasp. It seems to be a form of interoperability, to borrow a term from information systems research. Arguing from a broader perspective on IT and sociality, Star and Bowker have suggested to move away from a naturalizing, ahistorical perspective in describing the »double process by which information artifacts and social worlds are fitted to each other and come together«[32] and to rather speak of *convergence*. They argue that communi-

---

cial Worlds«, in: *Library and Information Science, Urbana-Champaign* (1998), http://www.sis.pitt.edu/ gbowker/converge.html [last accessed: 1.10.2010].

30 As Schneider has famously argued about modern American kinship perceptions: »If science discovers new facts about biogenetic relationships, then that is what kinship is and was all along, although it may not have been known at the time.« Schneider, *American Kinship*, op. cit. (note 10), p. 23.

31 For an excellent historical account see Lilly Kay, *Who Wrote the Book of Life? A History of the Genetic Code* (Palo Alto: Stanford University Press, 2000).

32 Star, Bowker & Neumann, »Transparency«, op. cit. (note 29), p. 4.

ties of practice[33] and information systems mutually constitute each other in forms of socio-material feedback loops, leading to the disingenuous perception that IT infrastructures (and the associated classification and ordering systems)[34] simply mirror the social worlds which they are part of: »Convergence here fits together the representation of knowledge and the phenomena which are being represented, through highly distributed knowledge systems.«[35] To highlight the historically derived and socio-material dimensions of this interoperability between Western perceptions of kinship knowledge and digital information technology I shall henceforth speak of a *convergence* between the two.

With more and more countries making non-anonymous sperm donation illegal (e.g. Sweden, Switzerland and Austria)[36] and court cases, wider regulatory debates, and public debates mainly centering on questions of human rights and identity formation,[37] one could argue that given the convergence of IT and kinship there is a more socio-material undercurrent to be taken into account – or story to be told: Even if *transparency* had not seemingly become a moral good in its own right in current Western societies (Strathern being one of the rare scholars to critically interrogate this tendency),[38] the idea of »the state« or rather its regulatory bodies and medical institutions keeping kinship information on donors (or siblings) away from families-by-donation, who want to pursue it, seems to have become practically impossible. Nor does it seem to be possible for a transnational corporation, such as Cryos, completely to contain such data. In my view,

33 The term »community of practice« has its origins in the anthropology of learning: Jean Lave and Etienne Wegner, *Situated Learning* (Cambridge: Cambridge University Press, 1991). It refers to a community, for instance a particular profession, which shares certain conventions, formal and tacit knowledge on certain tasks etc. The term has also found its way into parts of Science and Technology Studies, for instance through Bowker and Star: Geoffrey C. Bowker and Susan Leigh Star, *Sorting Things Out: Classification and Its Consequences.* (Cambridge, MA: MIT Press, 1999).

34 Bowker & Star, »Sorting Things Out«, op. cit. (note 33).

35 Star, Bowker &Neumann, »Transparency«, op. cit. (note 29), p. 12.

36 E.g. see Freeman et al., »Gamete Donation«, op. cit. (note 15), p. 505.

37 For instance the Rose & Anor versus HFEA court case in the UK in 2002, which proved to be the most significant legal step in paving the way towards non-anonymous gamete donation in the UK by ruling that donor anonymity was essentially a violation of the UK Human Rights Act (1998). Article 8 of the Act guarantees UK citizens the »respect for private and family life, including the right to form a personal identity.«

38 E.g. Strathern, »Refusing Information«, op. cit. (note 9).

it would thus be an important research topic to further explore the relationship between this convergence and the dominant, seemingly unrelated discourse concerning the »right to know.«[39]

The Imperative to Connect

Focusing more closely on the social actors involved, what shall we make of these IT afforded kinship practices, particularly of the apparent rise of what I have called wayward and horizontal connections? The underlying drive to use *genetic* connections as a trajectory for different modes of *social* connection making could easily – maybe too easily – be interpreted as a sign of a fairly straightforward geneticisation of society.[40] Instead, I want to point to an emerging line of research which takes a slightly different take on these phenomena: Both Michi Knecht and Jeanette Edwards see a wider cultural pattern, an imperative to connect, at work within contemporary kinship phenomena.[41] Edwards ethnographically describes the growing interest in »family treeing,« i.e. ancestry research, in the north of England, which »marries, amongst other things, the technological and the mystical, empirical research and imagination, kinship and class, thus connecting facets of human being that are often, in analysis, kept apart.«[42] Drawing on Green's, Harvey's, and Knox' work on information technologies and place making and extending it to kinship studies, she interprets her informants' detective work to unearth past genealogical connections and their strong reliance on IT infrastructures as part of an imperative to

39 Investigating this relationship will be one of the future research emphases of the Humboldt University research project »Kinship Cultures« (SFB 640, C4), of which the editors of this volume are all members.

40 E.g. Kaya Finkler, »The Kin in the Gene. The Medicalization of Family and Kinship in American Society«, in: *Current Anthropology* 42 (2001), 2, pp. 235–263.

41 Michi Knecht, »Der Imperativ, sich zu verbinden: Neue kulturanthropologische Forschungen zu Verwandtschaft in europäischen Gegenwartsgesellschaften«, in: *Österreichische Zeitschrift für Volkskunde* 112 (2009), pp. 28–51, and Jeanette Edwards, »The Ancestor in the Machine«, *CRESC Working Paper Series* 71 (2009), pp. 2–21, http://www.cresc.ac.uk/sites/default/files/wp%2071.pdf [last accessed: 18.5.2012].

42 Edwards, »Ancestor«, op. cit. (note 41), p. 18.

connect: where »making connections« becomes a moral good *in itself*, a social imperative – a joy and celebration of the serendipity moment.[43]

Knecht arrives at similar conclusions when observing activities of »transfamilial networking« between half-siblings, concerned groups, experts and genealogists within communities of families-by-donation or adoption.[44] She sees the imperative to connect implicated with the theme of fragmentation experienced by families where conception and parental roles have been distributed in nontraditional ways; it is a mode of »re-embedding« relationships and roles in newly defined family realms. Edwards suspects that the contemporary currency of the imperative to connect is both »inflected by a post-industrial landscape and recent experiences of social and economic upheaval« and »exercising some of the emotional capacities that would otherwise be exercised by organized religion.«[45] A common is established: Strathern's above mentioned notion of »the grand project of making society,« instituted along the old trajectory of genealogical connections, endorsed by what Edwards calls »an early 21st century complexion« of kinship through a contemporary convergence of IT infrastructures and relatedness.[46]

Edwards describes her surprise about how easily *her informants* are actually able to »family tree« herself, despite her giving away only very limited information on her relatives. Similar to my earlier conclusions, if not as closely interested in questions of IT technology, kinship, and digitalization, she states that this reflexive experience is »interesting in what it reveals about the increasingly diminishing domain of privacy, anonymity and ability to remain silent (unknown).«[47] She goes on to argue that this also reflexively puts into focus – and challenges – ethnological conventions of safeguarding the privacy of both researcher and informant. In a sense, this might just underline viewing fieldwork as an inherently relational pro-

43 Sarah Green, Penny Harvey, and Hannah Knox, »Scales of Place and Networks: An Ethnography of the Imperative to Connect through Information and Communications Technologies«, in: *Current Anthropology* 46 (2005), 5. Also see Strathern, *Kinship, Law and the Unexpected*, op. cit. (note 1), p. 11.

44 Knecht, »Der Imperativ«, op. cit. (note 41), pp. 49–50.

45 Edwards, »Ancestor«, op. cit. (note 41), p. 17.

46 Ibid., p. 5.

47 Ibid., p. 9.

cess, but for Edwards there is also something intrinsically contemporary at stake here: an »inherent overload of information.«[48]

Making and Cutting Connections

I would like to take up Edwards' moment of reflexivity (and Riles' insight that *the network* is an inherently recursive social form, both for her informants *but just as much* for herself as a social science researcher)[49] and explore how I, as a researcher, have become implicated in the imperative to connect and what analytical work my earlier introduction of field notes about more literal forms of connecting, namely making train connections, could do for the closing argument of this article. My interviewees regularly asked me to make horizontal connections for them, for instance, to pass on information about support groups and to encourage persons to get in touch or register on websites. I have become an active part of precisely those networking activities I am researching (to say nothing of my private Web 2.0 engagements or professional so-called networking), weaving the net of horizontal connections further. Like Edwards, I am faced with a dilemma of simultaneously wanting to honor my interview partners' wishes and interests and at the same time safeguarding their privacy and potential wish *not* to be connected (or not even to know about the mere possibility of being connected) and following the institutional ethical guidelines of a strict anonymity regulating my own research. Negotiating when to allow and encourage the making of connections and when to *hinder* them by not passing on certain information has become a complicated act, often decided on the spot after I have established a sense of my informants' general interest in meeting other DI families outside their social circle. This brings me back to my field notes, which do not convey a sense of proliferation or easiness regarding the more literal connections to be made, but rather give an impression of *hindrance*:

»As I travel from Koblenz main station to Cologne the train is ten minutes late. The announcement only comes when the train should already be arriving, causing

48 Loc. cit.

49 Riles, »The Network«, op. cit. (note 6), p. 172.

confusion with travelers who do not speak German. I translate for an Asian couple and engage in a conversation with an elderly woman about some of the problems Deutsche Bahn was recently having with punctuality.«

The impetus behind trying to make these literal connections is rather similar to what Knecht sees as the underlying impulse to the imperative to connect. If the imperative to connect is related to a fragmentation of conception and of parental roles and may be seen as a complicated countertactic, my attempts to make train connections are related to a form of fragmentation as well: a fragmentation of the classical ethnographic research process, in that I am not based in one permanent field site; a fragmented ethnography where I constantly dis-connect and re-connect with different informants and field sites, trying to still establish rapport by taking trains to see my interviewees face-to-face, while also juggling the obligations of my departmental position.[50]

But where are these reflexive analogies leading? Marilyn Strathern points out that applying the network metaphor (or, for that matter, my related metaphor of »making connections«) has many advantages in social science research, because it does not make assumptions about scale or hierarchy. However, it is also analytically problematic in the sense that it is potentially »autolimitless; that is, a concept which works indigenously as a metaphor for the endless extension and intermeshing of phenomena.«[51] Strathern argues that we need to introduce a second metaphor for the first one to do analytical work for us, a metaphor that can analytically cut the network. What is it, that is being disconnected, cut, limited – *hindered*, if one thinks of my own field notes? She introduces ownership and transactions as notions that help us grapple with the potentially vast proliferation of *the* network.[52] For instance, when envisaging a Latourian

50 Interestingly, Knox et al. link the theme of fragmentation and the theme of the network by pointing to the long history of »network thinking« in social anthropology as a »recognition of *fragmentation* and complexity [emphasis added]«; Knox, Savage & Harvey, »Social Networks«, op. cit. (note 6), p. 133.

51 Strathern, »Cutting«, op. cit. (note 5), p. 522. For a discussion of networks and questions of scale in ethnography also see Knox, Savage & Harvey, »Social Networks«, op. cit. (note 6), in particular p. 123.

52 For a critical discussion on how to recognise the actors comprising an actor-network, e.g. see Gesa Lindemann, »The Analysis of the Borders of the Social World. A Challenge for Sociological Theory«, in: *Journal for the Theory of Social Behaviour* 35 (2005).

actor-network involved in making a certain pharmaceutical appear, it is the moment of patenting in which a network length is determined and other parties are cut off. She argues: »So where technology might enlarge networks, proprietorship can be guaranteed to cut them down to size.«[53] Strathern also observes that within complex kinship systems it is most often the transactions of valuables, ritual objects, and money associated with different forms of kinship that establish more or less clearly restricted networks.[54]

Evidently, my attempt to focus on different modes of making connections in my research material and my research activities may be liable to a similar criticism of »autolimitlessness« as the one raised by Strathern with regard to the network metaphor. I have taken two ethnographic vignettes as a starting point to describe, discuss, and contextualize three contemporary transnational and Internet-based kinship phenomena to be found among kinship-by-donation: I have subsumed them under my guiding metaphor of *making connections*: horizontal, reproductive, and wayward. I have gone on to argue that embedded within a specific contemporary convergence of digital information technologies and kinship-related »connection making« there is a form of autolimitlessness, where kinship information becomes potentially uncontainable by a state or corporate monopoly and where making connections becomes a moral imperative in its own right. It would take further research to explore in detail whether ownership or transactions yield an »indigenous, Euro-American mechanism for cutting« within these kinship phenomena that is appropriate to my specific field of research.[55] As a preliminary step I have chosen to resort to a more reflexive and literary »mechanism« in order to keep this article from succumbing to the pitfalls of relational metaphors: the mechanism of juxtaposition.[56] While the examples of »connectivity« discussed above point to novel forms of doing kinship that surpass national regulation or information containment, one should not let get carried away in a dangerously simplistic and cliché proclamation of an increasingly smooth world in which basically everything is connected

53 Strathern, »Cutting«, op. cit. (note 5), p. 531.

54 Strathern, »Cutting«, op. cit. (note 5), p. 529.

55 Strathern, »Cutting«, op. cit. (note 5), p. 531.

56 E.g. James Clifford, »On Ethnographic Surrealism«, in: *Comparative Studies in Society and History* 23 (1981), 4, pp. 539–564.

to everything. While researching kinship-by-donation in the 21st century, some of the more mundane connections were not easy to make: trains were late, taxis lost without their sat navs, buses not expecting passengers, railway stations were for sale…

Juxtaposing these minor failures to connect to the seemingly easy feat of making kinship connections with the help of IT technology, foregrounds some important questions about the simultaneous unmaking and making of connections, the most obvious being: What specific character will those connections that I have termed horizontal kinship connections (i.e. the IT supported connections between half siblings, bridging two continents, in the case of Maria Lieb's daughter) or wayward connections (for instance the potential »tracking« of the Schneiders' anonymous Danish donor by their son) take on when more literal connections have to be made in order to actually meet face-to-face? What kind of sociality will unfold as an effect of making these connections? What kind of social relationships are established across large physical distances, when traveling cannot be afforded, seems too complicated, or cannot be integrated into the sociality of a different physical location? Furthermore, in the case of the Internet-based reproductive connection making of the Schneiders, one needs to ask how the actual physical flow of substances, such as the donor sperm ordered from Denmark – which will also have to make train or flight connections –, may be subject to »cuts« at national borders: because of the increasing enforcement of the 2004 EU Tissue and Cells Directive and the resultant tightening of controls on border-crossing human tissues, or because of the disappearance of nationally underregulated grey areas regarding the handling of gametes, such as apparent in the new German regulations.[57] A last and more distant trail I want to point out here, is related to the aforementioned rise of transparency and non-anonymity as moral obligations and the concomitant decrease of social domains of secrecy, not-knowing, silence and disconnectedness (Edwards quotes Deleuze on the potential »tyranny of expression/communication«[58] in this context): How will »Western« kinship practices change once the classical »kinship theme« – and the accompanying social practices – of the

57 E.g. the German Tissue Law (Gewebegesetz) of 2007.

58 Edwards, »Ancestor«, op. cit. (note 41), p. 9.

family secret[59] are becoming more and more dubious and outmoded by the convergence of kinship and communication technologies? Pointing to trains, sat navs, buses, and station buildings may not lead us out of this conundrum of questions, but it may indeed provide a first trail in.

59 For a discussion of this theme see, for instance, Leonore Davidoff, *Worlds Between: Historical Perspectives on Gender and Class* (Cambridge: Polity Press, 1995), or Carol Smart, »Families, Secrets and Memories«, in: *Sociology* 45 (2011), 4, pp. 539–553.

National Styles of Reproductive Governance and Global Forms

The Other Mother: Supplementary Wombs and the Surrogate State in India

Aditya Bharadwaj

Indian women offering commercial gestational services to a range of local and global consumers of assisted reproductive technologies (ARTs) have received unprecedented attention around the globe.[1] Actors and institutions as diverse as the mass media, academia (most notably anthropology and sociology), fertility clinics, law firms, brokers, and national governments have come to focus on *surrogates* for a myriad of political, intellectual, ethical, legal, and purely commercial reasons.

The notion of surrogate instantiates a host of significations: substitution, replacement, proxy, and stand-in. The conflation between the very act of surrogate substitution and motherhood is well established in the scholarly imagination[2]. This chapter further interrogates this conflation in the larger context of transnational surrogacy arrangements involving Indian women. In large part I wish to explore how we might better understand the existential predicament of Indian women who are seldom surrogate or substitute mothers but almost always an addition – supplement – to a transnationally located *mother in waiting.*

These concerns are embedded in years of ethnographic exploration focused on the bourgeoning rise of ARTs in India.[3] Thus far my en-

1 Cf. A. Gentleman, »India Nurtures Business of Surrogate Motherhood«, in: *The New York Times*, 10.3. 2008. http://www.nytimes.com/2008/03/10/world/asia/10surrogate.html?_r=1 [last accessed: 6.9.2010].

2 Helena Ragoné, *Surrogate Motherhood: Conception in the Heart* (Boulder, CO: Westview Press, 1994).

3 See (forthcoming) Aditya Bharadwaj, *Conceptions: Infertility and Procreative Modernity in India* (New York: Berghahn Books, 2011); Aditya Bharadwaj, »How Some Indian Baby Makers are Made: Media Narratives and Assisted Conception in India«, in: *Anthropology and Medicine* 7 (2000), 1, pp. 63–78; Aditya Bharadwaj, »Conception Politics: Medical Egos, Media Spotlights, and the Contest over Test-tube Firsts in India«, in: Marcia C. Inhorn & Frank van Balen (Eds.), *Infertility Around the Globe*

counters with »surrogacy« in India have remained confined to »altruistic« arrangements between family members who would routinely seek out specific private clinics to help arrange a quick surrogate pregnancy. I use the term surrogate here to signal the role of kinship in achieving conception through substitution or proxy. This mode of »non-commercial« family-forming creates different but equally important sets of relations of exploitation, piety, kinship, and support. However, the rapid proliferation of commercial gestational services and global fertility travels in the new century demonstrates how swiftly the Indian fertility industry has assumed a transnational dimension. Since 2005, a few scholarly accounts on global reproductive travels in search of »surrogate wombs« and the gendered commercial underbelly of »surrogate conception« in India have emerged.[4] Whilst the ongoing empirical research on commercial surrogacy – most notably led by graduate students in the United States, Europe, and India – is continuing to provide rich data on gender and kinship, science and technology, labor markets and processes, global travel and local sourcing, ethically fraught and dubious practices in India and beyond, there are very few theoretical conversations, conceptual analyses, and, above all, political debates taking place.[5]

The chapter lies on the cusp of conceptual elaboration and political critique. In so doing, I attempt a tentative unravelling of critical issues central to the local politics of supplementary wombs in India. It is my belief that moves to accomplish political mobilisation and cultural critique require

(Berkeley: University of California Press, 2002); Aditya Bharadwaj, »Why Adoption is not an Option in India: The Visibility of Infertility, the Secrecy of Donor Insemination, and other Cultural Complexities«, in: *Social Science and Medicine* 56 (2003), pp. 1867–1880; and Marcia C. Inhorn & Aditya Bharadwaj, »Reproductively Disabled Lives: Infertility, Stigma and Suffering in Egypt and India«, in: Benedicte Ingstad & Susan Reynolds Whyte (Eds.), *Disability in Local and Global Worlds* (Berkeley: University of California Press, 2006).

4 Cf. Amrita Pande, »Commercial Surrogacy in India: Manufacturing the Perfect ›Mother Worker‹«, in: *Signs* 35 (2010), 4, pp. 969–992; and Kalindi Vora, »Indian Transnational Surrogacy and the Commodification of Vital Energy«, in: *Subjectivities* 28 (2009), pp. 266–278.

5 For a notable exception and political critique see Jyotsna Agnihotri Gupta, »Towards Transnational Feminisms: Some Reflections and Concerns in Relation to the Globalization of Reproductive Technologies«, in: *European Journal of Women's Studies* 13 (2006), 1, pp. 23–38.

conceptual and semantic (terminological) clarity. Adriane Rich rightly observed that in *the interstices of language lie powerful secrets of the culture.*[6] In order to achieve this clarity I turn to Jacques Derrida to produce a conceptual separation between the figures of a surrogate and a supplement. I further reflect on early feminist scholarship, which I describe as the *radical feminist challenge*, to sketch out the contours of the exploitative relations of (re)production at the heart of transnational gestational arrangements in India. This is mainly achieved through a sustained critique of normative and ideological processes that have shaped the experience of gender and its present day consequences for supplementary women in India. I conclude by interrogating the role of the Indian State. In brief, I wish to ask:

a) What is it to be supplementary, or rather, what is it to exist, persist in a state of supplementarity? b) What are the sexual genealogies and gendered ideologies (even archaeologies) of »surrogacy« in India? And, c) Where is the state: is it absent, »spectral,« or surrogate?

The Supplementary »Other«

The poor around the world inhabit biologies that are routinely construed as waste, as disposable and dispensable.[7] In many parts of the world, wombs, embryos, and kidneys – to name a few commodities – exist in states of exception, as »bare life.«[8] Who and what gets defined as »waste« in any given society, argues Scheper-Hughes, often has bearing on the lives of the poorest in countries with a ready surplus of »unidentified

6 Adrienne Rich. 1995, *Of Woman Born: Motherhood as Experience and Institution* (New York: W. W. Norton & Company; first edition Norton, 1976).

7 Cf. Nancy Scheper-Hughes, »The Global Traffic in Human Organs«, in: *Current Anthropology* 41 (2000), 2, pp. 191–224.

8 Cf. Giorgio Agamben, *Homo Sacer: Sovereign Power and Bare Life* (Stanford CA: Stanford University Press, 1998). Agamben resurrects the figure of the *homo sacer* as the one allowing the sovereign to resort to a state of exception in which the bare killable body becomes situated as one lying before the law; thus it cannot be sacrificed, as this positioning renders it outside the purview of divine law. In other words, certain bodies become killable as they get positioned by law as lying before the very institution of law.

unclaimed pauper bodies.«[9] Extreme forms of this notion were well-supported in specific totalitarian contexts throughout human history. In the post-war 20th century, a less severe and reformed relationship to waste and disposal emerged in capitalist social formations, one predicated on ethics of limitless cycles of demand and supply. From the end of the 20th century to the closing years of the first decade of the 21st, this modality has given way to newer forms of exploitation and ethics of consumption that demand a different relationship to disposal and waste. This new formation can be conceptualised as the *neo-liberal mode of production*. The poor in a neo-liberal world inhabit biologies that are not so much construed as »waste« but rather as »going to waste«; this notion, I would further argue, gains traction only when those »going to waste« can be recycled in any tangible, meaningful, and above all profitable sense. Charis Thompson (2005) argues that in the »biomedical mode of reproduction,« unlike the capitalist mode of production, waste is seldom a political or logistical problem but rather an ethical one of how to designate life material [embryos] as waste.[10] I am suggesting that there is another layer of complexity at work. In the neoliberal mode of production the problem of how to designate life materials as waste is frequently addressed by resorting to recycling socially/ethically defined waste or surplus that cannot otherwise be gainfully accumulated. For example, innovative theodicies are enabled that mark surplus embryos as better utilised for research or adoption as opposed to being wasted. Questions of ethics and morality in this respect become commercial decisions where ethical deliberations only facilitate the recycling of entities going to waste[11]. So, that which would have been formerly discarded is now made available for maximum accumulation, recycling, and perpetuation. The shift is both semantic and material: waste has become displaced/supplemented/ supplanted by what

9 Scheper-Hughes, »The Global Traffic«, op. cit. (note 7); or Nancy Scheper-Hughes, »The Ends of the Body: Commodity Fetishism and the Global Traffic in Organs«, in: *SAIS Review* 22 (2002), 1, pp. 61–80.

10 Charis Thompson, *Making Parents: The Ontological Choreography of Reproductive Technologies* (Cambridge, MA: MIT Press, 2005), p. 264.

11 Aditya Bharadwaj, »Assisted Life: The Neoliberal Moral Economy of Embryonic Stem Cells in India«, in: Daphna Birenbaum-Carmeli & Marcia C. Inhorn (Eds.), *Assisting Reproduction, Testing Genes: Global Encounters with New Biotechnologies* (New York: Berghahn Books, 2010).

is *going waste*. One can say that going waste now stands in a relationship of supplementation with 20th century waste. The neoliberal citizenship demands that waste must be supplanted and become viable through cycles of ethical, preferably legal, and above all optimal recycling.[12] We must therefore ask, what kind of supplement is the so-called surrogate? Does the poverty and do the material circumstances of some women in India turn their reproductive vitality – otherwise going to waste – into a commercially viable proposition? Most importantly, what is it to live a supplementary life, not so much in lieu of or in the position of (an)other but rather as an additional other?

Jacques Derrida (1998) tells us that »substitution distances from birth, from the natural or maternal origin.«[13] Derrida was of course addressing and deconstructing a very different semantic context. However, I wish to appropriate his notion of the supplement to suggest that a surrogate is better conceptualised as supplement especially given her temporal positionality vis-à-vis the biosocial mother as (an)other. To achieve this, let us first understand how Derrida invokes supplementation. »Supplement,« for Derrida, harbors two important cohabiting significations.

»The supplement adds itself, it is a surplus, a plenitude enriching another plenitude, the fullest measure of presence. It cumulates and accumulates presence.« For example, writing for Derrida »substitutes the plenitude of a speech whose deficiency and infirmity it nevertheless only supplements.«[14] A surrogate in this respect is not only a substitute for the biosocial signifier *the mother*, but she also, through recycling her pauper body into an innovative new permutation, becomes the tool and trope for bypassing a »deficient infirmity,« a pro-natalist inflection on the body of the *biosocial mother*, albeit via circuitous and supplemental detour.

»But the supplement supplements,« warns Derrida. It adds only to replace (although its destiny is temporal and fixed). It intervenes or insinuates itself *in-the-place-of*; if it fills, it is as if it fills a void. If it represents and makes an image, it is by the anterior default of a presence. Compensatory [*suppleant*], the supplement is an adjunct, a subaltern instance that

12 Aditya Bharadwaj & Peter Glasner, *Local Cells, Global Science: The Rise of Embryonic Stem Cell Research in India* (London & New York: Routledge, 2009).

13 Jacques Derrida, *Of Grammatology* (Baltimore, MA: Johns Hopkins University Press, 1998), p. 199.

14 Derrida, »Of Grammatology«, op. cit. (note 13), p. 144.

takes-(the)-place. As a substitute, it is not simply added to the positivity of a presence, it produces no relief as its place is assigned in the structure by the mark of an emptiness. Somewhere, something can be filled up of *itself,* can accomplish itself, only by allowing itself to be filled through sign and proxy. »The sign is always the supplement of the thing itself.«[15]

The surrogate becomes a mother by supplementing. This transactional motherhood is achieved in the semantic and the enunciatory realms. A surrogate knows her place in the patriarchal, pro-natalist structure as compensatory, as both brought in and bought to fill the empty, womb-like void and delegated to supplant this void left un-full-filled by the biosocial mother. The dual quality of supplement is *replacement* and an *addition.* That which is deficient and replaced by the supplement is not merely substituted but rather is added to and in so doing a new structure is produced that cannot be reduced to the entity being replaced or supplanted.

According to Derrida this second signification of the supplement cannot be separated from the first. But the inflexion varies from moment to moment. Each of the two significations is by turns effaced or becomes discreetly vague in the presence of the other. Thus the first erasure is that of the biosocial mother, followed by the eventual erasure of the surrogate or the supplement. And, every now and again, one mother becomes discreetly vague in the presence of the other. But their common function is shown in this: whether it adds or substitutes itself, the supplement is *exterior*, outside of the positivity to which it is super-added, alien to that which, in order to be replaced by it, must be other than it. Unlike the complement (the biosocial mother), the supplement (surrogate mother) is an »exterior addition.«[16]

In other words a supplement is always doubly articulate: it fixes a fault, deficiency, absence or something missing and in so doing it adds something which is different and cannot be reduced to that which has become supplanted. A supplement in this respect cannot be a surrogate as that presupposes mere proxy ignoring the addition through supplementation. A supplementary woman like the surrogate only *substitutes* the missing, absent gestational potential of the biosocial mother. But in so doing she – the supplement – also substitutes the mother by *adding* her gestational

15 Derrida, »Of Grammatology«, op. cit. (note 13), p. 145.
16 Derrida, »Of Grammatology«, op. cit. (note 13), p. 145.

fecundity for the duration of the contract to enrich and enhance the social career of the biosocial mother. A supplement therefore remains an addition replete with her own biographical structure thus allowing new readings and interpretations of what it is to be the other mother.

The »Other« Mother: Sexual Genealogies, Gendered Ideologies

The title of this chapter, »The Other Mother,« is a provocation. It is a provocation and an invitation to question and (re)locate the figure of »the mother« in transnational surrogate transactions. Mother therefore is a misnomer. The conflation of mother and surrogate is in fact a fine illustration of the gendered cultural imprints that saturate thinking across a spectrum of institutions, such as biomedicine, state, law, family, marriage, or religion, in a stratified global reproductive topography.[17] Strathern argues that, for Euro-Americans, a surrogate mother makes explicit the relationship between gestation and other factors in childbirth. She, the surrogate substitute, is »acting on behalf of another woman, she represents a facet of motherhood but is not herself the real mother.«[18] This »stand-in« function, »metonymically occupying« the place in reference to another person who by implication is always the »real parent,« is how the »modernist Euro-American« sees the relationship between what I have been describing following Derrida, the complement and the supplement.[19] However, the category of real parent or real mother – even in the modernist »ethnoscape«[20] of Euro-Americans – needs cautious conceptualisation. The so-called real biosocial mother's erasure from the process of gestation – her privileged Euro-American position notwithstanding – remains poorly understood and articulated in transnational surrogate

17 Cf. Heléna Ragoné & France Winddance Twine, *Ideologies and Technologies of Motherhood: Race, Class, Sexuality, Nationalism* (New York: Routledge, 2000).

18 Marilyn Strathern, »Surrogates and Substitutes: New Practices for Old?«, in: James Good & Irving Velody (Eds.), *The Politics of Postmodernity* (Cambridge: Cambridge University Press, 1998), p. 185.

19 Strathern, »Surrogates and Substitutes«, op. cit. (note 18).

20 Arjun Appadurai, *Modernity at Large: Cultural Dimensions of Globalization* (Minneapolis: University of Minnesota Press, 1996).

transactions. This temporal slippage of the imagined real parent into the realm of *other mother* needs more nuanced empirical and conceptual elaboration.[21] Nevertheless, this process ensconces the substitute womb in the domain of fictive kinship that designates the supplanting womb *»as if« that of the real mother.*[22] Strathern (1998) argues that what makes the surrogate »like a mother« and not the real mother is that she helps the real mother to achieve motherhood.[23] In the case of transnational gestational surrogacy, for instance as currently being practiced in India, where the biogenetic *connect* with the *parents* of an evolving foetus and the biogenetic *disconnect* with the supplementary womb is almost always complete, a surrogate's nine-month-long motherhood is often figurative, a simple figure of speech that is routinized, normalized, and naturalized in media, policy, and clinical discourses. These *stratified reproducers*[24] seldom become »like a mother« given the racial, class, and ethnic differences between the supplanted mother and the *other mother*.

Throughout the 20th century the *cultural* penetrated deeper into the realm of the *cellular*.[25] From metaphoric postulations about women's bodies as ancient sites for/of reproduction to the gendered inscription of reproductive tissues,[26] motherhood could not only be objectified as preordained, encrypted natural destiny, but also »enterprised up« to fulfil

21 A recent ethnographic account by Elly Temen produces just such a nuanced narrative of a very specific case of »surrogate bodies« in Israel where surrogates and intended mothers negotiate and cooperate in bringing forth new life that produces both a deep and lasting bond between the surrogate and biosocial mother. Elly Temen, *Birthing the Mother: The Surrogate Body and the Pregnant Self* (Berkeley: University of California Press, 2010).

22 I borrow the formulation of fictive »as if« kinship principally from the work of Judith Modell (1994), who in the context of American adoptive kinship showed how bonds created through adoption are made »as-if« genealogical and natural. See Judith Modell, *Kinship with Strangers: Adoption and Interpretation of Kinship in American Culture* (Berkeley, CA: University of California Press, 1994).

23 Strathern, »Surrogates and Substitutes«, op. cit. (note 18).

24 Faye D. Ginsburg & Rayna Rapp, *Conceiving the New World Order: The Global Politics of Reproduction* (Berkeley, CA: University of California Press, 1995).

25 Evelyn Fox Keller, *Refiguring Life: Metaphors of Twentieth-Century Biology* (New York: Columbia University Press, 1995).

26 Both of these aspects were brilliantly described by Emily Martin. See Emily Martin, »The Egg and the Sperm«, in: *Signs* 16 (1991), 3, pp. 485–501; Emily Martin, *The Woman in the Body: A Cultural Analysis of Reproduction* (Boston: Beacon Press, 1987).

the fecund remit.[27] The feminist critique, especially the radical feminist challenge of the early 1980s, is in this respect not only noteworthy but also accidentally prophetic in its vision of the future. Long before invocations to the manifesto of the cyborg and techno-feminism became commonplace feminist activists like Andrea Dworkin (1983), Gena Corea (1985), and many others were (re)drawing the battle lines.[28] Now in great measure these early political encounters were received with guarded caution as either untenable in a globalized world or too Eurocentric to be fit for purpose in »other cultures.«[29] However, this critical distancing would only ring true if the radical feminist challenge of the 1980s is viewed from a discursive universe that equates the empirical with the experiential, epistemological positioning and ontological spectating as generative of *the real* and *truthful*. Thus viewed, arguments around agency, structure, and resistance can have displacing effects for these early feminist concerns. However, the radical feminist challenge was always unashamedly located on the edge between producing rhetorics of persuasion and manifestos for rebellion. Its vitality was of a different order, it was confrontational, it spoke in the projective future tense and re-conceived the world order in a different gendered configuration. It had the idealized purity of a revo-

27 See Gaylene Becker, *The Elusive Embryo: How Women and Men Approach New Reproductive Technologies* (Berkeley: University of California Press, 2000); Sarah Franklin, »Deconstructing ›Desperateness‹: The Social Construction of Infertility in Popular Representations of New Reproductive Technologies«, in: Maureen McNeil, Ian Varcoe & Steven Yearley (Eds.), *The New Reproductive Technologies* (London: Macmillan, 1990); Sarah Franklin, *Embodied Progress. A Cultural Account of Assisted Conception* (London: Routledge, 1997); Sarah Franklin & Heléna Ragoné (Eds.), *Reproducing Reproduction: Kinship, Power and Technological Innovation* (Philadelphia: University of Pennsylvania Press, 1998); Arthur L. Greil, *Not Yet Pregnant: Infertile Couples in Contemporary America* (New Brunswick: Rutgers University Press, 1991); or Marilyn Strathern, *Reproducing the Future: Anthropology, Kinship and the New Reproductive Technologies* (New York: Routledge, 1992).

28 Andrea Dworkin, *Right-Wing Women* (New York: Perigee Books, 1983); Gena Corea, *The Mother Machine: Reproductive Technologies from Artificial Insemination to Artificial Wombs* (London: The Women's Press, 1985b). I am grateful to the editors for reminding me that Haraway's Manifesto of the Cyborg and the radical feminist critiques were in fact contemporaneous; Haraway's Manifesto was first published in 1985, and republished in 1991 when it truly rose to global prominence.

29 Cf. Michelle Stanworth (Ed.), *Reproductive Technologies: Gender, Motherhood and Medicine* (Cambridge: Polity Press, 1987).

lutionary: naive but infectious, shrill but sincere, sensational but equally trite. It was passion out of control and anger devoid of discipline. A good illustration of this genre of politics can be found in what Dworkin (1983) and Corea (1985) passionately described as the »reproductive brothel.«[30]

Agitating against male control over women's reproductive destinies, Dworkin predicted a shift away from the »farming model applied to motherhood,« where men plant seeds and proceed to harvest the crop (a metaphoric postulation very much alive in India to this day), to a brothel model where women are collected together and held, thus reducing women to what »she sells.« The diatribe went on to conjure horrific scenarios that likened the later model to animal farming. However, when describing the possible future permutations of surrogacy arrangements, Corea almost predicts an uncanny and now familiar face of international surrogacy, albeit in 1985. Quoting social commentator Vance Packard, Corea argued:

»If the ›mercenary mother‹ were to gestate an embryo conceived with another woman's egg, the job should not require much of the surrogate ›in the way of education, family back-ground, good looks, or even skin color. If the woman is simply to be an incubator, the price would certainly be lower than if she contributed half the baby's heredity.‹ In south Texas, he wrote, ›pleasant conscientious Mexican-American girls‹ might leap at a fee of 5000 dollars for bearing a child and girls (sic) south of the border might leap at half that fee. ›If lawyers can arrange Mexican divorces for Americans,‹ wrote Peckard, ›they surely can arrange Mexican gestations.‹ Fees paid to ›host mothers‹ would probably vary with the country, as several commentators have suggested. Mexican women would do it for less. When it becomes possible to transfer human embryos routinely from one women to another (and it has already been done experimentally), then the way opens to use Third World women to gestate babies for wealthier Westerners. The president of a US foundation which helps arrange surrogate pregnancies told me: »If we could cross international lines, then 1000 dollars is a significant sum of money, where as (in the US), it's just a week or month's wages. Asked what countries he had in mind he replied: ›Central America would be fine.‹ It is ›inevitable‹ that the United States go to other parts of the world and ›rely on their support‹ in providing surrogate mothers, he thinks. Comparing United States to

30 Dworkin, »Right-Wing Women«, op. cit. (note 29); Gena Corea, »How the New Reproductive Technologies Could be Used to Apply the Brothel Model of Social Control over Women«, in: *Women's Studies International Forum* 8 (1985a), 4, pp. 299–305.

the city and Central America to the country, he pointed out that ›the cities are always supported by the country.‹«[31]

What seemed plausible in 1985 has become an empirical reality. The possibility of arranging »Mexican gestations« has given way to the surety of acquiring Indian gestational surrogacy. What are the implications for India?

In India today, assisted conception has become a visible, viable, and veritably thriving industry.[32] Some unconfirmed estimates go as far as to suggest that there are more IVF clinics in India than in all of Western Europe (some media reports put the total upwards of 500 clinics). The reproductive segment of the Indian medical tourism market is currently valued at over 450 million dollar per annum, and the Indian Council of Medical Research (ICMR) predicted this to grow to a 6-billion-dollar market by 2008.[33] There are no assessments currently available about whether indeed this whopping figure has now been reached or surpassed. It is within this commercial context that the global extent of India's burgeoning surrogacy industry has become well-known, if not terribly well understood. However, let me trace these developments in the context of India's fertility industry and the many cultural patterns that frame its spectacular rise. My point of departure is yet again conceptual. Let us return momentarily to a »critical event« in India's history, the partition of the sub-continent into India and Pakistan that left scores of women violated, abused and abducted.[34] There was a lot of *patriarchal waste* to sift through. In fact, the nature of violence and its focus on women's bodies was tantamount to violating and polluting the source of reproductive purity. Not surprisingly therefore, thousands of women were left unclaimed by families and networks of kin as, what I would like to conceptualise and politicise as *patriarchal waste.* When such tainted bodies were claimed, as Veena Das shows, the injury to normative concepts like purity and honour (of abducted/sexually violated women) could only be absorbed within the

31 Corea, »How the New Reproductive Technologies Could be Used«, op. cit. (note 30).

32 Bharadwaj, »Conceptions«, op. cit. (note 3).

33 Usha Rengachary Smerdon, »Crossing Bodies, Crossing Borders: International Surrogacy between the United States and India«, in: *Cumberland Law Review* 39 (2009), 1, pp. 15–85.

34 Veena Das, *Critical Events: An Anthropological Perspective on Contemporary India* (New Delhi: Oxford University Press, 1999, 3rd edition).

normal structures of family and marriage so long these breaches were subsumed in silence.[35] Das begins her account with the voice of Mitro, a character in Krishna Sobti's novel *Mitro Marjani*. Mitro articulates the strangeness of a world in which the sexual act is seen as a religious deed when a woman is impregnated by her husband and a sin if the man is a stranger.[36] The strangeness of this world lies not so much in the sacred and sinful nature of the impregnation, but rather in Mitro's inability to comprehend why this is indeed the case when in either situation she has no role in consenting to the brutal consummation. The difference between the consecrated »seed« and the sinful »weed« has a long cultural history on the Indian subcontinent.[37] Women are at best seen as »barren« fields incapable of bringing the planted seeds to fruition but by the virility of the seed itself, which is never questioned. In certain communities in India, surplus and dispensable bodies of women range from »barren« bodies conceived as empty vessels incapable of bodying forth life to bodies of widows reduced to a life of »living death.« The normative solutions resorted to in order to contain/discipline such transgressing/unyielding bodies are even more harrowing. An archaeology of these problematic bodies takes us back thousands of years to the customary laws that enjoined women to remain under male control and supervision, ranging from the father to the husband and, eventually, in old age the all-important son.[38] Here we encounter another pattern born within the domain of patriarchal semantics. In parts of north India, the term used to denote a widow and a prostitute remains the same to this day. Like a prostitute, a widow threatens control and ownership entitlements. Condemned to lead an austere life of self-denial and religious contemplation in the memory of a dead husband, young widows are sometimes literally recycled as prostitutes or forced to lead lives punctuated by sexual violence, social exclusion, and

35 Veena Das, »National Honor and Practical Kinship: Unwanted Women and Children«, in: Faye D. Ginsburg & Rayna Rapp (Eds.), *Conceiving the New World Order: The Global Politics of Reproduction* (Berkeley: University of California Press, 1995), p. 215.

36 Das, »National Honor and Practical Kinship«, op. cit. (note 365, p. 212.

37 Leela Dube, »Seed and Earth: The Symbolism of Biological Reproduction and Sexual Relations of Production«, in: Eleanor Leacock & Shirley Ardener (Eds.), *Visibility and Power. Essays on Women in Society and Development* (Delhi: Oxford University Press, 1986).

38 Bharadwaj, »Why Adoption is Not an Option in India«, op. cit. (note 3).

exploitation.[39] The normative and ideological reception and understanding of surrogacy arrangements in India exhibits a similarly fractal pattern, and the story of Nirmala is a good example.

On 11 June 1997, long before India gained notoriety as a commercial surrogacy destination, India woke up to a startling piece of news. Nirmala, a 30-year-old woman from Punjab in the north west of India, had decided to rent out her womb for 50,000 rupees to an infertile couple. The media frenzy was unprecedented. Overnight Nirmala became a household name, a woman who was renting out her womb so that she could pay her paralyzed husband's medical bills. What shocked people was not her decision to rent out her womb, but the terms of agreement with the couple – a retired Air Force officer and his wife for whom she worked. Nirmala was to have sexual intercourse with the husband, conceive a child, and, after it was born, hand over legal rights to the couple. The fear of being prosecuted under the Suppression of Immoral Traffic Act forced Nirmala to turn to the legal system to legitimize and recognize her right to rent out her womb. The sub-judge in Chandigarh, the capital of Punjab state, issued requests to the government of India and the union territory administration to decide if the renting of Nirmala's womb was legal and constitutional. Her lawyer, in turn, openly declared that because she was a Hindu, he would seek sanctions from the scriptures for her stance and called for testimonies from religious leaders like the four *Sankaracharyas* and the *Arya Samaj* on whether a woman could become a surrogate mother. Nirmala's ability to use an instrument of the state – the legal system – to assert her »cultural rights« as a Hindu by drawing on a shared cultural memory (*niyoga:* an ancient practice of surrogacy/levirate) to challenge her potential criminalisation under the law exposed yet another instance of »creative tensions« underlying the relations between individuals, communities, and the state in contemporary India.[40]

---

39 For more on the status of widows in India see Martha Alter Chen (Ed.), *Widows in India: Social Neglect and Public Action* (Delhi: Sage, 1998); P. Adinarayana Reddy, *Problems of Widows in India* (New Delhi: Sarup and Sons, 2004).

40 Das, »Critical Events«, op. cit. (note 34). Veena Das has shown that the relations between the state and (religious) communities in India are fraught with creative tensions on the issue of cultural rights. She draws on the case of a divorced Muslim woman – Shah Bano – who appealed for maintenance under section 125 of the code of criminal procedure in India, and how the involvement of the state came into conflict with the

The past invoked by Nirmala's defense by alluding to the practice of *niyoga* provides extremely fractured evidence, even in the realm of myth. Surrogacy in the Hindu worldview was never a preferred solution for female infertility (the patriarchal order had simpler solutions such as abandoning the »barren« waste), but was rather a cultural accommodation of an absence of male seed. Like intracytoplasmic sperm injection or ICSI, *niyoga* was a technology applied to the fertile body of a woman to treat male infertility. How common it was as a historical practice is unclear, but there is growing anecdotal evidence of its practice to this day as a means of bypassing infertility within the private realm of the family. In counter distinction to the historical practice of *niyoga* informal surrogacy arrangements between sisters or sisters-in-law within a family are reportedly quite common in India. A woman either conceives a child with her partner for an infertile sister to adopt, or, more recently, women have resorted to Intrauterine Insemination (IUI) or IVF using their brother-in-law's semen to conceive a child for an infertile sister. In the summer of 2005 I met a 24-year-old pregnant woman who had undergone an IUI using her father-in-law's semen. The fertility expert at the Delhi clinic where I encountered the pregnant daughter-in-law and donor father-in-law »couple« told me how very common this was, particularly in the Jat community in the neighboring state of Haryana. Insemination or donor IVF allowed them to practice the ancient custom of levirate. Unlike Nirmala, sexual intercourse in the present-day variant of »Jat levirate« was substituted by intercourse of a clinical kind. While Indian media is replete with reports

---

Muslim community and the assertion of cultural rights to practice its personal law. The second case she examines is that of a Hindu woman – Roop Kanwar – who in 1987 was forced to ascend the funeral pyre of her husband to commit *sati*. The state intervention was met with resistance from a section of the Rajput community asserting the cultural right to practice its religious customs. In both cases, the breakdown of the private and public distinction is crucial to the way communities asserted their »rights« as lying separate (and hence private) from the public domain occupied by the state. The definition of the community itself in both these cases came to centre around the »organization of memory« (especially the glorification of *sati* in a mythic/historical mode), thus memory becomes, as Das puts it, »both an archive and a history« (p 115). The Nirmala case is an interesting site to witness how reference to a »cultural memory« (*niyoga*) recreates tensions between Hindu ideals of procreation as sacred and confined to the institution of marriage and its commercialization that Nirmala is seeking to legitimize by turning to the institutions of the state.

of surrogacy arrangements, Nirmala's case stands out as unusual due to its non-clinical nature. To drive this point home, the media accounts drew on popular culture by establishing parallels between the Nirmala story and a film, *Doosri Dulhan* (The Other Bride, released in 1983), based on a true story of a couple in the Dadar Hindu Colony in Mumbai who paid their maid to bear them a child. In the film, however, the couple hires the services of a prostitute who is impregnated by the man, resulting in further emotional complications. Similarly, in 2000 another »Bollywood« film, *Chori Chori Chupke Chupke* (Secretly and Quietly), addressed the same theme. The protagonists – a married couple – hire the services of a prostitute to conceive through sexual intercourse. The reference to prostitutes in these films is interesting, as it likens such surrogacy arrangements to prostitution, a link that Nirmala sought to challenge. The interference patterns these diffracted dimensions produce bring into view the lives and bodies of women – both normatively compliant and transgressive – within the highly charged ideological zone of sexuality, reproduction, and control. In this zone the hierarchy and distinction between the Madonna and the Whore is continuously under threat. The Whore in this worldview epitomizes the absence of male control; she represents the market and invades the Habermasian (1989) »male public sphere«[41] with impunity.[42] Diffracted interference patterns of the Madonna and the Whore leave the attendant binaries of control and its absence, public and private, fertile and »barren« similarly compromised. Both prostitutes as surrogate wombs as depicted in popular culture and Nirmala's subjugated subject position challenging such cultural conflations engender tensions that challenge not only the patriarchal sense of control, but also force the use of one's pauper body and fertility as the »commodity of last resort.«[43] There are other subject positions to be considered here, such as the fertile young brides inseminated by their infertile husband's brothers and fathers or the emas-

41 Jürgen Habermas, *The Structural Transformation of the Public Sphere: An Inquiry into a Category of Bourgeois Society* (Cambridge, MA: MIT Press, 1989).

42 Cf. Seyla Benhabib, »The Pariah and Her Shadow: Hannah Arendt's Biography of Rahel Varnhagen«, in: *Political Theory* 23 (1995), 1, pp. 5–24; Nancy Fraser, »Rethinking the Public Sphere: A Contribution to the Critique of Actually Existing Democracy«, in: Craig Calhoun (Ed.), *Habermas and the Public Sphere* (Cambridge: MIT Press, 1992), pp.109–142.

43 Scheper-Hughes, »The Ends of the Body«, op. cit. (note 9).

culated existences of such infertile men. As one clinician told me: »People bring family, the father of the [infertile] man, brother of the man. I don't know how it affects their personal life!«

Marica Inhorn (1996) in her book *Infertility and Patriarchy* reminded us of the »classic patriarchy« model, where within the context of patrilineal, patrilocally extended households the senior male has authority over everyone else, including younger men.[44] Historically, the practice of *niyoga* or levirate was a way of bypassing an absence of male seed, sometimes on account of infertility but mostly in cases of death. In the context of a brother-in-law, this either meant a privileged sexual access or an obligation to marry a widowed sister-in-law. In using a sibling's semen for IVF or indeed the semen of the patriarch himself (as in the example above), the family members of an infertile man literally acknowledge his socio-genetic death in the age of high-tech conception.

Surrogate women in India often voice their concern about the social and media conflation of prostitution and surrogacy.[45] Perhaps this anxiety emerges from within this broader cultural pattern that views weak or absent male supervision as the reason for illicit and unauthorized pregnancies. The protestations and theodicies of these women, who hold up the scientific and clinical modality of their conception as proof of purity, are yet another kind of substitution, one between the phallus and the surgical syringe (most graphic and noteworthy in ICSI procedures). However, these attempts fail not because these women cannot disprove that surrogacy has nothing to do with prostitution, but rather because their substitution places them in the space occupied by similar subaltern subjects, some of whom are indeed prostitutes. The pollution, stigma, dirt, and aspersion of illegitimate sexuality are not the delegitimating causes in themselves: it is the very process of supplementation itself, the process of becoming the »other mother.«

---

44 Marcia C. Inhorn, Infertility and Patriarchy: *The Cultural Politics of Gender and Family Life in Egypt* (Philadelphia: University of Pennsylvania Press, 1996).

45 Pande, »Commercial Surrogacy in India«, op. cit. (note 4).

The State: Absent, Spectral, Surrogate?

What role has the Indian state played in the rise of transnational surrogacy in India? I wish to ask: Is the state absent or surrogate?

Cohen (2004) argues that to be »supplementable is to be able to receive a gift from the sovereign state in the form of another's body.«[46] Cohen's work describes in vivid detail how citizenship in India is (re)made through the trope of surgical interventions. The gift from the state in the quote above is a mythic gift. This present from the state is predicated on the creation and harnessing of diverse populations on the margins of society: populations imagined as endowed with passions but not reason. The supplementability becomes the price of citizenship itself, where by renouncing a part of one's body a redemptive, modern, and ethical contract with the state is forged. These imaginary subject citizens are supplementary in the state's calculations, their supplementary bodies in effect become their savior. Commenting on organ transactions, Cohen observes:

»The bureaucrat-physician [an extension/representation of the state itself] identifies with the buyer's need and alternatively ignores the seller or – particularly if the seller is female – imagines the sale of an organ as the minor exception preventing her from the more traumatic violation of prostitution. Again and again, nephrologists on and off the committee suggested that if people were not allowed to sell their kidneys, they would have to sell their entire bodies.«[47]

Surrogates are captured in the slightly different supplementary logic of the »neoliberal calculus of the Indian state.«[48] Whereas a surrogate is purchased for the contracted period of time, more than her womb is owned for the contracted period. Pande's study of Surrogate women in Anand, Gujarat shows that women's labor becomes an exploitable resource, the creation of the perfect mother-worker, and her autonomy and control over her body are selectively suspended for the duration of the contract.[49] She, the substitute, is now continuously enjoined to eat, take medication, and

46 Lawrence Cohen, »Operability: Surgery at the Margin of the State«, in: Veena Das & Deborah Poole (Eds.), *Anthropology in the Margins of the State* (Santa Fe: School of American Research Press, 2004), pp. 165–190, in particular p. 167.

47 Cohen, »Operability«, op. cit. (note 46).

48 Bharadwaj, »Assisted Life«, op. cit. (note 11).

49 Pande, »Commercial Surrogacy in India«, op. cit. (note 4); see also Vora, »Indian Transnational Surrogacy«, op. cit. (note 4).

sleep whilst confined to the surrogate hostel, a holding facility that oversees and surveys surrogate pregnancies and (in)valuable gestating life. The prevailing legal vacuum in India renders the whole process restricted to the private commercial sphere, where the surrogate workers are not so much enveloped in an ethic of care but rather caught up in concerns dictated by commercial profit and enterprise.

Guidelines such as the Indian Council of Medical Research's (ICMR) guidelines on surrogacy and assisted conception technologies demand, perhaps necessitate interpretation. Even the proposed law, as and when rendered enforceable, would inevitably fall in this gray zone of legal interpretation.[50] For instance, Sunder Rajan has shown how clinical trials in India are not conducted in the absence of ethical framing but rather in a space of »hyperethicality,« where trials are tightly regulated under some of the strictest clinical trial laws in the world.[51] The structural violence in this scenario is not embedded in the realm of a lack of regulation, enforcement, or oversight, but rather in the ethically informed and »merely risked subjects« partaking in a gold-standard, clinical-research-organisation-sponsored (CRO), ethically monitored and legally supervised clinical trial.[52] Such displacing effects of legal oversight render the intention of the state open-ended and supplemental. The state in this respect is either rendered absent, silent, or comes to enunciate through surrogate organs, constituents, and intermediaries. The state, in the words of Veena Das (2004), comes to have a »spectral presence.«[53] Through the disciplinary modality of guidelines, for instance, the state ensures the optimal utilisation and harnessing of the reproductive vitality of the surrogate wombs. Clinical mediations, brokers, semen banks, law firms, and middlemen all begin to have a supplementing effect as the state

50 ICMR, *The Assisted Reproduction Technologies (Regulation) Rules* (India: The Ministry of Health and Family Welfare, 2010).

51 Kaushik Sunder Rajan, »Biocapital as an Emergent Form of Life: Speculations on the Figure of the Experimental Subject«, in: Sahra Gibbon & Carlos Novas (Eds.), *Biosocialities, Genetics and the Social Sciences: Making Biologies and Identities* (London: Routledge, 2008), pp. 157–187, in particular p. 179.

52 See also Kaushik Sunder Rajan, »Experimental Values: Indian Clinical Trials and Surplus Health«, in: *New Left Review* 45 (2007), pp. 67–88.

53 Veena Das, »The Signature of the State: The Paradox of Illegibility«, in: Veena Das & Deborah Poole (Eds.), *Anthropology in the Margins of the State* (Santa Fe: School of American Research Press, 2004), pp. 225–278.

further withdraws from regulating, controlling, and morally defining the contours of commercial exploitation of its citizens. The discursive mediation facilitated by physicians, law firms, and semen banks through tropes and incantations of »the ethical« »legal contract« and the »invocation and interpretation of ICMR guidelines« further evokes the »spectral presence of the state.«[54] The visible presence of the physician or lawyer is not so much one that can be relegated to the register of a middleman/broker between commissioning couples and supplementary wombs, but rather he is the mediator between the state and the local and global citizens. In so doing, the clinical space, for example, the purveyor and surveyor of the »surrogate hostels« that Pande describes in her research, becomes a substitute of the state by taking over the function of defining, interpreting, and enforcing surrogacy contracts: a veritable state of the surrogate state.

The recent ICMR ART draft regulation bill (2010) proposes setting up ART banks registered as an independent entity under the provisions of the proposed Act. The bank is enjoined to source, store, handle, and keep records for gametes, embryos, and surrogates. All screening and provision responsibilities for the above entities would remain with the banks, which would operate independently of any ART clinic in the country. All ART-banks should have »standard, scientifically established facilities and defined standard operating procedure for all its scientific and technical activities.«[55] *Surrogate banks* will be solely responsible for advertising, procuring, and supplying surrogates to clinics and their clients. The provision of such a facility displaces the *surrogate hostel* with a *surrogate bank*, a veritable mirror-opposite *holding space* for supplementary wombs. The bank, privately set up under the provisions of the Act, would be delegated to supplement the clinic as the site of optimal control, circulation, and accumulation of reproductive tissues and *bankable* supplementary wombs. This state of the surrogate state becomes possible in precisely such contexts where »the state becomes illegible.«[56] The readability of its rules and regulations becomes open to interpretation as they diffuse further through surrogate intermediaries, organs, and institutions. Inevitably oscillation between the state and surrogate state becomes the defining feature.

54 Das, »The Signature of the State«, op. cit. (note 54), p. 234.

55 ICMR, »ART Regulation Rules«, op. cit. (note 51), pp. 20–21.

56 Das, »The Signature of the State«, op. cit. (note 54).

Addendum

It is doubtful that an account of India's ongoing tryst with technologies of procreation and transnational fertility travels in search of gametes, wombs, and technicians delivering conception and gestation at a fraction of the global prices in a highly stratified, competitive, and buoyant global market will ever be possible. The problem is both one of scale and limit to what ethnographic production can achieve in a rapidly globalising market. Herein lie the true implications for knowledge production and political activism. How do we critique and resist that which escapes the ethnographic gaze? I have only sketched in broad stokes some crucial issues in need of conceptual and empirical unravelling as well as urgent political mobilization. Several other concerns lie scattered in the transnational terrain of supplementary gestations. The potential for exploitation and coercion by family members, brokers, middlemen and now, increasingly, »ex-surrogates« acting as brokers – alone or sometimes in cahoots with other interested parties – can have a severe impact on women's ability to choose, agree, or challenge the terms of gestational agreements. Global media reports on »surrogacy in India« (currently a staggering 134,000 returns on Google's search engine alone) often narrate accounts of financial hardships, of women stepping in to pay off familial debt or to bail out their husbands' bad debts or investments. Just how such a state of social, familial, and financial depredation can become the basis for a liberal contract with the neoliberal state under the sign of informed choice and consent continues to remain both deeply problematic and untenable.

Elsewhere I have shown that a »moral economy« is on the ascent in India.[57] I argued that the unprecedented ethical quagmire created by emerging life forms under the neoliberal formation also creates states of exception where capital, profit, accumulation, production, consumption, and circulation by (market-dictated) necessity become aligned to local/global ethical and moral registers.[58] The search for ethical and moral standards is in turn inextricably linked to the creation of standardized

57 Bharadwaj, »Assisted Life«, op. cit. (note 11); Edward P. Thompson, »The Moral Economy of the English Crowd in the Eighteenth Century«, in: *Past and Present* 50 (1971), pp. 76–136.

58 Bharadwaj, »Assisted Life«, op. cit. (note 11), p. 242.

research, assembly and production protocols, routinized manufacturing practices, the purchase and procurement of raw materials, and the expertise contained in standardized supply chains around the globe. Although research practices, manufacturing processes, labor markets, quality controls, and moral, ethical, and governance protocols are mobilized to create a standardized entity (e.g., a human embryo, surrogate womb, stem-cell line, or a pair of shoes!), political formations and businesses are seldom able to achieve the »ethical end products« without invoking states of exception. This neoliberal condition I described as a *moral economy*. That is, a moral economy allows us to witness what kinds of regimes of exploitation, tropes, and technologies of obfuscation and processes of unproblematic, guilt-free consumption are facilitated if one literalizes the »moral« in the economic calculation of new invention, experimentation, and globalization. For the moral economy to flourish, the state of exception must either remain systematically misrecognized or become a feature of the autonomous, rational, informed, and freethinking ideological calculus of neoliberal citizenship.[59] Thus argued, the Indian state can recycle the pauper bodies of its many millions of citizens and reinvest the »reproductive viability« of its formerly going-to-waste citizens in the service of a booming *neo India*.[60]

The enactment of laws in India to control surrogacy would only have a displacing effect. As argued earlier, under the new proposed ICMR-sponsored law, surrogate women would find themselves removed from the clinical context and »held,« surveyed, and supplied through dedicated holding facilities that have legal recognition. This legal oversight renders moral and ethical any procurement of supplementary wombs alienated from the real person and her biological and social experience of pregnancy. Whilst the focus stays on the gestating life in the supplementary womb, the legal control remains on the entire body held under contract for the duration of the pregnancy. The structural violence and material circumstances, not to mention a woman's ever-depleting agency and control on her circumstances for the duration of the contract, remain in a state of

59 Bharadwaj, »Assisted Life«, op. cit. (note 11), p. 242–244.

60 Cf. Aditya Bharadwaj, »Reproductive Viability and the State: Embryonic Stem Cells in India«, in: Carole Browner & Carolyn Sargent (Eds.): *Reproduction, Globalization and the State* (Durham, NC: Duke University Press, 2010), pp. 113–125.

exception. The body of the supplement can now be imagined as relocated and held in a private bank. These new facilities or surrogate organs of the state under the proposed new law curiously perform the necessary work of making the entire process legal, moral, and ethical. The legal context bestows and restores much more than commercial gestation, as now supplementary wombs become legally accessible and guilt-free. The moral »taint of commerce«[61] is removed in and through the fine print of the neoliberal, legally enforceable contract, and the very modality of *stratified reproduction* – via the supplementing detour – is thereby misrecognized.

The margins of the state in India appear frayed and illegible. At these margins the state is made and unmade, added to and withdrawn from, or, as Derrida would remind us, forged in a relationship between the complement and supplement. In this analysis there are two key entities in the transnational topography of fertility travels: The *Indian State* and the *Other Mother.* The two are hugely different in scale, power, agency, and ability. Nevertheless, the surrogate state and supplementary wombs curiously underscore the everyday, mundane generation of gestating life in a state of moral, ethical, and legal exception.

61 Eric Hirsch, »Negotiated Limits: Interviews in South-East England«, in: Jeanette Edwards, Sarah Franklin, Frances Price & Marilyn Strathern (Eds.), *Technologies of Procreation: Kinship in the Age of Assisted Conception* (Manchester: Manchester University Press, 1993), p. 88.

Assisted Reproductive Technologies in Mali: Asymmetries and Frictions

Viola Hörbst

In the francophone West African region, the first baby conceived through in vitro fertilization (IVF) was born in 1998 at the Biasa private clinic in Lome, Togo. In the following decade, clinics in Cameroon, Ivory Coast, and Senegal followed suit. Since 2003 insemination (IUI) and in vitro fertilization (IVF) have also been offered at a private clinic in Bamako, Mali – one of the poorest nations in the world. But assisted reproductive technologies (ARTs) in Mali did not develop in a socio-cultural, biomedical, economical, or political vacuum. Nor did they travel there in an inter- or transnational vacuum: rather they were either pushed or blocked by diverse actors and forces. This article seeks to identify these actors and forces in their local, global, and transnational contexts. How do local handlings of infertility (in socio-cultural, religious, political, and economical terms) affect the use of ARTs in Mali? How do transnational and international ideologies, forces, and actors influence what forms of ARTs are made available (or not) in Bamako?[1] Which dynamics, asymmetries, and frictions do these complexities re-shape or bring about?

To reflect on the complex and dynamic configurations that impact on infertility and ARTs in Mali, I will use the concept of »medicoscapes«[2] to

1 Following Steven Vertovec, the term *international* in this article is used to refer to interactions between national governments or to aspects of different nations' policies. The term *transnational* is instead applied to »linkages and ongoing exchanges among non-state actors based across national borders – business, non-government-organisations, and individuals sharing the same interests.« Steven Vertovec, *Transnationalism* (London: Routledge, 2009), p. 3.

2 Viola Hörbst & Angelika Wolf, »Globalisierung der Heilkunde: Eine Einführung«, in: *Medizin und Globalisierung. Universelle Ansprüche – lokale Antworten*, ed. by Angelika Wolf & Viola Hörbst (Münster: LIT, 2003), pp. 3–30, in particular p. 4; Viola Hörbst & Kristine Krause, »›On the move‹ – Die Globalisierungsdebatte in der Medizinethnologie«, in: *Curare* 27 (2004), 1+2, p. 55; at the conference *IVF as a Global Form*

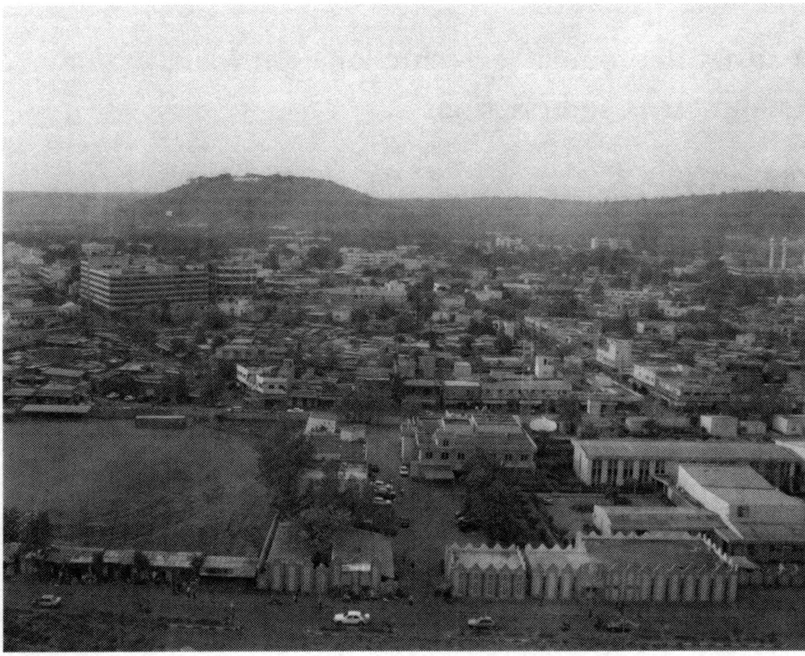

Figure 1: Partial view of Bamako, Mali's capital city (March 2007). Photo by Viola Hörbst

depict the entanglement of various unequal actors in health-related fields. Inspired by Arjun Appadurai, the metaphor of medicoscapes connects heterogeneous actors related to health care (such as individuals, states, transnational institutions), diseases, treatment practices, and things that are present in different localities. The metaphor of medicoscapes thus links spatially distant localities as well as the different perspectives, activities, knowledge regimes, ideas, ideologies, and interests related to the actors and breaks down the dichotomy of local and global. Following specific actors' interconnections and power arrangements within medicoscapes al-

that preceded this anthology, various participants drew on the Appaduraian concept to grasp the global entanglements in reproductive spheres. They used similar terms and ideas such as »reproductive scapes« (Sven Bergmann), »transnational scapes of reproductive technologies« (Stefan Beck, Maren Klotz, Michi Knecht), or »reproscapes« (Marcia C. Inhorn).

lows to pin down aspects of global medical transnationalization and their entanglements with infertility and ARTs in Mali.[3]

Based on these thoughts, I will explore ARTs in Mali within a broad netting of social orders and regimes, where different actors, ideologies, practices, and interests intersect and interact on several levels. These relationships necessarily display asymmetries and »frictions,« which Anna Lowenhaupt Tsing defines as »… the awkward, unequal, unstable, and creative qualities of interconnection across difference.«[4] The first section of this article[5] will reflect on how fieldwork with patients and experts in a transnational context can influence the anthropological role and the ethnographic production of knowledge. Based on the fact that global forces only become tangible in localities,[6] I will then describe a Malian gynecologist's efforts to locally provide ARTs. This is put into the context of the Malian policy on infertility and its entanglement with transnational and international ideologies of the (health-related) development arena. These views will then be contrasted with the value of making children in Bamako before focusing on gender-specific perspectives in the local handling of infertility. Referring to the experience and prospects of three couples suffering from infertility (Kadidya and Tomas, Ndeye and Abdou, Fanta and Amadou), I describe how they ponder the locally available technical and social solutions to their reproductive aims and how gendered asymmetries are deepened and new conflicts arise. After this patient-centered passage I return to the gynecologist, now focusing on his experiences with the process of establishing treatments with ARTs, the resulting appropriations of its use, and how these are influenced in the doctor's contention with local, international, and transnational dynamics. The article closes with a final synopsis of the different perspectives, layers, and levels of frictions and asymmetries that have been explored.

3 Hörbst & Krause, »›On the move‹«, op. cit. (note 2), in particular p. 59; see also Viola Hörbst, Kristine Krause & Angelika Wolf, »On the move – Medical Anthropology, Transnationalism and Mobility«, paper presented at the V. Nordic Conference in Medical Anthropology, *Medical Anthropology in the 21*st *Century: Scope, Theory and Practice,* 2007.

4 Anna Lowenhaupt Tsing, *Frictions. An Ethnography of Global Connection* (Princeton, MA: Princeton University Press, 2005), in particular p. 4.

5 I want to thank Babette Mueller-Rockstroh, Angelika Wolf and the editors, in particular Michi Knecht, for their inspiring comments on former versions of this article.

6 Lowenhaupt Tsing, »Frictions«, op. cit. (note 4), in particular p. 1.

Fieldwork with Transnational Experts and Patients

In this article I draw on data resulting from long-term fieldwork on infertility and ARTs done from 2004 to 2008 mainly in Bamako, Mali.[7] To grasp the processual character of experiences with ART treatments, I worked with a relatively small sample (15 individuals and 7 couples). I conducted repeated (in)formal interviews with most of them, visited them at their homes, and accompanied their search for a solution for several years. With socially devastating topics such as infertility, trust and discretion are of enormous importance, and regularly returning to the field facilitated my relations with patients and doctors. In time, the long-term perspective of the research also led to the narration of more profound and ambivalent aspects of fertility treatments. Different moods and happy or negative events determine how experiences, feelings, and plans are differently evaluated and communicated at different stages of the search for a solution, which may last for several years.

Only a few patients from less affluent milieus initially mistook my research as a support project from an NGO and hoped to gain access to treatment that they could not otherwise afford. They, as well as the majority of patients who could loosely be associated with the middle and lower upper class talked with me rather openly. They seemed to take me as a neutral person within the highly complex Malian social order with whom they could share secrets, facts, and feelings without jeopardizing their social standing. They also used me as a counselor and mediator of information on ARTs and for psychological support, as well as for support on decisions and contacts when planning to go overseas for treatment. Two of them even visited me in Germany.

7 The field research in 2004 and 2005 was financed by a scholarship from the women's representative at the Ludwig-Maximilian University of Munich within the framework of the *University and Science Program (Hochschul- und Wissenschaftsprogramm)* and completed by a donation from the *Friends of the Ludwig-Maximilian-University of Munich (Freunde der LMU München).* The research from 2006 to 2008 was financed by the German Research Foundation (DFG). I am most grateful to these three institutions. Moreover, I want to especially thank those people who worked for me during these research periods. I am also most indebted to all women, men, institutions, and practitioners with whom I worked during my research in Bamako and Lomé. With respect for their privacy, personal names in this article have been changed.

My experience with gynecological *experts* in Mali was fairly similar: They allowed me open access to their consultations and interventions concerning fertility treatments in their clinics. By giving me a lab coat they integrated me into the experts' side, and, over time, started to increasingly discuss patients' cases with me. They also facilitated the recruitment of patients for my research, for which I am very grateful to them.

Concerned as they were about issues of confidentiality, patient interests, and their own reputation, doctors to some extent used their gatekeeping position to pre-select which patients talked to me and which opinions were communicated. They mostly proposed patients who held fairly liberal views, and most of them had also had some transnational experience. Patients from less educated or very religious milieus were kept away from me and so were, to some extent, patients undergoing IVF with donor ova.[8]

To some extent these constraints were balanced by my work with couples thinking about treatment with ART whom I met by coincidence, through my own social network in Bamako or through the small Malian community in Munich. Moreover, cross-checking information with (focus-group) interviews with non-afflicted persons from different backgrounds (such as social science students, medical students organized within a fundamentalist Islamic organization, women's and men's neighborhood networks, as well as religious stakeholders, members of the ethics council, and members of the ministry of health) further broadened my information base.

While in a research cooperation informants often ask for reciprocity and mutual profit in the forms of gifts or payments, neither patients nor practitioners (mostly from the middle or upper class) in Mali asked for a financial contribution. Reciprocity took place by providing access to information and connections to relevant fields. For instance, my chief expert informant Dr M made it clear in our very first meeting that he was not interested in money but in contacts. As I had done a one-week field internship at one of Munich's fertility clinics before going to Mali, I offered

8 For the dynamics of channeling research by biomedical practitioners see also Marcia C. Inhorn, »Privacy, Privatization, and the Politics of Patronage: Ethnographic Challenges to Penetrating the Secret World of Middle Eastern, Hospital-Based In Vitro Fertilization«, in: *Social Science and Medicine* 59 (2004), pp. 2095–2108.

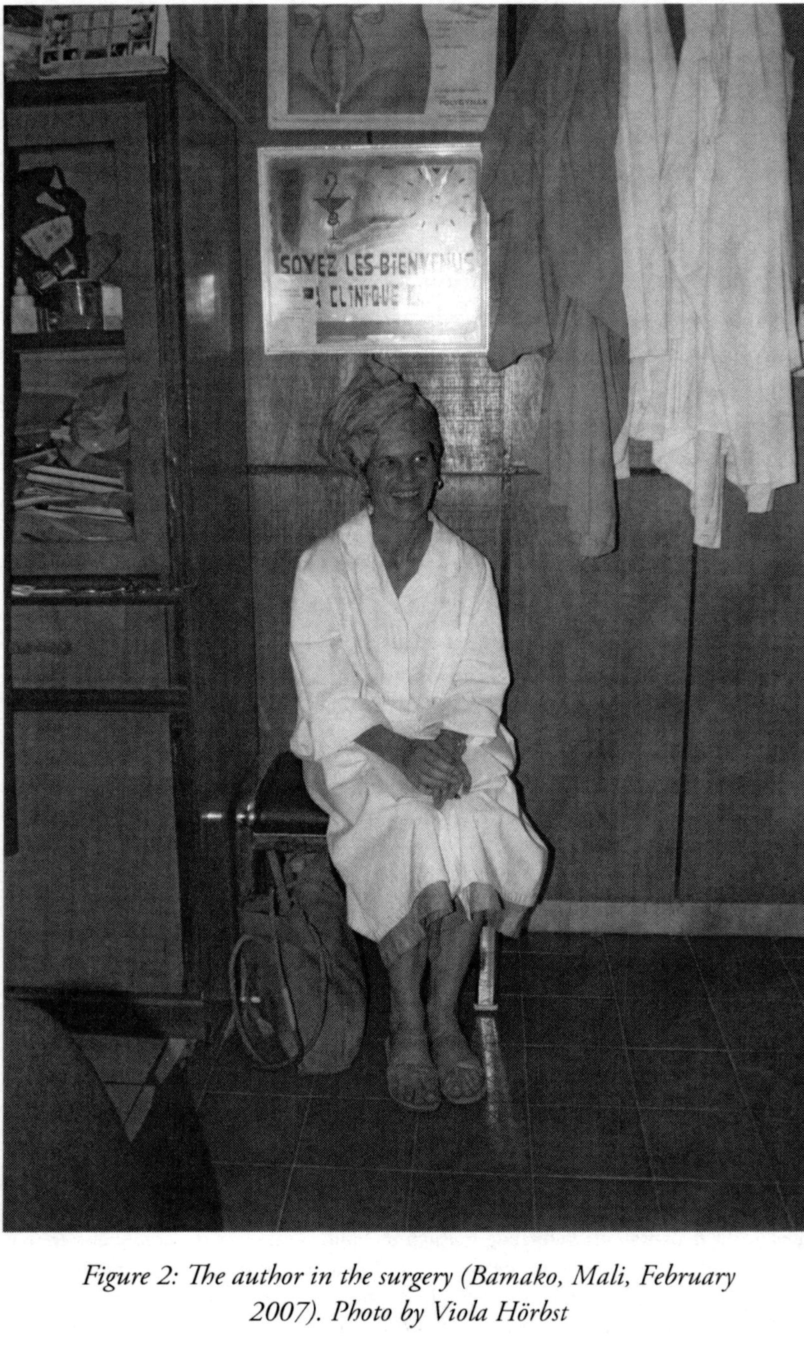

Figure 2: The author in the surgery (Bamako, Mali, February 2007). Photo by Viola Hörbst

to arrange an internship for him and his biologist there – which they carried out in 2005. Particularly Dr M, but also some patients integrated me into their transnational networks as a mediator of connections and a supporter of their different aims and the introduction of ARTs in Mali. Some of the persons participating in my research also asked me to create a developmental project with an NGO to support infertile couples.

Anthropology is one of the transnationally mobile careers par excellence. When anthropologists do research with equally transnationally mobile experts and patients, who can afford to travel to Germany for treatment, for training, and for buying lab devices, borders between the anthropological »here« and »there« get blurred. The anthropological field can no longer be neatly separated from the daily life of the anthropologist. This situation renders anthropologists more likely to become involved as transnational brokers, helping to overcome the many barriers for experts and patients in the South trying to get access to ARTs. In this way the borders between research and active engagement are also blurred. This again is related to the fact that all information and data received in fieldwork are bound to personal contacts and based on mutual confidence, which is essential for continuing research. Moreover, patients and particularly biomedical experts mobile in transnational fields are highly aware of transnational differences and asymmetries, such as the fact that they often only have access to inferior technological devices. Many of them are very familiar with the ideals and interests of donors in development aid arenas, and know how to mirror and emphasize an image of themselves that accords with these aims. It also becomes very complicated and expensive for researchers to follow mobile informants to other places and experience and observe them as they switch between transnational fields in order to analyze their various frames of reference. In such an entanglement, a critical gaze on transnational biomedical practices and biomedical practitioners from West Africa remains to some extent incomplete and complicated. Furthermore, this transnational mobility of both researcher and researched experts and informants gives rise to ethical questions of how to handle the information collected from people in the field and the analysis of biomedical practitioners and practices. What, for example, should be withheld from publication in order to protect informant gynecologists from conflicts with models of »best practice«

in biomedicine (bound to specific localities) or with the convictions of religious stakeholders influential in their contexts of origin. These are all problematic points without any patent remedy at hand.

ARTs in a Private Clinic in Bamako: Transnational Linkages and Material Asymmetries

One of the main biomedical actors concerning ARTs in Mali is Dr M, whom I first met in his private clinic in December 2004. Dr M studied gynecology and obstetrics in Kiev with a grant from the Malian state. When he returned to Mali, he worked at a public hospital for one year before starting a small gynecological practice in 1993. Since then he has worked exclusively in the private sector. In 1998 he moved to his present location, situated in a rapidly expanding business area of Bamako. Medical doctors employed in his clinic offer services in general medicine, cardiology, urology, pediatrics, and general surgery. A medical laboratory with five lab assistants, headed by a Malian biologist who studied in Belgrade, also belongs to the clinic. Dr M himself is specialized in fertility treatments but also provides other services in gynecology and obstetrics.

In 2002 Dr M started to establish ARTs in Mali, due to what he anticipated would be a high demand for fertility treatments: according to Dr M, more than 60% of his consultations focus on unwanted childlessness, out of which, he assumes, one or two couples per week are in need of ART treatments. Until recently, he referred them to European clinics (mostly in France, Germany, and Austria) or to francophone African clinics (in Senegal, Cameroon, or Togo). But, as Dr M explained to me:

»More and more there are barriers between the West and the East, between the North and the South. There is the problem of getting a visa, and people are obliged to undergo treatment in their own countries. Thus it is necessary that the technology arrives here, this will facilitate things. The money you spend for a return ticket, the expenses for the hotel – you can invest this capital into treatment. For one single journey you can buy three attempts here [in Bamako], if my calculation is right. People are spending five to six million FCFA [around 7500 to 9000 euros] to go away and make one attempt. Well, with one and a half mil-

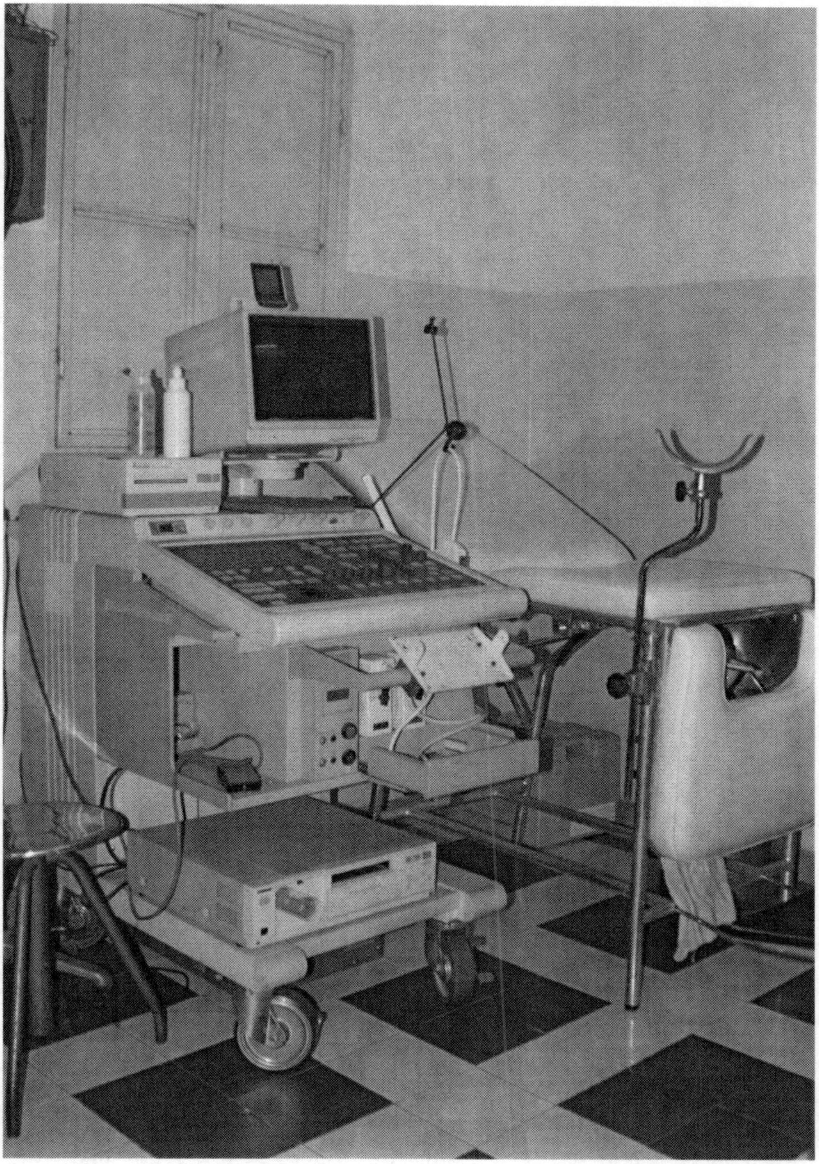

Figure 3: Ultrasound scanner and gynecological table in the practice (Bamako, Mali, January 2005). Photo by Viola Hörbst

lion FCFA [fees and medicine included; roughly 2200 euros] one can make an attempt here. This is what people have to be made to understand.«

Whereas mobility is usually emphasized in globalization processes, Dr M referred to political forces that increasingly force immobility upon Malians. He explained that this dynamic is a reason why sophisticated and cost-intensive technologies consistent with current international standards should be provided in Bamako. Dr M also stated that he was not yet breaking even in his ART venture, but he calculated that his investments would pay back in the future: providing ARTs in Bamako at a lower cost than in Europe would attract Malian elites, who still sought such treatment predominantly in Europe. It would also enlarge his spectrum of clients, as Malians who could not afford the travel expenses and higher costs of treatments outside Mali might be able to finance the lower costs of ARTs in Bamako.

Dr M has only been able to organize access to medical technological know-how and skills as well as technological and pharmaceutical equipment via his transnational connections. Dr M and his biologist arranged an internship training in Canada (2002) and two in France (2003, 2004), both of which were mediated by a Togolese colleague. Additionally, the lab assistants locally received special training. In 2003, Dr M created a »unit for ART« in his clinic by dedicating one room (including a bathroom) to these activities. The room is equipped with a gynecological table, an ultrasound scanner, an incubator, a centrifuge, two microscopes, a heating plate, and a monitor linked by a video camera to the microscope.

Because of his limited budget, Dr M had to purchase all devices second hand – partially from a retiring French gynecologist whom Dr M met by coincidence at a conference, and partially from different wholesale distributors in France and Mali, who specialize in second-hand medical equipment. While reagents for sperm and ovocyte treatments are purchased directly from a Danish producer and sent via airmail to Bamako, Dr M brings some equipment back from his regular visits to conferences, mostly in France, e.g. special needles for punctuation that are offered for free at the conferences by pharmaceutical companies.

As there are no specific laws or regulations on ARTs in Mali to date, the management of ARTs is left up to individual doctors, and Dr M is bound only by his biomedical and moral convictions, his entrepreneurial

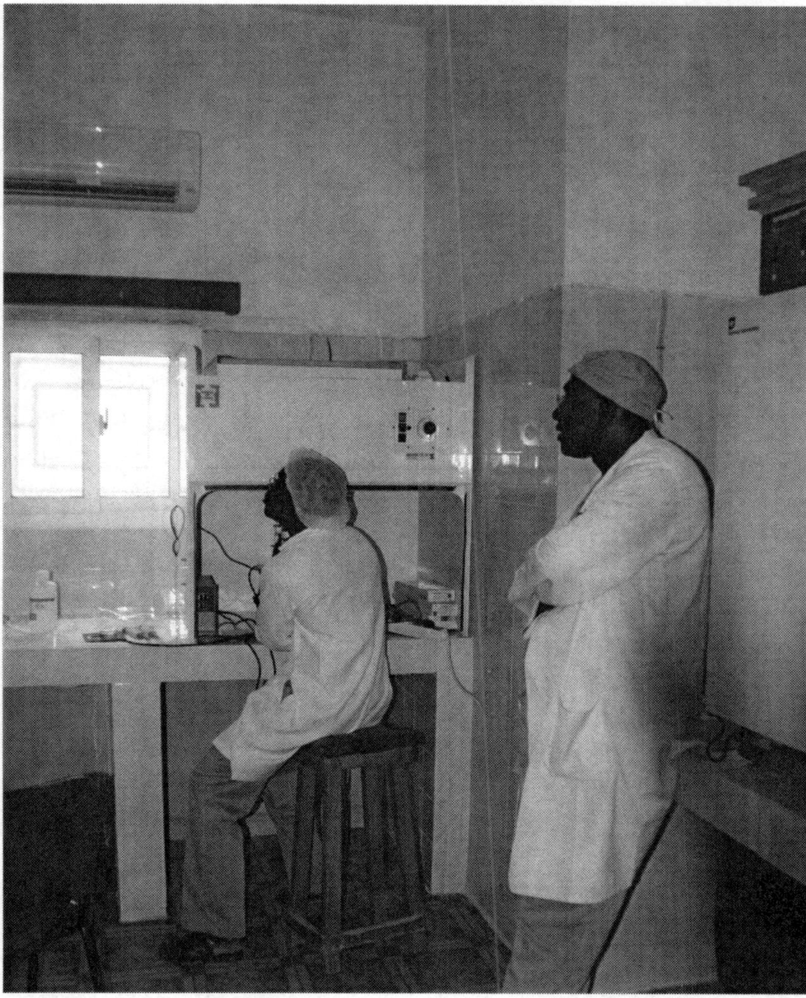

Figure 4: The fertility lab in a private clinic (Bamako, Mali, November 2007). Photo by Viola Hörbst

considerations, and his reputation among his patients. In one of our first conversations in 2005 Dr M told me that he did not aim to realize any form of ARTs with donor sperm or donor ova, as this is considered to be out-of-bounds according to Islamic moral regulations.[9] However, his opinion and practice of this procedure changed during the course of my fieldwork and by 2008 he had started to use donor ova in specific circumstances.

For hormonal stimulation he used various protocols and he transferred up to three fertilized eggs. Not having ICSI at his disposal Dr M. explained that, unlike in Europe, he would also carry out intrauterine insemination (IUI) if one fallopian tube was blocked or in cases of severe oligospermia and specific forms of azoospermia. While both these latter cases, according to him, would be subject to ICSI in Europe, he applied homologous IUI (using the couple's gametes) in such cases after treating the man with hormones (from one up to several months) in order to increase his sperm quality.

Being situated in the private health sector, Dr M receives no support from the Malian state for his ART program. The modest onset of ARTs in Bamako is tied to transnational professional networks where individual support is given through private contacts. However, Dr M's practices of ARTs relied on technical devices that have been purchased second hand, or, in the case of ICSI, were simply not available (see footnote 45). Both aspects also affect how ART treatments are applied and whether they are successful. The access to pharmaceuticals is another issue that shows asymmetrical power relations in the medical field. In order to lower costs, Dr M used to purchase the pharmaceuticals needed for hormonal stimulation in France. By doing so, he circumvented the import taxes, interest rates of Malian pharmacists, and transportation charges that render these goods more expensive in Mali – another fact that underlines asymmetrical economic connections in global medicoscapes.

9 Nominally, 90 percent of Mali's 10.6 million inhabitants consider themselves to be Sunni Muslims, about 9 percent practice African religions and 1 percent belong to the Catholic church, see John L. Exposito, »Mali, Islam in«, in: *Oxford Dictionary of Islam,* ed. by John L. Esposito (Oxford: Oxford University Press, 2004), p. 189.

National and International Fertility Policies: Frictions and Ideological Asymmetries

The prevalence of infertility in Mali is high – currently an estimated 10.4 percent of women suffer from primary infertility and an estimated 23.6 percent from secondary infertility.[10] Although these numbers are problematic, they provide at least an idea of infertility's dimensions in the region.[11] Up-to-date ARTs in many cases represent biomedicine's most adequate treatment of severe oligospermia, azoospermia, or blocked fallopian tubes.[12] However, there is no ART program in the public sector in Mali, although Mali signed the agreements resulting from the International Conference on Population and Development (ICPD) in Cairo in 1994 where reproductive choice was assigned the quality of a human right[13] and the access to adequate treatment was expressed as a major ob-

10 Shea O. Rutstein & Iqbal H. Shah, »Infecundity, Infertility, and Childlessness in Developing Countries. DHS Comparative Reports No. 9«, (Calverton, Maryland: ORC Macro and the World Health Organization, 2004), pp. 15–25. In comparison, 11.3 % is the estimated infertility rate in Europe (Jacky Boivin, Laura Bunting, John A. Collins & Karl G. Nygren, »International estimates of infertility prevalence and treatment-seeking: potential need and demand for infertility medical care«, in: *Human Reproduction* 22 (2007), 6, pp. 1506–1512; in particular p. 1508) and 7,5 % of sterile couples with desire for children are estimated to be infertile in Germany (Wilfried Karmaus & Sven Juul, on behalf of the European Infertility and Subfecundity Study Group, »Infertility and subfecundity in population-based samples from Denmark, Germany, Italy, Poland and Spain«, in: *European Journal of Public Health* 9 (1999),3, pp. 229–235; in particular p. 231. For explanations of higher numbers of infertility in sub-Saharan Africa see Sylvie Schuster & Viola Hörbst, »Introduction«, in: *Reproductive Disruptions: Perspectives on African Contexts, Curare special issue* 29 (2006), 1, ed. by Viola Hörbst & Sylvie Schuster, pp. 5–16, in particular p. 6.

11 For specific discussions on definitions of infertility and resulting effects on estimated rates see Lone Schmidt, *Infertility and Assisted Reproduction in Denmark. Epidemiology and Psychosocial Consequences* (Copenhagen: Laegeforeningens Forlag, 2006), in particular p. 19, 33 et. seq.; Ulla Larsen, »Research on Infertility: Which Definition Should We Use?«, in: *Fertility and Sterility* 83 (2005), pp. 846–852.

12 These afflictions have especially high prevalence in West Africa, see Philippe Mayaud, »The Role of Reproductive Tract Infections«, in: *Women and Infertility in Sub-Saharan Africa: A Multi-Disciplinary Perspective*, ed. by J. Ties Boerma & Zaida Mgalla (Amsterdam: Royal Tropical Institute, 2001), pp. 71–108, in particular pp. 75, 87.

13 Marcia Inhorn & Aditya Bharadwaj, »Reproductively Disabled Lives: Infertility, Stigma, and Suffering in Egypt and India«, in: *Disability in Local and Global Worlds*, ed. by Benedicte Ingstad & Susan Reynolds Whyte (Berkeley: University of California

jective. Malian state activities regarding fertility emphasize the prevention of pregnancy and disease: They inform about the risks of abortion and sexually transmitted diseases (STDs) and the need of biomedical treatment in such cases, and they advocate the use of condoms to prevent STDs.

Neither the general topic of fertility treatments nor ARTs in particular seem to be important issues on the national health policy agenda, as interviews with representatives of the Malian Health Ministry have shown.[14] Although the head of the gynecological ward in one of Bamako's university hospitals has been telling me for more than three years that an ART program with state funding will soon be established, nothing has happened by the time of this article's publication. The director of another public hospital in Bamako explained the non-engagement of the Malian state simply as »a lack of political will.«

However, the lack of governmental commitment to ARTs is not surprising as it is linked to several Malian specificities. With a gross domestic product (GDP) of about 414 euros per capita in 2007,[15] Mali is currently ranked one of the poorest countries in the world.[16] At the same time Mali has an average birth rate of 6.7 children per woman, one of the highest in sub-Saharan Africa.[17] Mali's general health system is in a miserable condition, and has difficulties with providing access to basic health care for its population. The Malian government must manage a highly fertile state with few resources and is dependent on international donors for expenditures in the health sector. Thus it is under pressure to *reduce* fertility rates

Press, 2007), p. 78–106; Abdallah Daar & Zara Merali, »Infertility and Social Suffering: the Case of ART in Developing Countries«, in: *Current Practices and Controversies in Assisted Reproduction. Report of a Meeting on »Medical, Ethical and Social Aspects of Assisted Reproduction« WHO Headquarters, Geneva, Switzerland, 17–21 September 2001*, ed. by Effy Vayena, Patrick J. Rowe & P. David Griffin (Geneva: WHO, 2002), pp. 15–21.

14 See Hamadou Konate, Mamadou Ballo & Yéya Maiga, *Analyse de la situation de la santé de la reproduction au Mali* (Bamako: Ministère de la Santé, 2002).

15 http://www.auswaertiges-amt.de/diplo/de/Laenderinformationen/01-Laender/Mali.html[lastaccessed:10.6.2009].

16 In 2005 Mali was ranked 173 out of 177, see: http://web.worldbank.org/WBSITE/EXTERNAL/COUNTRIES/AFRICAEXT/MALIEXTN/0,,menuPK:362193~pagePK:141132~piPK:141107~theSitePK:362183,00.html[lastaccessed:20.11.2008].

17 http://www.usaid.gov/pubs/cbj2003/afr/ml/[last accessed: 10.9.2009].

and to spend its scarce resources for what in many donor states are seen as more pressing diseases and higher priority problems like HIV/AIDS, malaria, and tuberculosis. International opinions also add to reluctance towards a Malian ART program, even in the private sector. Euro-American institutions seem to regard infertility (in Africa) as an individual problem, a »trivial« condition or even as a »natural« means of countering overpopulation.[18] Moreover, infertility is not a contagious affliction, and although it may lead to severe social suffering it does not lead to biological death.

Consequently, infertility and its treatments are overlooked by national, international, and transnational governmental organizations as well as non-governmental ones (NGOs). This holds as true for Mali as for Africa in general: Although there are a variety of non-governmental organizations in Bamako engaged in several topics (e.g. circumcision, HIV/AIDS, malaria), there is not a single one that is active in the field of infertility providing information and/or funding for fertility treatments or even for ARTs. There are also no self-help groups for Malians suffering from infertility. The president of a Malian NGO explained to me that she sees a pressing need for a project to fight against infertility, but she also asked, »Who in the international donor community would finance such a project?« She therefore thinks it would be an unfeasible aim.

The frictions occurring in the international debate about ART programs in Africa had clearly come to the fore by the beginning of the new century. The World Health Organization (WHO) held a symposium in 2001, where controversial opinions on the feasibility and reasonability of ARTs for sub-Saharan countries were brought forward by international experts – including African ones. Some African physicians and social scientists argued against the introduction of ARTs to sub-Saharan countries,[19] mostly focusing on the overpopulation and scarce financial resources of African states. Several other issues were also addressed: the problem of poorly trained practitioners, the lack of regulatory mechanisms to detect dishonest or incompetent ones, the legal vacuum that opens the door to

18 Marcia Inhorn, »Global Infertility and the Globalization of New Reproductive Technologies: Illustrations from Egypt«, in *Social Science & Medicine* 56 (2003), pp. 1837–1851, in particular p. 1844.

19 Friday Okonofua, »The Case against New Reproductive Technologies in Developing Countries«, in: *British Journal of Obstetrics and Gynaecology* 103 (1996), pp. 957–962; Inhorn, »Global Infertility«, op. cit. (note 18).

the unregulated application and abuse of ARTs,[20] as well as the priority of more pressing health problems (see above).[21] »Traditional social« solutions such as adoption or child-fostering were suggested by social scientist Tangwa as solutions for childless sub-Saharan Africans.[22]

Those who argued in favor of ARTs in sub-Saharan Africa found »governmental support for non-profit organizations« to be vital »in providing affordable access to infertility care,« and called upon state activities to lower the costs of ARTs »by bulk purchase of drugs, consumables and equipment.«[23] Others put emphasis on public-private partnerships to make ART accessible for the majority of the poor in low-resource countries.[24] Where public funding is insufficient,[25] it was recommended that the costs of ARTs be shared »between the countries, private sectors, individuals and international agencies such as WHO, the Rockefeller Foundation, the Ford Foundation, and the Bill Gates Foundation.«[26] Six years later, »progress towards the attainment« of these recommenda-

20 Ruth Macklin, »Reproductive Technologies in Developing Countries«, in: *Bioethics* 9 (1995), 3+4, pp. 276–282; Godfrey Tangwa, »ART and African Sociocultural Practices: Worldview, Belief and Value Systems with Particular Reference to Francophone Africa«, in: Vayena, Rowe & Griffin, »Current Practices and Controversies in Assisted Reproduction«, op. cit. (note 13), pp. 55–59, in particular p. 58.

21 Daar & Merali, »Infertility and Social Suffering«, op. cit. (note 13), in particular p. 15.

22 Tangwa, »ART and African Sociocultural Practices«, op. cit. (note 20), in particular p. 58.

23 Daar & Merali, »Infertility and social suffering«, op. cit. (note 13), in particular p. 20; Friday Okonofua, »New Reproductive Technologies and Infertility Treatment in Africa«, in: *African Journal of Reproductive Health* 7 (2003), 1, pp. 7–8; Osato F. Giwa-Osagie, »ART in Developing Countries with Particular Reference to sub-Saharan Africa«, in: Vayena, Rowe & Griffin, »Current Practices and Controversies in Assisted Reproduction«, op. cit. (note 13), pp. 22–27, in particular p. 26.

24 Daar & Merali, »Infertility and Social Suffering«, op. cit. (note 13), in particular p. 20; cf. Sylvie Schuster & Viola Hörbst, »Introduction«, op. cit. (note 10), p. 8.

25 Vayena, Rowe & Griffin, »Current Practices and Controversies in Assisted Reproduction«, op. cit. (note 13); cf. Willem Ombelet, Ian Cooke, Silke Dyer, Gamal Serour & Paul Devroey, »Infertility and the Provision of Infertility Medical Services in Developing Countries«, in: *Human Reproduction Update* 14 (2008), 6, pp. 1–17, in particular p. 11.

26 Giwa-Osagie, »ART in Developing Countries«, op. cit. (note 23), p. 26.

tions remains slow and the WHO's programs for fertility treatments in developing countries still focus on prevention.[27]

The question of whether or not to support ARTs in developing countries like Mali is shaped by an international atmosphere in which transnational institutions in politics and biomedicine are predominantly ruled by doubts about its adequacy and economical feasibility. Investments in fertility treatments are judged to be less worthy than investments in fighting other diseases that are evaluated as being more disastrous and exigent. As a result, the neglect of the topic of infertility by both international and national policy makers is a daily occurrence in developing countries. Without support from the Malian state or from international state and transnational non-state agencies active in health-related development fields, patients in need of ARTs are left by these actors to gain access to ARTs by their own private means – meaning that most of them are excluded from such a treatment. This situation shapes the operationality of Dr M and his possibilities of locally providing ARTs. Besides using his private capital, he is dependent on individual professional networks to follow his objective of successfully providing ARTs in Bamako.[28]

Local reproductive policies in Mali are thus intimately entwined with transnational and international reproductive governance. They are also linked to the struggle against other diseases. The limited international capital and transnational financial resources for supporting health care in Africa are used to fight other diseases that are given higher priority. Therefore reproductive technologies (like other biomedical areas) cannot be looked upon without regarding their linkage to other diseases, which all are competitive and interactive agents in international ideologies, economic activities, and power arrangements covered by medicoscapes.

27 Ombelet, Cooke, Dyer, Sevour & Devroey, »Infertility and the Provision of Infertility Medical Services«, op. cit. (note 25), p. 11.

28 Viola Hörbst, »IVF in Bamako: Globalizing Technology, Mobile Knowledge, Reinterpreted Practice?«, in: *Transnational Medicine, Mobile Experts: Globalization, Health and Power In And Beyond Africa*, ed. by Hansjörg Dilger, Abdoulaye Kane & Stacey Langwick (Indiana University Press, in press).

Local Reproductive Governance: Gendered Asymmetries

Information on ARTs has already reached many Malians by way of French TV broadcasts on test-tube babies, talks with friends and migrants, or rumors about Malians who are assumed to have undergone treatments. Dr M also disseminates information on ARTs, as do his patients through mouth to mouth propaganda. For Malians who are facing marital childlessness, an assisted reproductive intervention is a tempting option – at least in theory – as it promises to produce the parents' own genetic/biological children.

Not »having children,« but rather »making children« in the sense of bodily producing them is a social necessity in Bamako.[29] As part of the expected Malian biography it is simply taken for granted and no issue to decide about. Apart from their personal desires, for many Malian women producing children represents the fulfillment of a duty towards the extended family of the husband, for children are considered to belong to the father's patrilineage. In mainstream familiar and popular narratives, the wives are made responsible if children fail to appear. In addition to their own disappointment, many childless women are subjected to teasing and provocations by neighbors and their wider social networks, for example at the wedding or baptism ceremonies frequently held in Bamako. Simultaneously, they often encounter insinuating remarks and hurtful insults from their husband's family – as my interview partner Kadidya explains:

»Here, if you are married and you don't manage to have children, the sisters of your husband say: ›Ah, really, we didn't marry you so you could eat like this – you have to make children. We are in need of them, or we will marry a second wife to your husband, one who will have children.‹«[30]

29 See Marcia C. Inhorn & Aditya Bharadwaj, »Reproductively Disabled Lives: Infertility, Stigma and Suffering in Egypt and India«, in: *Disability in Local and Global Worlds*, ed. by Benedicte Ingstad & Susan Reynolds Whyte (Berkeley: University of California Press, 2007), pp. 78–106.

30 It seems a recurrent pattern that in extended families where there are several cases of childless marriages, the degree of stigmatization is less than in families where only one couple is childless. Equally, the duration of childlessness, the living arrangements, and the wife's economic position can be important factors in determining the degree of stigmatization by family members in daily life, how childless women are affected by it, and how they handle the situation. See: Viola Hörbst »Infertility and In Vitro-Fertilization in Bamako, Mali: Women's Experience, Avenues for Solution and Social

I met Kadidya, 31 years old, and her husband Tomas, aged 39, during their consultation at Dr M's clinic in 2007, where Tomas was diagnosed with absolute azoospermia. Tomas, a filmmaker, was brought up in France where his parents and siblings are still living. 8 years ago he decided to go to Mali to start his own business. He met Kadidya and they married at the end of 2005. Together they live in a small villa apart from their extended family. Besides housework, Kadidya is engaged in the informal selling of cloth.

Like Kadidya, many Malian women whose husbands are infertile are continuously stigmatized. Male factor infertility is one of the greatest imaginable causes of shame and disgrace for men. Thus, the mainstream narrative is used to conceal male factor infertility and adverse results are frequently hidden from the family. This was the case with Ndeye and Abdou, whom I met in 2007 in Dr M's practice. Ndeye was 33 years old, had studied computer sciences in France, and held a good job in one of Bamako's banks. Since 2003 she had been married to Abdou, 33, who also worked at a bank. When five months after the wedding ceremonies Ndeye was still not pregnant, she started to consult doctors. Abdou was diagnosed with severe oligospermia and finally Dr M suggested a hormonal treatment for Abdou followed by an IUI. While Abdou did not talk with anyone from his family about his diagnosis, Ndeye informed her mother and her sister. However, she kept Abdou's secret from her husband's extended family, thus protecting him from humiliation.

In contrast, Tomas told his parents in France about his diagnosis. But although he was raised in France and considers himself more Western-oriented, even Tomas has not informed any member of his extended family in Bamako. Kadidya in turn keeps her husband's secret as well.

These two examples from fieldwork show how the local social handling of infertility in Mali is pervaded by patriarchally shaped gender asymmetries that bring about various conflicts.

As biomedicine can also assign the cause of marital childlessness to men, biomedical diagnostics contradicts the gendered popular narrative that mainly blames women for infertility. However, many couples use this mainstream narrative to protect husbands diagnosed with sub- or

Contexts Impacting on Gynaecological Consultations«, in: Hörbst & Schuster, »Reproductive Disruptions«, op. cit. (note 10), in particular p. 39.

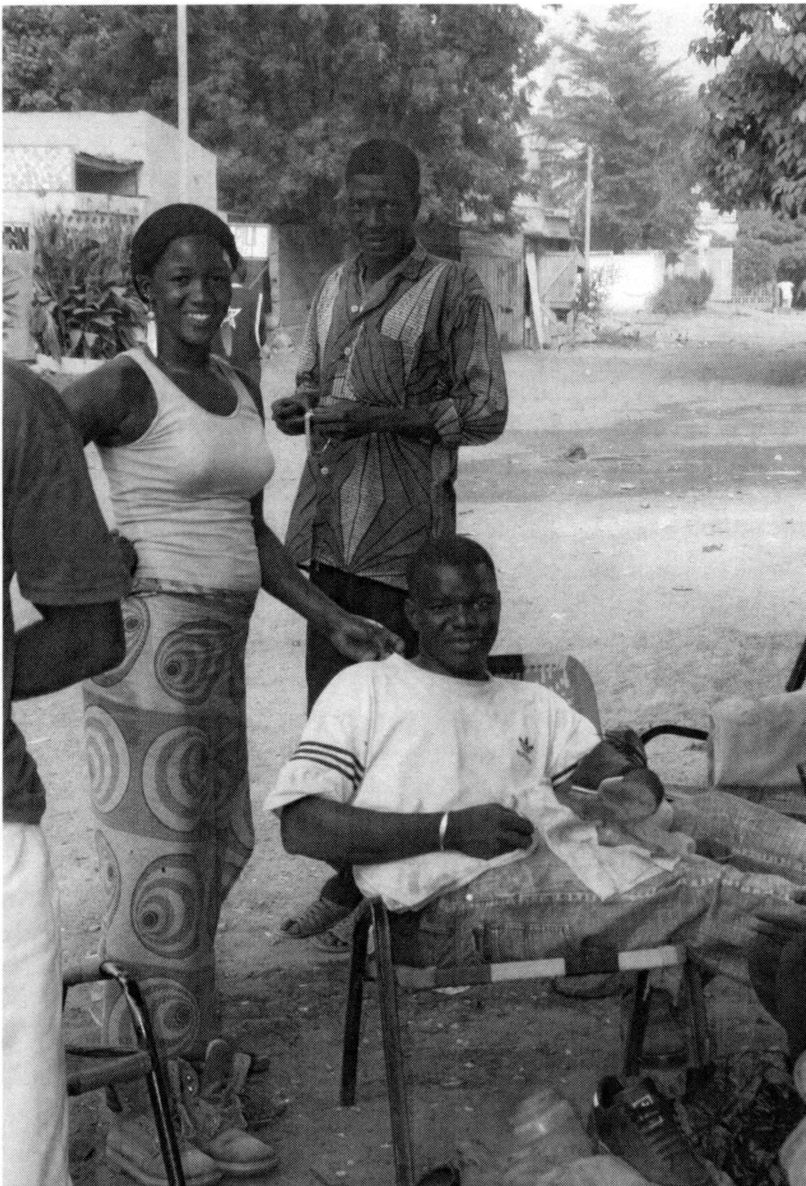

Figure 5: Young Malians gathering to exchange information in the street (Bamako, Mali, November 2008). Photo by Viola Hörbst

infertility, thus helping to constantly reproduce this narrative. This paradox becomes understandable when considering the patriarchal Malian marriage and family setting where, according to family laws, women are subordinate to their husbands. It is crucial for women not to damage their husband's virile reputation, which is intimately intertwined with his respectability and authority.[31]

Thus the stigmatization of childless women is persistent. Their social suffering, together with the local necessity of making children, create strong pressures and specific needs that contrast the prevailing perception of the international and transnational public that infertility in Africa is an individual and trivial problem. How these forces – these local and international asymmetries – are tied up with and co-shape treatment decisions will be the focus of the next section.

Biomedical-Technical vs. Social Assistance: New Asymmetries

For many Malian men and women, polygyny seems to be an ideal social solution to marital childlessness. While only monogamy is allowed for the Christian minority, the Muslim majority in Mali is legally allowed to marry up to four women. While several wives increase the status of the husband and his family, some, particularly older men told me that a second wife in the household only triggers problems that in the end will be carried out on the back of the children. Some men stay monogamous, while many others have a »second office« (*deuxième bureau*) – as extramarital lovers are called – even though this is forbidden according to Islamic and Christian morals.

Depending on the kinship position of a woman in relation to a man, female perception of polygyny may vary and can even be contradicting. From their perspectives as wives, the majority of women fear receiving a co-wife. In case their husband wants to marry anew, women with affluent husbands will try to negotiate that the second wife must live in another

31 For more information on this point, see Viola Hörbst, »Focusing Male Infertility in Mali: Impacts on Gender Relations and Biomedical Practice in Bamako«, in: *Muslim Medical Ethics: Theory and Practice*, ed. by Jonathan Brockopp & Thomas Eich (Indianapolis: Indiana University Press, 2009), pp. 118–137.

villa – if possible at the other end of town. However, for women in the position of sisters and mothers, it seems attractive to receive a further sister or daughter-in-law by the second marriage of their brother or son. While a second wife limits claims on the brother's or son's financial support, she increases her mother- and sister-in-law's sphere of influence and domination, as they are the ones who will demand work from the second wife and her children.

Although (female) members of the extended family might push towards polygyny, for couples afflicted with childlessness the decision for or against polygyny also depends on whom infertility has been attributed to. In case of the husband being diagnosed sub- or infertile, polygyny does not promise the husband an easy way out. On the contrary, polygyny would aggravate the situation of both partners and complicate the chances of becoming parents with ARTs some day, as two women would have to be treated. Nevertheless, in some cases, especially when childlessness continues, the husbands marry second wives even though they know their diagnosis. This might result from a mixture of family pressures, social norms and stigmatization, religious beliefs in miracles, disbelief in the diagnosis, and also love and desire.[32] Mainly younger couples in my sample entertain notions of a relationship that is more oriented towards Western ideals of partnership and love, confidentiality, and discussing and sharing decisions. To some extent they try to keep their relationship away from external influences, especially by family members, thus relieving the pressure to marry a second wife. In the case of the wife being diagnosed sub- or infertile, religious and social pressures must not necessarily lead to polygyny, especially if there is still hope that a child will be conceived one day.

In discourses on infertility and ARTs in African contexts, social solutions are proposed as alternatives to ARTs. Polygyny, although a »traditional African practice,« is never suggested as a solution. Instead, other social practices such as foster children, extramarital sex with a husband's relative, or formal adoption are introduced by the Cameroonian philosopher Tangwa as »traditional African« possibilities for solving infertility. He argues that »in most parts of Africa, biological parenthood is deempha-

32 See Hörbst, »Focusing Male Infertility in Mali«, op. cit. (note 31).

sized to the advantage of social parenthood.«[33] While this might be true for raising and educating children after they are born, biological motherhood is a key aspect for unwanted childless women in Mali. They consider the option of social parenthood to be inappropriate to their problem since a foster child, as Ndeye states, »… is not your own child, you haven't had the pregnancy […].« Moreover, Kadidya points out:

»Well, in the end you give all your love to this child, she will grow up and then she will go to her own mother to tell her ›she made me do this, she made me do that.‹ Or she will take her things and leave you. If she would be your own child – anybody else can leave you, but your own child cannot leave you.«

Similar convictions were communicated to me by many other women – fertile or not. They emphasized recurrent aspects with regard to foster children: First, they are difficult to handle in daily life. Second, they are not as reliable as biological children as they can go back to their biological parents. Third, the women do not go through a pregnancy. First and foremost, pregnancy is the socially visible bodily proof of the couple's capability of making children and the only means to end stigmatization.[34]

Adoption (with the transfer of name and rights of inheritance) is forbidden by Muslim regulations, thus for most Muslim Malians it is not considered as an option. For women, the lack of pregnancy that disqualifies foster children as being an adequate solution to their problems plays a similar role with regard to adoption, as the case of Kadidya, a Muslim, and Tomas, an atheist, shows: Tomas, who lived in France for 25 years, regards himself to have acquired a more European understanding and worldview. While he is reluctant to engage in heterologous interventions with ARTs, he favors social parenthood by adopting a child. Instead of adoption, Kadidya prefers ARTs with sperm donation:

»All this, I am prepared to go through, but not adopting a child. […] All this [ARTs with sperm donation] is better; like this you will be pregnant, even if it

33 Tangwa, »ART and African Sociocultural Practices«, op. cit. (note 20), in particular p. 57.

34 Cf. Bernhard Hadolt & Viola Hörbst, »Problemlagen, Anwendungskontexte, Nutzungspraktiken: Assistierte Reproduktionstechnologien in Mali und Österreich«, in: *Medizin im Kontext: Krankheit und Gesundheit in einer vernetzten Welt*, ed. by Hansjörg Dilger & Bernhard Hadolt (Frankfurt am Main: Peter Lang Verlag, 2010), pp. 95–116, in particular p.102, 110.

won't be from the husband, nevertheless you will be pregnant. Well, all this is more reasonable than adopting a child.«

Kadidya continues to explain that by whatever means they try to get a child, in the end she wants that »people will say I am a real woman.« In order to be acknowledged as a »real woman« by her social surroundings, Kadidya needs to prove her bodily capability by pregnancy. Thus, for many women who are either infertile themselves or married to infertile husbands, the promise of pregnancy is a powerful argument for both homologous ARTs (using the couple's own gametes) or even heterologous ARTs (using donor ova or sperm). Ndeye, who had born a child after intervention with IUI after her husband was diagnosed infertile, reflected on ARTs by ova donation and explained:

»In my opinion, if you undergo the pregnancy, it is like it is your child; you don't consider that it is the ova of someone else. [...] It is a bit on an abstract level that the ovum comes from you or from someone else. It can make you afraid if you don't know the person, you can ask, ›This child there, how will it develop, and will there be some traits in his character that I can't cope with?‹ This can be perhaps disturbing. But besides that, if the ovum comes from you or from someone else, from the moment you have gone through the pregnancy, really, you have all succeeded, according to my view; you will perceive this child as your own child.«

Like Ndeye and Kadidya, 41-year-old Fanta, who works as a nurse in the public health sector, also argues with the bodily process of pregnancy. For eleven years she has been married as a second wife to Baba, a relatively affluent economist working as an entrepreneur. While Baba has children with his first wife, his marriage with Fanta has remained childless due to an occlusion of one fallopian tube. Fanta has known about the option of undergoing ARTs in France for years, but she has been reluctant. Now she feels under pressure, as her time for having children may be running out. A friend told her about Dr M offering ARTs in Bamako. Fanta found this option convenient, as local ARTs would be cheaper than in France and more feasible as her husband must be present in Bamako due to his business. In 2007 Fanta consulted Dr M, who in contrast to his statements in 2005 by then had changed his mind and started to provide IVF with ova donations. Dr M discovered that Fanta's ovarian reserve had aged and offered to do IVF with ova from her sister. On ARTs with ova donation, Fanta told me:

»If I carry this child until the end, I will say that it is mine. I will think perhaps 10 or 15 percent is from my younger sister.«

Linked to religious regulations but also to aspects of biological fatherhood, male interview partners expressed much more resentment towards ARTs than women.[35] Some men afflicted with infertility argued that Islam would forbid ARTs in general – a notion that is not correct, as Malian religious leaders have unanimously stated that only heterologous forms of ARTs are considered illegitimate.[36] Other infertile men were afraid of gametes getting mixed up in the lab. However, most men participating in my study found homologous ARTs acceptable – at least in theory. But the majority of them rejected the idea of heterologous forms of ARTs. Both fertile and infertile men argued on the basis of Islam.[37] Some infertile men reasoned that a child resulting from donor sperm would not fulfill their aim of having their »own« child. However, one of them explicitly compared the usage of donor sperm with social solutions like taking a foster child from a brother: both children would not be his own biological children, but with a foster child, he reasoned, it would at least originate from the patrilineage and thus ensure its continuity.[38]

35 For more information on men's problems with biomedical interventions in reproductive processes see Viola Hörbst, »Male Perspectives on Infertility and Assisted Reproductive Technologies (ART) in sub-Saharan Contexts«, in: *Facts, Views & Vision in ObGyn. Issues in Obstetrics, Gynaecology and Reproductive Health. Scientific Journal of the Flemish Society of Obstetrics & Gynecology. Monograph VIII: Social Aspects of Accessible Infertility Care in Developing Countries*, ed. by Willem Ombelet & Frank Van Balen (2010), pp. 22–27.

36 For a discussion of heterologous and homologous ART and Islam see Marcia C. Inhorn, »Religion and Reproductive Technologies. IVF and Gamete Donation in the Muslim World«, in: *Anthropology News*, February (2004), pp. 14–15; Marcia C. Inhorn, »Middle Eastern Masculinities in the Age of New Reproductive Technologies: Male Infertility and Stigma in Egypt and Lebanon«, *Medical Anthropology Quarterly* 18 (2004), 2, pp. 162–182.

37 Viola Hörbst, »Islamische Grundsätze und die Handhabung assistierter Reproduktionstechnologien in Bamako, Mali«, in: *Reproduktionsmedizin bei Muslimen: säkulare und religiöse Ethiken im Widerstreit?*, ed. by Thomas Eich (2009), pp. 48–64 (http://tobias-lib.uni-tuebingen.de/volltexte/2009/3785/pdf/Tagung_Islamische_Medizinethik_2008.pdf [last accessed: 27.8.10]).

38 Only two infertile men (both Christian) were open towards ART with donor sperm.

The issue of involuntary childlessness and the resulting quest for a solution clearly shows that biological parenthood is of high importance for Malians. They have to prove their bodily capacity to make children. As pregnancy is visible for their social surroundings it is a key factor for childless women to end stigmatization and social exclusion. Fanta, Kadidya, and Ndeye view ART with donor gametes as a worse solution than conceiving a child biologically originating from both spouses. But contrary to their husbands' point of view, the inclusion of pregnancy makes even heterologous forms of ARTs more attractive than adoption, foster children, or polygyny, as these options do not satisfy the necessity of being pregnant. For men, to have biologically related offspring is important, but through ART this is only possible if their own sperm can be used.

Only certain other social forms, such as getting a divorce and marrying a new husband, clandestine extramarital sex with a lover, or the discretely organized coupling with a husband's younger brother (communicated to me as being the »traditional« solution to cases of male infertility) can enable fertile women to become pregnant – but only with another partner. However, love, social control, fear of being discovered, and religious morals are named by the majority of women as reasons not to make use of such strategies (at least at this stage of their lives).[39] For a fertile husband, polygyny seems to be an intriguing strategy due to its socially acknowledged status and its option to grant him his »own« biological/genetic children. Based on children's biological relation to their parents and on gender-specific reproductive aims, it seems that women find (even heterologous) ARTs more appealing than men.[40]

Financial considerations play an important role when comparing ARTs with locally available social strategies of having a child. In the case of ARTs, access to financial resources through spouses and their families are crucial for these high-cost interventions, as health insurances are rare in Mali. No state support is available to (co-)fund such treatments and patients have to shoulder the expenses themselves. Many infertile couples already have

39 Only one woman told me that extramarital sex could be an option for her. It is very unlikely, however, to find women who have discretely chosen this solution and who are prepared to talk about it, as they all have reasons to conceal their actions and will not take any risk by telling an anthropologist about it.

40 For more on the translation of legitimate relations into biological substances, see Hörbst, »IVF in Bamako«, op. cit. (note 28).

difficulties covering costs for consultations, ultrasounds, and hormonal analyses. In private clinics these cost from 10 to 35 euros each, although consultation fees are cheaper in public hospitals.[41] Nevertheless, many try to consult the private sector whenever they have the financial means, due to its higher reputation. Many of them spend huge amounts of money over the years for repeating the same treatments with different doctors.

Given the lack of state subsidies, ARTs are only accessible to a relatively small minority. Paying between roughly 1,000 and 2,000 euros for an insemination including pharmaceuticals or between 2,500 and 3,000 euros for a single IVF cycle for most Malians is an insurmountable barrier. Even for those who have larger financial resources, the costs of ARTs are high. Some make bitter accusations against Malian politics for not caring well for the population, especially those who cannot raise money to fund a treatment with ARTs. Others demand funding from the international community as they view fertility problems in Mali as a serious public health issue.

According to local common sense, raising money for treatment belongs to the responsibilites of the husband, who is also in charge of deciding whether, when, and what treatments are to be carried out. An ART treatment becomes possible if one or both of the spouses are employed with good salaries, which is rare in Mali, or if they have (additional) incomes from informal activities (business, negotiations, etc.), which is often the case in Mali. Moreover, various networks are approached for raising money, but the real objective – an ART treatment – is covered up and often medical interventions (an operation of the fallopian tubes or something similar) are used as a pretext to explain the need of money. These networks usually include informal savings groups. Both men and women are generally members of one or several such groups, where the monthly contribution can range from 5 euros to 150 or more. Depending on the number of members (roughly 5 to 20), the total monthly sum will be given to a different member each month. Family members and friends are also approached. This often involves transnational social fields through the remittances from family members living outside Mali. The larger the net-

41 This is not true for hormonal analyses or ultrasound sessions, as some public hospitals cannot offer these services themselves and have to send patients to the private sector for them anyway.

works and the higher the person's affluence within them, the greater the possibility to find the money needed. The more infertile women can contribute to ART treatments, like in Fanta's case, the more likely it is that the husband will agree to spend the money on an IVF even if he himself already has children with another wife.

Again, various asymmetries come to the fore that affect the local attractiveness of ART. Even if money is available, sometimes different claims from other network members (for instance school fees, expenses for other family members' diseases, or emergencies) must be prioritized by the head of the household. The non-existence of supportive measures for patients from the Malian state deepens existing asymmetries between richer and poorer people's access to ARTs. This non-existence is also linked to the prevalent neglect of infertility in trans- and international health interventions, as well as the depletion of inter- and transnational funding resources in fighting other health problems. These frictions deepen existing asymmetries between developed and less developed nations and their respective availabilities in overcoming unwanted childlessness with ARTs. At the same time, specific forms of ARTs deepen existing asymmetries in local gender-specific reproductive aims and trigger new ones when considering the social alternatives available in Mali.

Five Years of Experience with ARTs: Modifications, Frictions and Persisting Asymmetries

Coming back to the physician Dr M, it is interesting to note that he worked for six years to establish ARTs in Bamako. As of 2009 he had made some forms of ARTs available: homologous IUI had been successful, homologous IVF or IVF with donor ova have not. Due to a lack in resources, ICSI could not yet be provided. In anticipation of his patients' preferences, Dr M has made neither insemination nor IVF with donor sperm locally available. According to his understanding these procedures contradict local Muslim moral codes. Nevertheless, the clinic allows men to bring the sperm needed for treatment from home. Thus it is left up to the husband to discretely bring in a younger brother's sperm for use in the intervention. According to Dr M's observations this happened in several cases as in some cases the quality of the sperm brought in was very different from the first sperm analysis.

In 2008, Dr M told me that his greatest handicap was his lack of contacts to international clinics or reproductive practitioners who could provide medical equipment at lower cost and thus increase the amount of IVFs he could carry out. This would be a way of enhancing his competence and skills with such treatment and in his view could particularly contribute to finally producing a baby with IVF. Already rumors have been spread by envious colleagues that he is not capable of managing IVF. Thus a further delay of success with IVF would damage his professional reputation and in the long term undermine his business. As much as his patients need a baby to prove their capability of »making a child« to their social surroundings, Dr M himself must prove to his professional surroundings his ability to »make a child« with IVF.

For the physician, new ambivalences are emerging that are embedded in ongoing processes of commercialization in both public and private health care sectors worldwide. In Mali, these processes seem to partially be the result of structural adjustment programs demanded by the World Bank and the International Monetary Fund (IMF).[42] Without governmental, transnational, or international options to fund the pharmaceuticals needed for ARTs, Dr M tries other ways of lowering costs for him and his patients. He collects several patients in need of IVF and IUI and treats them at the same time in order to save expensive lab reagents that only have a short shelf life. It is still a risk for Dr M to purchase these devices, as some people will then decide not to undergo treatment with ARTs. This also affects the pharmacists, who stock hormonal products and

42 Since then, health care is no longer free in the public sector and bad salaries are prevalent for health care personnel, including doctors. Nevertheless, people often wonder how professors and doctors who earn around 300 euros per month in the public sphere can afford to drive Mercedes or Range Rovers and live in villas. Even employees of public health facilities complain about widespread corruption – of others, of course. Moreover, people speak about under-the-table fees frequently demanded in Bamako's public hospitals when a good or urgent treatment is needed. Besides, doctors working in public structures are allowed to work in private clinics as well. It is an open secret that some of them are rarely at hand in the public hospital. Cf. Yannick Jaffré & J.-P. Olivier de Sardan (Eds.), *Une médecine inhospitalière. Les difficiles relations entre soignants et soignés dans cinq capitales d'Afrique de l'Ouest* (Paris: Karthala, 2003).

run the risk that they won't be bought before expiration date. To avoid such problems, Dr M now cooperates with a local pharmacist who stocks hormonal drugs and offers them at a discount for Dr M's patients. By coincidence, Dr M met a French reproductive practitioner in 2007 who offered him his surplus hormonal drugs that his patients return to him after treatment. This enables Dr M to offer one or two IVF cycles to patients at lower costs every six months. In addition, he gives discounts on the second and third attempts of both IUI and IVF. He provides some services like ultrasound examinations for free and in some cases reduces his fees. But these private efforts are insufficient to substantially reduce costs for patients, while the amount of products Dr M currently needs is not large enough to negotiate discounts with producers.

Dr M also adapts ART applications to local specificities. Summarizing his experiences and results, in early 2009 he told me that IUI is working quite well, with 60 attempts made and 15 children born as a result. He suggested that one reason for the attractiveness of IUI may be that IUI is cheaper than IVF and that this is mostly done when men are sub- or infertile. In such cases, he argues, men have a high motivation to pay for the treatment, as there are no appropriate social strategies at hand. But, he continues:

»If the husband hears that the fallopian tubes are blocked, than he will rather marry a second wife than spend money for an IVF on his first wife.«

As already mentioned above, there are some exceptional cases where the husband is willing to invest in IVF for his wife, but according to Dr M's observations, this is not the norm. Thus, Dr M no longer believes in success with homologous IVF, as couples who will pay for it are rare. Cases are too few to allow him to gain enough experience and skill to successfully carry out fertilization and nidation and to finally achieve an IVF baby's birth. Furthermore, he continued to explain, in most cases in which couples are ready to pay for an IVF, the women are already in their forties with complicated clinical histories. Age and clinical background drastically limit the chances of success for IVF. In contrast to his original plans in 2004 not to use donor gametes, he adapted his activities according to his anticipation of female agreement and now offers women IVF with ova donated from a younger sister, cousin, or niece. As much as this procedure increases the women's chance of success, it also clearly increases Dr M's chances of making an IVF child.

For IVF with ova donation, Dr M has personal guidelines: He only offers these proceedings to women who have no child at all, who are »serious« in their desire, and who, in Dr M's opinion, follow Malian norms of respect and good education. This latter aspect is intimately linked to his own need to keep his activities with heterologous ARTs concealed from the public. To avoid conflicts with colleagues or religious representatives, this option remains an internal agreement between him, his lab, and the afflicted woman.

Nevertheless, by 2008 no attempt with IVF had been successful. Until then, he explained, his biomedical guidelines for hormonal stimulation recommended that ova production not be triggered too much. But after talking with French and Togolese colleagues, he started to use higher doses of hormonal stimulation to receive more mature eggs, thus increasing his chances of creating more embryos. His colleagues, Dr M explained to me, told him that they did the same in the beginning in France. In addition, he bought a new (not second-hand) incubator because his former second-hand one could not reliably control temperature and CO^2 concentration. At the moment, the next step on his clinical »obstacle course«[43] to an IVF baby is a successful nidation after transfer.

In order to come to terms with lacking national and transnational support and the financial and social specificities of his clients, Dr M tried to activate his professional transnational fields and contacts[44] as much as possible to meet his and his patients' needs and lower costs. However, he customized his offers to the preferences of the husband as the one who – at least officially – decides about the treatment and is responsible for financing it. He has extended his ethical principals and adapted them to local demands and his own interests in order to succeed with this challenging treatment. While patients benefit from these strategies, Dr M also aims to attract more IVF patients and thus, at the same time, to (potentially) increase his chances of meeting his own professional need: the birth of an

43 Sarah Franklin coined the term »obstacle course« for the experience and process of women handling the different stages of ART treatment. See Sarah Franklin, *Embodied Progress: A Cultural Account of Assisted Conception* (London: Routledge, 1997).

44 Hörbst, »IVF in Bamako«, op. cit. (note 28).

IVF child.[45] Thus Dr M's medical activities blur the boundaries between best medical solution for infertile patients and best solutions for his own objectives. This fact is again closely linked to the national, transnational, and international lack of financial support for the introduction of ARTs and reveals how transnational and international reproductive policies can be awkwardly connected to local biomedical practices.

ARTs in Mali: Limited by Persisting Asymmetries – Triggering New Ones

Medicoscapes connect heterogeneous actors, ideologies, and practices scattered around the world with local health practices. Focusing on infertility and ARTs in Mali, in this article I tracked their interrelations to several heterogeneous actors, knowledge regimes, and practices, as well as their positioning in various power arrangements on local, inter-, and transnational levels. These arrangements influence in a subtle or more direct way how ARTs are used and applied in Mali.

The high value of having children in African societies is interpreted by local and transnational NGOs, by transnational and international development institutions, and by funding agencies in health-related fields in terms of a danger for overpopulation and development. While high birth rates in Mali seem to make the problem of infertility insignificant for attention outside Mali, living in a society with many children renders childlessness and infertility for many Malians even more visible. However, the problem of infertility in Mali competes with other problematic health conditions for the scarce resources of inter- and transnational funding for adequate treatments, while the Malian state is dependent on external donations for its expenditures in the health sector. Many stakeholders within the inter- and transnational health donation community give priority to

45 In 2009 Dr M and his biologist received a bank loan. They re-shaped and enlarged the ART unit and they purchased all lab devices anew, including the micro-injectors for carrying out ICSI. Since the end of 2009 they provide all forms of ARTs (including third party donation of gametes). At the moment of this article's revision for publication, several pregnancies after IVF or ICSI intervention are on their way, and the first baby after IVF carried out in Mali was born in August 2010.

diseases that disrupt biological health and life, whereas infertility is »only« seen as an – albeit severe – threat to social health and life. It thus has no platform with transnational philanthropic organizations or international development agencies. As a consequence of this paradoxical and awkward constellation, there is no significant support from trans- or international organizations for the implementation of ARTs in Mali. Some experts argue for a »social fix« of infertility by relying on »traditional« African solutions (e.g. foster children, adoption). As shown in my case studies, most of these solutions do not match Malian women's necessities. In order to get a hold on ARTs, »being transnational« is a crucial prerequisite for Dr M as well as for other Malian providers interested in realizing ARTs in the private health sector. Only if they have an individual transnational network with reproductive practitioners at their disposal can they access the training and technical equipment needed for treatment. Relationships in these networks are not balanced: biomedical experts from Mali rely on gifts from their biomedical counterparts in other countries. They are also dependent on low-price technical equipment. To some extent these are donated by various European gynecologists or clinics, however, they might lack the necessary quality and only partially fulfill their tasks.

Situated in the private health sector, Malian gynecologists have only scarce access to either national state-based or transnational non-governmental or (inter)national governmental forms of support. However, in developing countries such as Mali, excluding private doctors from economic support may encourage biomedical protagonists to give in to dynamics of commercialization and professional goals, which blur the boundaries between the best medical solution for patients and the physician's own need for success with treatments such as IVF.

The disinterest of most inter- and transnational organizations in the advancement of fertility treatments in developing countries and the lack of systematic support directly and indirectly complicate both providers' and users' access to ARTs. In order to overcome these barriers, Dr M uses his individual transnational connections to reduce both his personal expenses and the prices for his patients. Simultaneously, he adapts IUI and IVF treatments to existing social forces in order to increase patients' access and his own chances of success. He is caught between local gender-specific social strategies and the neglect of trans- and international organizations.

The cheaper and technologically less sophisticated IUI is provided and used more frequently, as it mainly applies to cases of male factor infertility, for which there are no appropriate social solutions available. In contrast, IVF is mostly realized when wives have their own financial means or access to such means. Infertile women up to now seem to profit less from ARTs provided in Mali, thus existing gender asymmetries are to some extent strengthened through the complex constellations of ideologies and forces that have an impact on this field.

During the years of my fieldwork, Dr M has adjusted his practices and now provides ova donation (which is technologically more complicated) but no sperm donation (which is technologically easier). While this is in line with Muslim views of the more important role of sperm in making a child and establishing a legitimate relation to its father's family, this adaptation also supports the gynecologist's interest in achieving a birth via IVF: whereas offering sperm donation would lead mostly to IUI and would not allow Dr M to achieve this goal, ova donation increases his chances because the younger women's ova he uses are easier to fertilize.

While information about ARTs and its promises has reached many Malians through TV and communication with Malian emigrants, the great majority of Malians in need of ARTs has no access to it. Those who have the financial means and the mobility to cross international borders can profit from ARTs provided in European or other African states. Others can benefit from the already successfully provided IUI in Bamako. If they are in need of IVF, they will have to cooperate with the local pioneers of this treatment. Although ARTs have reached Mali through the transnational activities of individuals, the venture of Dr M as well as the effort to undergo such treatments by his patients are permeated by various asymmetries and barriers on local, national, transnational, and international levels. Globalization and transnationalization not only entail the unrestricted flow of people, goods, practices and ideas, but also the reinforcement of already existing (national, political, and ideological) boundaries and power asymmetries and the creation of new ones. Political and economic forces actively contribute to these demarcations, while they may also, at least partially, contribute to their dissolution. Although there is some mobility and transnational linkage by individuals engaged in the dissemination of ARTs to Mali, the situation is still mostly shaped by the restricted mobility of people, artifacts, technologies, knowledge and skills as well as ideological, political, and economic barriers along persisting asymmetries between North and South. ART in Mali is a zone of conflict and dissent, where local reproductive governance is always at the same time deeply entangled with transnational and international reproductive governance active in medicoscapes that span the globe.

Concerned Groups in the Field of Reproductive Technologies: A Turkish Case Study

Nurhak Polat

Introduction

Sibel Tuzcu of Istanbul had suffered childlessness for years, undergoing multiple fertility treatments in Turkey. In 2000 she launched an Internet exchange portal: she wanted to speak about her experiences with involuntary childlessness and fertility treatments. She wanted to share her experiences with others *who had the same problem.* The organization ÇİDER (*Çocuk İstiyorum Dayanışma Derneği* – the *I Want a Child-Association*) resulted from the success of the Internet portal (www.cocukistiyorum.com), and was the first of its kind to raise the issue of Turkish infertility and involuntary childlessness from the point of view of affected female or male individuals and couples.

The Internet offers various ways of networking and making connections for individuals and groups. In the case of ÇİDER, the Internet is a tool to establish and weave connections between persons affected, but it also enables involuntarily childless individuals to contact medical professionals online. However, ÇİDER does not only operate on the Internet. It also connects professionals and »patients« *(hastalar)*[1] by way of information meetings *(bilgilendirme toplantıları)* in various locations all over Turkey. These meetings must be seen in the context of changing notions

1 In this paper I put the term »patient« in quotation marks because of the ambiguity of the term in the field and particularly in the Turkish health context. In everyday usage of the word *hasta* (plural *hastalar*) has several literal meanings such as »sick,« »il,l« and »patient.« However, given the changing position of »patients« in encounters with professionals, particularly in the field of assisted reproductive technologies, it is impossible to distinguish between the categories of »patient« and »consumer.« The quotation marks are meant to make this ambiguity explicit.

and representations of »patients« within Turkish modernization processes, especially the recent massive privatization of the Turkish health sector.

The main goal of this article is to understand how ÇİDER has created a space for itself as an institutional actor. ÇİDER takes a specific position vis-à-vis the private and the national public health sector as well as vis-à-vis nationally and transnationally operating entities such as concerned groups, the pharmaceutical industry, and doctors' associations. At the same time, it must also take into account changing perceptions and roles of individual »patients« and »patient« groups. In this position, the organization has developed a specific set of services based on knowledge and experience that is clearly structured by the market of reproductive medicine, by supply and demand, by local infrastructures, by perceptions, by social conventions and by cultural norms.

In this paper I discuss a series of ethnographic vignettes from my fieldwork[2] in Turkey, which represent the role of the concerned group[3] ÇİDER in the field of reproductive technologies as a knowledge producer and manager, as a support group, and as a national and transnational actor

2 The data used here are based on my ongoing ethnographic research with the concerned group ÇİDER that I am carrying out in Istanbul and other locations in Turkey for my dissertation at Humboldt University, Berlin. The dissertation is located in the context of a project at the Collaborative Research Center »Representations of Changing Social Orders,« funded by the German Research Foundation. Here, my project is part of a larger research endeavour on »Kinship as Representation of Social Order and Practice: Knowledge, Performativity, and Legal-Ethical Regulation.« Since October 2008 I have interviewed employees, volunteers, members, and website users of ÇİDER at different locations in Turkey and done participant observation at the ÇİDER headquarters, its information meetings, and at international conferences. Interviews with doctors and observation in clinics and at medical conferences have further helped to better understand ÇİDER's work.

3 The term used here is borrowed from studies by Michel Callon und Vololona Rabeharisoa, who have examined the emergence and establishment of *concerned groups* in numerous publications (see for example Michel Callon & Vololona Rabeharisoa, »The Growing Engagement of Emergent Concerned Groups in Political and Economic Life: Lessons from the French Association of Neuromuscular Disease Patients«, in: *Science, Technology, Human Values* 33 (2008), pp. 230–261). I prefer this term as it accentuates the complexity of the relationships and interactions between different actors in this field. However, it must be mentioned that my interview partners and others involved in the field refer to organizations (locally or globally) active in this field as »patient associations« (*hasta dernekleri*). This holds for ÇİDER employees and members as well as for medical professionals.

operating in diverse relations and constellations. The first such vignette illustrates the career of the personal narrative of the female founder of ÇİDER, Sibel Tuzcu, which may be seen as indicative and exemplary for mobile narratives. Such narratives have the capacity to travel or bridge differing social domains, connecting media representations with science discourses and intimate personal spheres. The second vignette focuses on a group of involuntarily childless women who first met each other in the forums of the ÇİDER website, but then translated their acquaintance into a specific local social form called *gün* (in Turkish literally »day«), a kind of rotating savings meeting mainly common with urban middle-class women in Turkey. In the third vignette I describe and analyze an exemplary transnational event held under the motto *Break the Silence* to show ÇİDER's transnational linkages and their impact on the position of the organization at the national level.

In all these vignettes I focus on the local and transnational interconnectedness of ÇİDER and allied organizations in the field of ART. The paper presents two arguments. First, both the emergence and establishment of *concerned groups* are embedded in local circumstances. Local circumstances play a central role in the relations between members of *concerned groups* and thus also for the positioning of the organizations themselves in diverse relations, interrelations, and interactions with »environing fields« such as the media, medical, legal, or parliamentary fields.[4] At the same time there occurs a »simultaneous production« and interlocking of the local/translocal and transnational,[5] for example when the organization demonstrates its engagement in both local and global networks. The second argument holds that, due to contemporary technological, medical, and political developments, concerned groups become important new actors intervening in existing social relationships between doctors and »patients,« creating new ones, and inventing new forms of knowledge practices and a whole spectrum of what I call »new services.« These new services are based on emerging forms of educating and mobilizing lay participants in medical and economic sectors; these forms

4 Nick Crossley, »The Field of Psychiatric Contention in the UK, 1960–2000«, in: *Social Science & Medicine* 62 (2006), pp. 552–563.

5 Michi Knecht, »›Vor Ort‹ im Feld? Zur Kritik und Reakzentierung des Lokalen als europäisch-ethnologischer Schlüsselkategorie«, in: *Österreichische Zeitschrift für Volkskunde* LXIV/113 (2010), pp. 23–49, here p. 23.

are not limited to local or national configurations, but they still operate within local and national discourses that frame the national health system and social norms and circumstances.

The Proliferation of Knowledge Spaces and Concerned Groups

In recent years, interdisciplinary science and technology studies have paid much attention to the transformation of the relation between society, science, and economy. One of the important analytical and empirical outcomes of studying this transformation has been the notion of a *switch* from a *public understanding of science* to a *public engagement*,[6] leading to a pluralization of knowledge production and to an expansion and diversification of actors involved in the health sector, paralleled by an increasing activation of patients/consumers. Nowotny, Scott, and Gibbons in *Re-Thinking Science* have proposed that the production of scientific knowledge in its historical development can be understood in two modes. In mode 1, science was considered »external« to society and the ways of knowledge production were more homogenous. In contrast to this, in mode 2 knowledge production is no longer homogenous and authoritative, but »internal« to society; this implies a proliferation of spaces in which scientific knowledge is produced and consumed.[7] Society »invades« science, but is also »invaded by science.«[8]

A crucial characteristic of this transformation is the mobilization of experience and experiential knowledge that leads to the development of self-help and patient organizations. In many Western countries such or-

6 Cf. Marilyn Strathern, »Robust Knowledge and Fragile Futures«, in: *Global Assemblages: Technology, Politics, and Ethics as Anthropological Problems*, ed. by Aihwa Ong & Stephen Collier (New York: Blackwell Publishing, 2005), pp. 464–481.

7 Helga Nowotny, Peter Scott & Michael Gibbons, *Re-thinking Science: Knowledge and the Public in an Age of Uncertainty* (Cambridge: Wiley-Blackwell, 2001).

8 Helga Nowotny, »The Changing Nature of Public Science«, in: *The Public Nature of Science under Assault. Politics, Markets, Science and the Law*, ed. by Helga Nowotny et al. (Berlin: Springer, 2005), p. 10. For further reading about the multilevel transformation of the relation between society and science, see Regula Valérie Burri & Joseph Dumit (Eds.), *Biomedicine as Culture. Instrumental Practices, Technoscientific Knowledge, and New Modes of Life* (New York/London: Routledge, 2007).

ganizations started to emerge as early as the 1940s, however, international connections among different national groups were only developed during the 1980s.[9] In this period, patient organizations found themselves in the process of making their concerns public, fighting for medical, political, and social rights, and choosing different forms of social and political mobilization in interaction with scientific research and knowledge.[10] Whereas self-help groups focus their activities on mutual support and education, other concerned groups focus their work on scientific activism. They interact with research institutions and professionals, participating in the production of scientific knowledge on the basis of their own experiences.[11] The characteristics of concerned groups can be examined within the context of the emergence of these organizations in interaction with biomedical expertise, with new forms of knowledge and technologies, and, last but not

9 Thomasina J. Borkman, »Introduction to the Special Issue«, in: *American Journal of Community Psychology* 19 (1991), 5, pp. 643–659; Thomasina J. Borkman, »Experiential Knowledge: A New Concept for the Analysis of Self-Help Groups«, in: *Social Service Review* 50 (1976), 3, pp. 445–455.

10 Vololona Rabeharisoa, »Articulating Rare and Orphan Diseases in Public Arenas: Biomedicine, Patients' Activism and the Politics of Causes« (Berlin: lecture manuscript, 2009).

11 Rabeharisoa, »Articulating Rare and Orphan Diseases«, op. cit. (note 10). Rabeharisoa and Callon identify three models of *concerned groups* based on their relationships to medicine and science: »auxiliary associations,« »partner associations« or »partnerships,« and »opposing associations.« The first model is based on the close cooperation between professionals and patients, key to this is the flow of information from one group to the other. The second model sees the patient as a partner in interaction and in the process of acquiring knowledge, assuming active participation and a co-productive role in research (See Vololona Rabeharisoa & Michel Callon, »The Involvement of Patients' Associations in Research«, in: *International Social Science Journal* 171 (2002), pp. 57–67; Vololona Rabeharisoa »The Struggle against Neuromuscular Diseases in France and the Emergence of the ›Partnership Model‹ of Patient Organization«, in: *Social Science & Medicine* 57 (2003), 11, pp. 2127–2136; see also Steven Epstein, *Impure Science. Aids, Activism, and the Politics of Knowledge* (Berkeley: University Press of California 1996) and »The Construction of Lay Expertise: AIDS Activism and The Forging of Credibility in The Reform of Clinical Trials«, in: *Science Technology and Human Values* 20 (1995), pp. 408–437. The third model excludes all possibilities of cooperation with medical scientist and researchers. Another example of a »militancy model« was developed by Janine Barbot in her analysis of activist groups and »active patients« in French AIDS organizations. Janine Barbot, »How to Build an ›Active‹ Patient? The Work of AIDS Associations in France«, in: *Social Science & Medicine* 62 (2006), pp. 538–551.

least, with regulatory and commercial entities. In an essay from 2008, Callon and Rabeharisoa elucidate this subject, defining a group as concerned group if

»its formation is strongly contingent on the existence of matters of concern shared by its members. Initially, there may well have been no particular relations between the members of the still inchoate groups. Then, owing to the activities of some of them and to the publicity given to difficulties that first seem to be individual, they gradually move closer to one another as they share their emotions, and develop common actions.«[12]

Assisted reproductive technologies represent a global form whose locally specific usages and characteristics are connected by translocal practices of cooperation, comparison, and regulation. Thus the practices of concerned groups are both locally embedded and translocally and transnationally interconnected. The American anthropologist Anna Tsing has demonstrated in a different context how social movements and NGOs now reach out globally and get actively involved in the globalization process. At the same time, globalization and the emerging global markets facilitate the emergence and development of such groups. As they interconnect transnationally, they must also work within and around the restrictions of nation-states, which is where they first must be politically active in order to gain a position of power in international and global politics. The engagement of people and groups with the health sector and in biopolitical debates is shaped by local conditions and linked to local contexts. The development of a globally operating network that is active on an international and transnational political level does not imply a dissolution of local contexts. On the contrary, medical professionals and »patients« in my interviews frequently argue that global forms present themselves in local differentiations: in distinct ways of accessing knowledge and financial resources and in distinct strategies of dealing with local structures and regulations.

12 Callon & Rabeharisoa, »The Growing Engagement of Emergent Concerned Groups«, op. cit. (note 3).

The Turkish Health System and Concerned Groups

The emergence of concerned groups in the Turkish context began comparatively late. In order to understand the role of patient groups, they must first be contextualized within the modernization and privatization of Turkey and its health system. During the early years of the Turkish republic, the development of a state-based health system was one of the most important aspects of the Kemalist process of modernization that was primarily based on an opposition between »modern« and »traditional.«[13] The health system was developed according to the ideals of the modernization project; within this, biomedical knowledge was considered to be one of the most important instruments for grasping modern ideals and transporting them into social life. It made the construction of subjectivity and citizenship according to modernist ideals possible. The elites of the republic were thought to be responsible for »leading« the »people« *(halkı)* and the population towards the modern ideals of the republic. Kemalism and its *grand social project (büyük toplumsal proje)* saw »the citizen« as »preceding the individual«[14] and constructed the citizen on the basis of his or her obligations towards the state rather than on his or her rights. The realization of a new society with its new modern citizens was based on discourses of rationality. However, it remains questionable how much »common citizens« were regarded as active actors in this phase of modernization. The establishment of social awareness and of the »educated patient« were at the center of modernization processes in the health sector.[15] Doctors were the main agents of this modernization process.

In the 1980s, however, neoliberal politics led to yet another far-reaching process of transformation in the nexus of state, society, and

13 Christoph Dole, »In the Shadows of Medicine and Modernity: Medical Integration and Secular Histories of Religious Healing in Turkey«, in: *Culture, Medicine and Psychiatry* 28 (2004), pp. 255–280. See also Maral Erol, »Tales of the Second Spring: Menopause in Turkey through the Narratives of Menopausal Women and Gynecologists«, in: *Medical Anthropology* 28 (2009), 4, pp. 368–396.

14 Ayşe Kadıoğlu, »Citizenship and Individuation in Turkey. The Triumph of Will and Reason«, in: Gerrit Steunebrink & Evert van der Zweerde (Eds.), *Modernization in Intercultural Context: Russia, Japan, Turkey* (Amsterdam: Edition Rodopi, 2004).

15 For a reading of the medicalization of menopause in Turkey that discusses the raising of awareness, consciousness, and the Kemalist ideal of a »conscious citizen« in the process of medicalization, see: Erol, »Tales of the Second Spring«, op. cit. (note 13).

economy.[16] As a result of the massive privatization of the health sector, the role of doctors and state-based health systems also changed.[17] Because health services were no longer restricted to the state, such services could now be bought by persons from the middle- and upper classes; a »patient/consumer« *(hasta/tüketici)* model was established.

Today, this model creates new challenges for hierarchical structures. But the dominant discourse of modernization still remains vital, particularly in the notion of »raising the consciousness of the people.« As a relatively new field of health, the field of reproductive technologies has become a space within which such discourses are reproduced and negotiated. A number of reproductive technologies have been available in Turkey since the middle of the 1980s.[18] A massive privatization of the reproductive medical sector has been going on since the end of the 1990s.[19] Since then, the reproductive medical sector has grown rapidly in Turkey. The establishment of concerned groups is affected by the proliferation and accessibility of reproductive technologies, as well as being also directly connected to the rapid expansion and popularization of information

---

16 See İlker Ataç, Bülent Küçük and Ulaş Şener (Eds.): *Perspektiven auf die Türkei. Ökonomische und gesellschaftliche (Dis)Kontinuitäten im Kontext der Europäisierung* (Münster: Westfälisches Dampfboot, 2008).

17 Since 2003, the »Health Transformation Program« has been at the center of a series of reforms designed to restructure and decentralize Turkey's health system. Health policies in Turkey are based on hierarchies of citizens according to their status in the national insurance program that regulate their access to health services. See Nazan Üstündağ and Çağrı Yoltar, »Türkiye'de Sağlık Sisteminin Dönüşümü: Bir Devlet Etnografisi«, in: *Avrupa'da ve Türkiye'de Sağlık Politikaları. Reformlar, Sorunlar, Tartışmalar*, ed. by Çağlar Keyder et al. (Istanbul: İletişim Yayıncılık, 2007), pp. 55–94.

18 Since then, reproductive technologies have been available solely for heterosexual and officially married couples, which means the whole institutional and regulative framework of application of this technology is based on heterosexuality and excludes other services like sperm, egg, and embryo banking, donor insemination etc. This is also the determining factor for the construction of discourses on ART and its representation on the local level. The locally dominant discourse and the acceptability of reproductive technologies are strongly rooted in the heterosexually defined accessibility of practices in the country. This also strongly affects the practices and discourses of the concerned group about the diverse ART practices.

19 According to records of the Ministry of Health (updated in January 2010), there are one hundred and eighteen clinics in Turkey including state clinics (www.saglik.gov.tr); however, most clinics are private.

technologies (Internet, media, etc.), particularly in urban areas, as the following story of Sibel Tuzcu illustrates.

The Career of a Story about the Desire for Children

The story of the personal experience of the founder of ÇİDER was decisive for the establishment of the first website of the organization and then of the organization itself. Tuzcu's experience with involuntary childlessness and with assisted reproductive technologies spans a period of more than 20 years. It was characterized by failures for many years until at the age of 42 she gave birth to her first and only daughter with the help of in vitro technologies.[20] She spread the news of her »success« to her social environment, where after years of hearing of failed medical fertility interventions skepticism prevailed. With the birth of her daughter she became a »focus of interest.« This was how she came to broadcast her story and share it with other people, »who had the same problem.« The number of visitors to her website gradually increased. When she thinks back to those early times, Tuzcu says,

> »What people here (on the Internet) were most interested in was my struggle, my surroundings, my belief in myself, while all of the doctors kept saying no. [I said:] I can cope with this matter by myself, I will never give up. I am sure that somewhere a child is waiting for me.«

But there is more than »suffering« and »success« to Sibel Tuzcu's story. With the launch of the website, her way of storytelling, which underlines the hero-like quality of trying and retrying, became exemplary to many in that it also offered a sense of hope. In her narrative, she underlines the importance of her will: »only my will« was responsible for the final »success« in having a biological child of her own. With her strong presence both on the Internet and in numerous reports and interviews about her

20 Sibel Tuzcu, the founder of the self-help organization ÇİDER, recalls that »infertility was an indecent word,« (in: *Verwandtschaft machen. Reproduktionsmedizin und Adoption in Deutschland und der Türkei*. Berliner Blätter. Ethnographische und Ethnologische Beiträge Bd. 42 (2007), ed. by Stefan Beck, Nevim Çil, Sabine Hess, Maren Klotz & Michi Knecht, pp. 168–174).

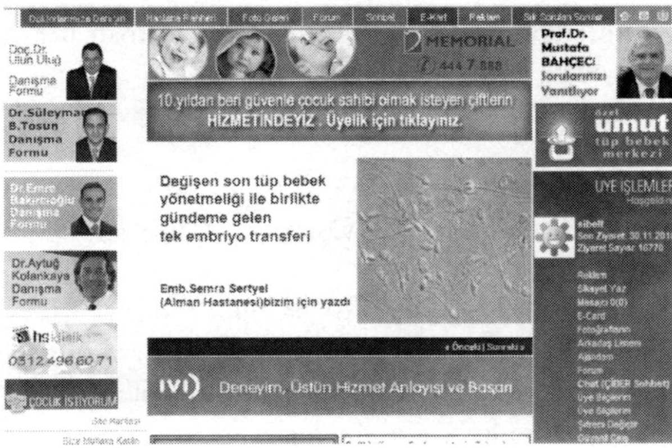

Figure 1: Website of the organization ÇİDER

experience in other media, Tuzcu primarily aims at giving hope to families who try to have children with the help of ART. The public reception and recognition of her narrative is based on her specific way of storytelling. The individual background is important: an ordinary woman in her mid-forties, with no higher education, from an ordinary urban family, with a husband and his first child from a former marriage, she was the first person ever to make her experience with IVF and involuntary childlessness public in Turkey.

Tuzcu's story eventually paved the way for the official foundation of a »patient organization« in 2002:

»[...] because the website was not able to increase its influence on the legislative level, we felt obliged to become an official institution in order to have more possibilities to talk. Because, in the end, the website is still an artificial place«[21]

as Kader Şimşek,[22] one of the founding members of the organization, pointed out.

ÇİDER's first Internet forum offered mutual emotional support for women, men, and involuntarily childless couples. In later years, with the

21 As becomes apparent in the excerpt from the interview, political demands and their necessity in the first instance were subservient to the exchange of shared experiences. Political issues became more important only as people began to realize that sufferers were not only united by the intersubjective (emotional) level of experience and that it was necessary to contribute to raising awareness at a social level.

22 All names in this article except for founder Sibel Tuzcu have been made anonymous.

founding of the official association, a social and political mission was established as well. Today ÇİDER, according to its own statements, has more than 40 000 users visiting its website, not all of them registered as official members of the organization.[23] Most of the users or the members are from different cities in Turkey, but there are also people from abroad, mostly ethnic Turks from other countries such as Germany, England, etc. As ÇİDER received increasing recognition in reproductive medical and national circles as well as among »patients,» its field of activity expanded, according to the mission of the organization, to include spreading consciousness (*bilinç*) about infertility and about assisted reproductive technologies in society at large.

Raising Consciousness *(Bilinçlendirme)* and Overcoming Shame

New information technologies and the massive increase in the participation of the media in forming public awareness, especially with regard to health issues and technological developments, has brought about a »new informed patient« who is capable of handling the available knowledge him or herself, of raising his or her *bilinç* independently of medical professionals. *Bilinç* refers in this context not only to increasing medical knowledge, but also to acting »consciously« in handling social pressure and taboos and as well as socially embedded individual perceptions of one's own situation. The modernization process has already created and circulated a notion of *bilinçli patient* in the Turkish health sector, but in recent decades this notion has gained a specific character which has been paralleled by a massive privatization of the medical sector and the popularization and expanded use of information technologies in the middle and upper classes. In the context of reproductive medicine narratives about personal experiences, popularized and mobilized by the media, have become a way of transport-

23 People usually only apply for official membership to ÇİDER when they want to profit from the organization's services, gaining a discount on treatment costs or the arrangement of appointments in clinics, etc. Therefore not all users of the ÇİDER website are official members of the organization. Some people never formally apply for membership, even though they have been in contact with ÇİDER for many years.

ing knowledge about reproductive medicine into society, as the story of Sibel Tuzcu demonstrates.

According to Sibel Tuzcu herself, when her organization was founded, many social milieus in Turkey were dominated by a »*great unconsciousness*« regarding reproductive technologies and the medical causes of male and female infertility. In her view, this situation by and large »*has remained the same*« until today.[24] Co-founder Kader Şimşek describes the main mission of their organization as follows:

»So what we've done to a certain extent with this organization is to raise awareness among the people, to make sure that they ask questions; that is, after all, the reason for our meetings. We travel from city to city [...] In the more closed social milieus we've managed to open the doors, even if only a just little bit [...] They need to find out, to inquire, to question, not blindly say ›yes‹ to everything: Why are you doing this to me, what is that, what is its goal? [...]«

On the one hand, the work of the organization aims at raising people's awareness, enabling them to have better access to the scientific knowledge available, and to know how to deal with it. As the phrase »*not blindly say ›yes‹ to everything*« indicates, the organization wants to create an attitude that enables the people concerned to challenge the relationship between doctors and »patients« with respect to their own treatment. On the other hand, Tuzcu and others do not only narrate their experiences with IVF, but also their role in raising awareness in society, which can be conceptualized as socially pioneering.[25] In their own understanding, they are breaking taboos about fertility problems enshrined in the social image of »barren-

24 Cf. Sibel Tuzcu, »Infertilität war ein Wort, das sich nicht ziemte,« op. cit. (note 20).

25 In her ethnography on the social influence of prenatal diagnosis, Rayna Rapp describes the experiences of mothers-to-be with PND in America and their individual decisions and strategies in dealing with this technology. She refers to these women as »moral pioneers« (p. 306) when faced with the option of having – or not having – a child with Down Syndrome. More important is the analysis of the technologies within their reach that make these women »moral philosophers of the private« (p. 306). For Rapp, the moral values used by these women to negotiate their private lives are important. Women who undergo amniocentesis and its consequences are moral pioneers because they must make »unprecedented decisions.« I have been inspired by Rapp's concept in my analysis of the narratives of my informants. However, I replace »moral« with »social,« because in the case of ÇİDER narratives are aimed at reaching a certain public; they are publicly mobilized on purpose. The members of ÇİDER are pioneers because they are involved in social education about infertility and ART. See Rayna

ness« (*kısırlık*) and involuntary childlessness; they are making society more sensitive to and aware of infertility and of the possibility of using technologies of assisted reproduction.

The meaning of the relationship to other affected people builds on the perception of raising individual awareness. It challenges individual and social boundaries related to social taboos and gender-specific norms in social and familiar environments, for example by talking about sexual intercourse, sexual organs, or reproductive cells. In an interview, Veli Kalem, one of the first male persons engaged with Tuzcu's webpage and later a co-founder of the organization ÇİDER, spoke of how the online communication with other people influenced his view on talking about infertility and how helpful it was to be aware of his own perception of »shame« *(ayıp),* which for him had its roots in the »ways of education« (in society) and in taken-for-granted forms of handling such issues in society».

»You see, if I can comfortably talk about this today then it's thanks to the website; otherwise I'd never have been able to talk about it like this [...] But that has something to do with the closedness of society (*toplumun kapalılığı*). When I started talking with these friends, that is to say, when we talked to each other online, I noticed that these people talked about it really comfortably. And in contrast I had to blush even talking about it online. That is to say, I could feel how I would turn red. And now you are sitting in front of me and we are talking about this live [...].«[26]

»The closedness of society« specifically refers to the perception of a lack of consciousness and intolerant social attitudes towards infertility in large parts of society. Although the establishment and accessibility of fertility clinics in various parts of the country shows that high-tech fertility treatments are gaining in social acceptability (cf. Gürtin, this volume) and becoming increasingly visible in public (TVs, newspapers, websites), it is still a topic burdened with strong social taboos in some parts of society. In this sense, the narratives reflect the meaning of shared experiences with regard to the same issue; they bring people to a shared perception of »being subject to the same conditions« and of creating or finding a specific space

Rapp, *Testing Women, Testing the Fetus: the Social Impact of Amniocentesis in America* (New York: Routledge, 1999).

26 This interview was conducted by Nevim Çil, former researcher of the »Kinship as Representation of Social Order and Practice« project (note 2).

of their own, such as ÇİDER, which offers a platform allowing people to talk about their experiences with infertility and reproductive technologies.

The Internet is not the sole means for communicating IVF experiences. *Bilgilendirme Toplantıları* (information meetings) are also spaces where different narratives of personal experience (success and failure stories) are mobilized to »break the taboos« and »raise consciousness« about the issues concerned. At these meetings, professionals communicate reproductive medical knowledge about infertility treatments, but they also function as spaces where the commercial interests of both parties, clinics and »patients,« can be negotiated. I will return to this point later, but let me first focus on how the narratives of IVF experiences are circulated and become shared stories.

Narrative Technologies of Hope and Success: Shared Stories

In the Turkish context, assisted reproductive technologies and their usages are connected to diverse strategies of both secrecy and transparency based on different personal, cultural, familial, and social logics. There is more than one strategy for dealing with infertility treatment processes by a wide variety of protagonists. For example, one interview partner told me in a conversation about secrecy that she had kept her treatments secret from her family and most of her friends because she did not want her treatment to become part of a *shared expectation* (*toplu beklenti*). However, there is also an opposite way of experiencing involuntary childlessness and infertility treatments connected to a non-secretive coping strategy or even a making-public of these narratives. Such shared expectations are created, connected, and fixed by the mobile narratives of a *common* experience of suffering, of hope, and of waiting for success. Fertility treatments are also closely aligned with *hope*, with the feeling of *having to try*,[27] with years of unsuccessful treatments, and in some cases utter failure.

27 Sarah Franklin, »›Having to Try‹ and ›Having to Choose.‹ How IVF ›Makes Sense‹«, in: *Embodied Progress. A Cultural Account of Assisted Conception* by Sarah Franklin (London: Routledge, 1997), pp. 168–197.

British cultural studies scholar Maureen McNeil, in her study of different kinds of narratives about the desire to have children in Great Britain, has identified strong similarities in these narratives. Despite individual variations, these stories all follow similar patterns of confrontation, suffering, and resolution.[28] Although I am more preoccupied with how these stories are exchanged, I also found certain parallels in my own research. What is of interest to me here is how hope and failure are transformed into collective issues, how they are constructed as shared stories, and how these narratives are communicated. In this sense it is important to ask what the role of the organization ÇİDER is in the construction of shared stories and expectations is. The narratives are often based on the assumption of a similar bodily, medical, or social situation. Thus, sharing such narratives not only means sharing medical and clinical experiences with IVF procedures, but also sharing emotions and important moments in people's everyday lives (their personal and social experiences with childlessness, but also the reaction of family and social environments to IVF treatments). In exchanging personal experiences participants develop their specific rationalities with regard to reproductive technologies that may well contradict the medical objectifications used by doctors. Shared experiences in these narratives function as symbolic resources that keep reviving the narrative techniques of instilling hope for success. The success story of Sibel Tuzcu (like similar »success stories«) is an excellent illustration of this search for »other« truths besides medical diagnoses, which form an essential part of the staging of ÇİDER's information meetings.

Almost immediately after its foundation, ÇİDER started to organize information meetings in cooperation with private fertility clinics in practically all Turkish cities, from the coast of the Black Sea to eastern and western Anatolia. Thanks to its status as an officially recognized patient association, ÇİDER often has access to local resources (assembly venues etc.) or receives support from the local administration in publicizing the event.

28 Maureen McNeil, »I Can't Have a Baby Stories: Telling Tales of Reproduction and Technosciences«, (Lecture Menuscript: Berlin, November 2004), p. 2.

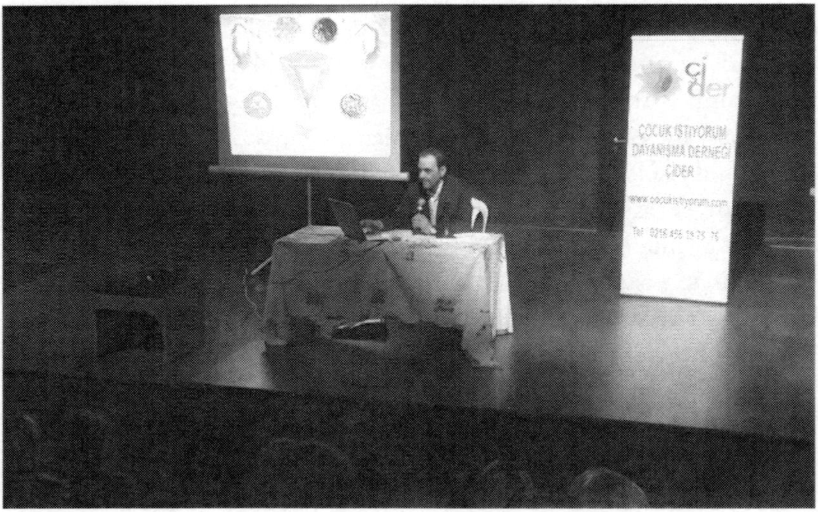

Figure 2: IVF-presentation by the doctor of a cooperating clinic during a ÇİDER meeting in Pendik, city of Istanbul, June 2009. Photo by Nurhak Polat

All information meetings I have participated in during my research[29] have followed the same uniform scheme: first comes the information about the activities of the organization itself (on a national scale, but also its international connections and memberships), then Sibel Tuzcu or other co-founders tell the story of the foundation of the organization and of their own personal experiences, which both serve to underline a strong message of hope in success (cf. below). Then one of the cooperating clinic's doctors explains the medical part of IVF treatments, often illustrated with pictures and slides. These presentations have some variation in style, but communicate very similar information, e.g. about different methods of artificial fertilization, their advantages and disadvantages, laboratory conditions, male and female infertility etc. After this, participants get the opportunity to ask questions, to relate their own experiences. This part often encourages participants to share their experiences and to very frankly

29 I took part as an ethnographer in some of the information meetings held in the western part of Turkey (in the Pendik district in Istanbul and the nearby city of Tuzla) and also in the northeastern part of the country in the cities of Ordu and Giresun on the Black Sea coast.

ask all the questions they would like to have answered. The intensity and the course of these public conversations strongly depends on the participants, on the city in which the meeting is held, whether there are mostly couples or single women and men attending, whether the lecturing doctors are renowned experts in a particular field of reproductive medicine, and similar factors.[30] Afterwards, a staff member of the clinic gives some more detail about treatment costs and discounts for ÇİDER members and, should anybody inquire, about the possibilities of financing treatment with the help of public health insurances. At the end of the formal part of the event there is a lottery for bargain treatments in the clinic.[31] I will come back to this point later, but first I want to discuss the importance of these meetings for producing and shaping IVF experiences and narratives, as spaces for performing such narratives, and for feeding the feeling of hope.

As in all other meetings, during a meeting in Tuzla (a small town, a suburb of Istanbul) the founder Sibel Tuzcu tells her own story[32] of fertility treatments and says, »I was told that I can't be a mother, and the doctors told me this. They stood in front of me and said that it was too late. […] At age 42 I became a mother.« She then continues, »Whether this was a miracle or the result of belief (in myself), everyone of you must decide for themselves. For me it was both.« That she hadn't given up and continued to believe is what had »made her a mother.« Tuzcu continues by talking about the natural powers of the body and the limits of medical knowledge:

30 Only relatively rarely do men participate in these meetings without their wives. This again may partly be due to where the meeting takes place. For example, more men attended the Black Sea meetings, possibly because of a prevalence of male infertility in this region.

31 »Lotteries« (*çekiliş* or *kura*): During the information meetings organized by ÇİDER and clinics, couples can win discount treatments at the participating clinics. Until recently ÇİDER provided a free clinic treatment for one couple at every information meeting.

32 If the founder Tuzcu is not able to participate in the information meetings, the speech is given by one of the co-founders of the organization. In this case, the structure, subject, and message of the speech remains very similar, except for the change of the storyteller, who tells both her own story and the story of Tuzcu. In one of my interviews Tuzcu told me she no longer felt comfortable about speaking in public and preferred one of the co-founders, who was very proficient at holding public speeches, to take over this part of the meetings.

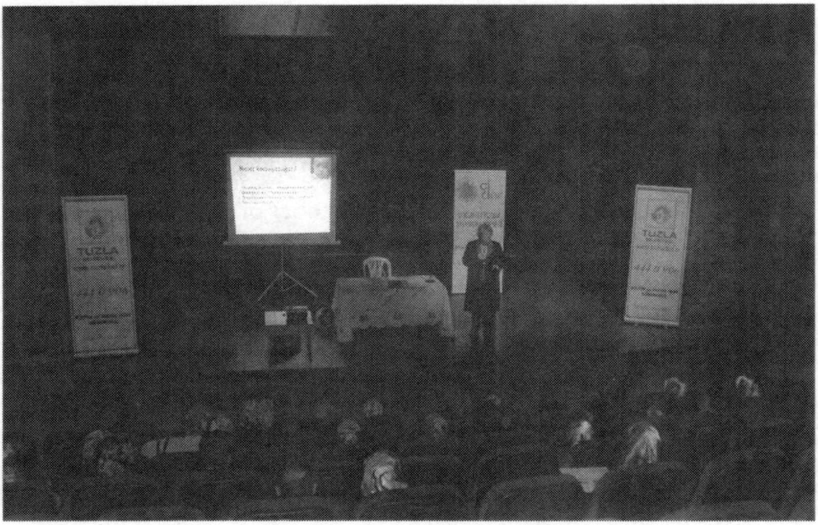

Figure 3: Sibel Tuzcu speaking during a ÇİDER information meeting in the region of Tuzla, Istanbul, March 2010. Photo by Nurhak Polat

»The doctors, for all their knowledge, don't always have an explanation or a solution – and then it happens anyway. So, what I'm trying to say is that you mustn't give up hoping (*Umutsuzluğa kapılmamak lazım*).«

Usually ÇİDER invites local women or couples who have become pregnant with the help of ÇİDER or in the participating clinic to join these meetings. These people, who have succeeded in conceiving a child with assisted reproductive technologies, frame and support the message and underline the promise of both the clinics and the technology. Everything is welded together in the one message *»never to give up hope.«* The representation of success thus is strongly imbued with individual strength and will.

Keeping hope alive is thus also an effect of the face-to-face interactions between members of the organization who are in a close relationship with one another. As I will show in the next chapter, members eventually will become familiar with one another to such an extent that they know all about their emotional changes and the details of IVF treatments they had.

These personal experiences are individual and intimate, but they are also connected to representations of commonly shared stories.

Friends by Destiny *(Kader Arkadaşı)* and »Gün« (Women's Gatherings)

The Internet is one of the most important media for the mobilization of personal and intimate stories. The *intimate machine*,[33] as Sherry Turkle has called it, makes networking via the Internet possible, and computer-based communication opens up new ways of making connections. As in the case of ÇİDER, the desire for children can be shared, produced, and reproduced in all its nuances via the Internet. The communication options of forums and chats serve to mobilize the stories of involuntarily childless persons from different backgrounds in newly created relationships of solidarity. For example, through ÇİDER I came into contact with a women's group from a large city near Istanbul. For over a year these women shared their experiences on the ÇİDER website, where they opened a regional chat forum under the name of their city and built up intimate relationships to other women. They then translated this relationship into a specific form of women's gathering known as *gün,* usually practiced by urban middle-class women for whom the group is a specific social arena. These *gün* meetings take place at one of the members' houses and function as a kind of rotating savings plan: at every meeting, all participants pay an equal contribution, the sum of which is given to the hostess, who thus receives a large amount of money. The group negotiates who may func-

33 Turkle explored the concept of an intimate relationship between people and machines in her earlier work, on the basis of which she dubbed computers »intimate machines.« See Sherry Turkle »Computational Reticence: Why Women Fear the Intimate Machine«, in: *Technology and Women's Voices*, ed. by Cheris Kramarae (New York: Pergamon Press, 1986) pp. 41–61. In one of her later works Turkle further develops this notion, stating that with the establishment of the Internet new possibilities of the *intimate machine* are produced. She maintains that people project their own dramas onto computer screens of which they are producer, director, and star, dramas of private nature that still involve other people (see Sherry Turkle, *Life on the Screen. Identity in the Age of the Internet* (New York: Simon & Schuster, 1995).)

tion as hostess and when a meeting is held, according to the needs of the women.[34]

For the *gün* of the ÇİDER women, the priorities negotiated are related to upcoming IVF treatments or births that require money. Special to these meetings is the fact that all participating women have been confronted with involuntary childlessness and have come into contact with reproductive technologies; some have had successful treatments and bring their children to the meetings, while others are currently undergoing fertility treatment. They thus see themselves as having a *shared problem* and as being connected by a similar experience. The realization of these similarities finds expression in the often heard phrase »I was surprised to find I am not the only one« *(bir tek ben değilmişim).* Or in statements like the following:

> Because we've gone through the same thing, we can understand each other better. For example, when we start we don't talk about things like why can't you have children, why doesn't it work, how was it and so on. When we talk, our conversations take their own routes. We never ask each other straight out; perhaps we figure things out when someone is talking and lets something slip without noticing. But outside, in society, it is not the same thing. Maybe you want to keep things secret; maybe you don't want to be asked because you get sudden reactions like ›aah, you can't have a child – well, don't you worry, it will work out!‹ But here [in the context of ÇİDER relationships, NP] we know that we have all gone through the same experiences, that we have lived though the same feelings. Here, it's easy to talk about it, we don't have to force anyone.«

Since what brought them together is the fate of childlessness and infertility, these women call theirs a »friendship by destiny.« In their social environments, the experience childlessness is often associated with taboos, exclusions, and social pressures leading to emotional, social, and financial

34 This form of middle class women's gatherings in urban spaces only started in Turkey in the 1980s. The contributions paid for the meetings are often made in foreign currencies such as Euros or dollars in order to increase the efficiency of the savings. However, there are also other forms such as *Paralı Gün* (money day) or *Altın Günü* (gold day), when the contribution is made in gold. For more information on *Gün* see Berna Ekal, »How *a kaynana* Should Behave? Discussions on the Role of Mothers-in-Law in Two *Gün* Groups«, in: *European Journal of Turkish Studies*, Thematic Issue N°4 (2006) *The Social Practices of Kinship. A Comparative Perspective*, retrievable at http://www.ejts.org/document619.htm; Ferhunde Özbay, »Gendered Space: A New Look at Turkish Modernization«, in: *Gender & History* 11 (1999), p. 3.

difficulties that make hopelessness and feelings of loss and failure a part of their everyday lives. Shared notions of *success* (successful treatments, pregnancies) and *loss* (non-successful treatments, miscarriages, a loss in the quality of egg cells, or a total incapacity to produce egg cells) form the basis for close friendships characterized by confidentiality and similarity of experiences. By communicating their lived experiences, members of a group produce a kind of shared intimacy that at the same time constitutes a kind of a semi-public space. Within these expanded boundaries of intimacy they develop an interest in the bodily rhythms and functions of the other women – the type of fertility problem they suffer from, their bodily or medical parameters (markers, blood test results), the process of stimulation of ovarian hormone levels e.g. with the help of a follicle stimulating hormone *(FSH)*, the number of fertilized eggs, the results of sperm analyses, the number of embryos transferred, of frozen cells, of embryos, etc. Relations of mutual evaluation between the members emerge as they accompany each other through the process of »living with assisting reproductive technologies,« providing checks and balances as well as encouragement and enabling the distribution of knowledge.

Topics of everyday life, married life, relationships with friends and family are also touched upon, uniting these women beyond involuntary childlessness and fertility treatments. The implications of these friendships are wide. The women are able to re-define their identity in many settings and constellations. In their new social environment they are no longer somebody's wife *(birinin karısı),* somebody's daughter-in-law *(birinin gelini)*, or the marginalized, pitiable, quiet, childless woman in need of protection. Almost all of them conceive of themselves as women who can free themselves from the influence of their usual social environment and who, within the social spaces of their own making, can live involuntary childlessness in their own way, at least for a certain time. For some of the women, the key motivation for participation in such a group is the quest for possibilities and model cases that keep the hope of »becoming a mother someday« alive.

As Ceyda Bitkin, who has years of fertility treatments behind her, described the meaning of her relationship with the women's group:

»Every time I come to a meeting, when I come to our gün meeting, I become a mother for a couple of hours. For a couple of hours – I get goose bumps – for a few hours it feels like I've become a mother. They let you feel it, the women who are mothers already and those who will soon be mothers. I have begun to say that I can become a mother.«

The experiences of other women and couples are taken in by other persons concerned and affect their decision whether to continue with the reproductive treatments or not. Hope is »kept awake,« »kept alive,« and »made felt« by sharing and collectively communicating medical as well as experiential knowledge. The reception of the experiences of others naturally focuses on »successful« treatments, which function as a proof of the belief that the intensity of willing can supercede medical findings and explanatory models. Personal experiences thus turn into a kind of knowledge that is negotiated among the group concerned and acquires a validity of its own. By contrasting medical knowledge with »shared experiences,« a new type of knowledge is »extracted.« The group socialization allows for a new form of personal truth that can be »systematized«[35] in a pragmatic way. During the negotiation process, medical »truths« and collective »truths« are welded into an idiosyncratic pragmatic logic, the systematizations of which permanently call medical knowledge into question and try to complement medical practices and practitioners.[36]

In the next chapter I will discuss how this kind of experience-based knowledge expands into market relationships and brings forth a new form of services.

35 The ideas of an »extraction« and »systematization« of experiential knowledge are borrowed from Stefan Beck, »Die Mobilisierung der Erfahrung. Anmerkungen zu Translationen para-ethnografischen Wissens«, in: Ina Dietzsch, Wolfgang Kaschuba & Leonore Scholze-Irrlitz (Eds.), *Horizonte ethnographischen Wissens* (Köln: Böhlau Verlag, 2009), pp. 221–238. Beck develops his perspective in the context of serious diseases. He maintains that laypersons want to »exert« the experiential knowledge they have developed and »feed it back into science.«

36 »[…] Alluding to personal experience does not imply a truth claim that would be universal or generalizable in the sense of scientific knowledge. On the contrary, perspectivism, relationality and situatedness are exerted and used as a resource.« The question then remains whether »universalistic claims of (natural) scientific knowledge are partially invalidated, limited or (only) amended,« Beck, »Die Mobilisierung der Erfahrung«, op. cit. (note 35), p. 227.

Hizmet and »*New Services*«

In order to understand the role of the concerned group ÇİDER, it is necessary to look into the complexity of interactions within the field of assisted reproductive technologies. Economic markets are sociotechnical arrangements[37] that play a crucial role in the design of concerned groups. In the Turkish case, the privatization of the service of assisted reproductive medicine highlights the importance of newly emergent actors. In the following I will show how local circumstances and economic market structures combine with the practices of both individuals and ÇİDER. I will also show the importance of the activities of the said organization with respect to what I call »new services.«

To begin with, the expression »service« is the translation of the Turkish concept of »*hizmet.*« The usage of this term in my research field cannot be reduced to an economic, profit-based dimension since sometimes it also encompasses a social mission. It is exactly this multidimensionality of the idea of *hizmet* that characterizes the present field. On the one hand, *hizmet* is imbued with the perception of a voluntary charitable mission and duty, the will to »serve« other human beings. On the other hand, the term means something like »knowledge work,« as when it represents awareness raising and helping others to find orientation in the medical sector. So *hizmet* has very positive connotations.

As indicated before, the cooperation with doctors and private clinics encompasses a wide spectrum of services, from written online consultations to live chats with doctors in chat rooms to organizing information events in various locations, the costs of which are invariably covered by the respective clinics. The »doctors' forums«[38] on ÇİDER's website, for example, offers people the possibility of writing directly to the doctors

37 Callon & Rabeharisoa, »The Growing Engagement of Emergent Concerned Groups«, op. cit. (note 3).

38 The »doctors' forums« are set up to enable concerned people to get a consultation via ÇİDER's website, where they can address »voluntary« doctors registered with ÇİDER. By filling in an online form they give all the medical information they have about themselves, details about diagnosis and prognosis, and about the operations and treatments both partners have already received, and are advised accordingly. Often both parties (doctors and »patients«) use these forums to make first contact, and notably »patients« frequently use them to get a first impression of doctors (and the clinics, in which they work).

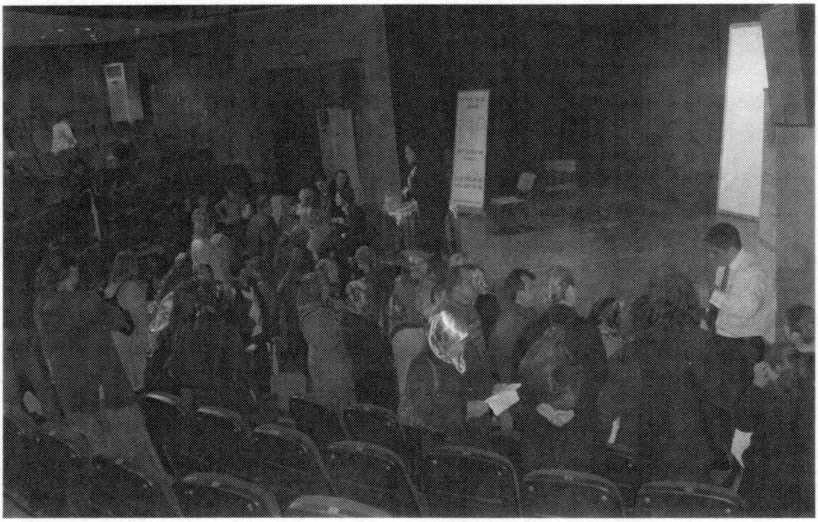

Figure 4: Talk with the doctor after a lottery, city of Ordu, April 2010. Photo by Nurhak Polat

to ask them for their professional opinion. In all these cooperations with doctors and/or clinics, information about the treatments offered by the cooperating clinics are made available on the homepage next to commercial advertisements appealing to the possible future consumers. A specific type of cooperation between ÇİDER and the clinics offers people a free first consultation in cooperating clinics if they become a member of the organization[39].

It is necessary to examine the situatedness and the asymmetries in the relationships of three actors: patient organizations, clinics/professional medical scientists, and »patients.« These complex relationships form part of a commercialized medical system directed towards »new forms«[40] of participation of laypeople and of medical consumerism. In the specific

39 The annual membership fee in 2010 is about 150 Turkish Lira. If a couple is not able to pay this fee, they may, on request still get a free first consultation in one of the associated clinics.

40 Adele E. Clarke, Janet K. Shim, Laura Mamo, Jennifer Ruth Fosket, Jennifer R. Fishman, »Biomedicalization: Technoscientific Transformations of Health, Illness, and U.S. Biomedicine«, in: *American Sociological Review* 68/2 (2003), pp. 161–194. See also Beck, »Die Mobilisierung der Erfahrung«, op. cit. (note 35).

context at hand, experience is seen as a knowledge resource and an interest-based resource that mobilizes medical and everyday contexts. It is important to note here that the experiential knowledge[41] of some of the laypeople is transformed into a multifaceted *concept* containing entangled political, social, and commercial aspects.

The rapidly growing access to knowledge blurs the boundaries of traditional actor positions in the medical sector (boundaries that for long have been viewed as robust) and affects social and institutional relationships. On the one hand, the position of the doctors is changing: in a highly capitalized and privatized area they become commercial actors themselves, follow commercial interests, and engage in directly commercial relationships with other doctors, institutes, and with their clients. On the other hand, the position of »patient« vis-à-vis doctors is also transformed in various ways. The growth of highly commercialized relationships in the field brings about a skeptical attitude of persons seeking medical help in the private sector and undermines older forms of trust characteristic of healing relationships. This change in patient-doctor relationships cannot be explained within the context of privatization and consumerism in medical encounters alone. It is also due to the changing position of biomedicine and to the increasing importance of scientific experts' knowledge in the daily lives of laypeople.

This changing position of laypeople leads to a distinction between ordinary laypersons and so-called lay experts, who in acquiring medical knowledge become »experts« on their own issues. It must be underlined that to a certain degree they are able to operate with both medical and experiential knowledge. They thus come into a position that is primarily seen as positive by other laypeople.

According to Callon and Çalışkan in their study about economization and marketization, socio-technical arrangements serve to »objectify« and »transform« objects, entities, or services »into packages, ›things‹ which can be valued.«[42] This can be read from the perspective of inequalities and asymmetries in the markets, which is important in the analysis of exclusions and inclusions, but also from the perspective of a domination based

41 Thomasina J. Borkman, »Experiential Knowledge«, op. cit. (note 9).

42 Koray Çalışkan & Michel Callon, »Economization, Part 2: A Research Programme for The Study of Markets«, in: *Economy and Society* 39 (2010), 1, pp. 1–32, here p. 7.

on »the gaps between unequal agencies.« To further illuminate this process, Callon proposes the French notion of *habilitation*, which »proffer[s] a capacity to act to someone who lacks it«: »The equipment required, for instance, for a liberal subject (either collective or individual) – who should be capable of interacting, defining objectives, calculating interests and even entering into sophisticated cooperative games – to be able to exist and act is particularly costly to obtain and is not equally distributed.«[43] The lack of such capabilities may then be filled by other agencies.

The notion of *habilitation* may be fruitful in examining the role of the concerned group ÇİDER, who became a new actor in the market. The group brings together providers of techno-scientific services and consumers. It creates its own network with marketing and managing strategies. It generates knowledge-based services in order to help people exist in the networking structures of contemporary markets. While building this network, ÇİDER positions certain actors like Sibel Tuzcu and the other founders of the organization as well as some of the active members as lay experts who take the lead role in building up close, emotional, and trust-based relationships with persons in need of or searching for advice and support. This implies a hierarchy amongst laypersons, some of whom have acquired the status of lay experts.

By networking and »knowledge work,«[44] ÇİDER generates new services that fulfill the needs of all parties concerned: Clinics (and also doctors) gain access to consumers by collaborating with the concerned group and by engaging in its social mission. Clients often need financial, social, emotional, and informational support in order to navigate the health system, especially in its privatized sectors, and »new« areas of knowledge. ÇİDER's relationship to clinics is not an unimportant reason to become a member, especially for people with insufficient financial resources.[45] The

43 Çalışkan & Callon, »Economization, Part 2«, op. cit. (note 42), p. 13.

44 Stefan Beck, »Mobilisierung der Erfahrung«, op. cit. (note 35), p. 237.

45 In a different context, Stefan Beck maintains that laypersons »inform themselves by way of antagonistic resources; [they must] consider [their options] on the basis of incomplete knowledge and make decisions.« This can lead them to the establishment of their own strategies. In the present context this should translate into conscious strategies of people who want to have children rather than individuals »controlled« by clinics and other interest-based organizations. They are acting as individuals guided by self-interest.

increasing dominance of the private sector in the area of reproductive medicine at the same times creates need and demand for these services. The great bureaucracy in the public sector and frustrated expectations in dealing with it often bring individuals or couples unable to cope with these structures to call upon the private sector where, however, costs of one treatment regularly exceed the average yearly income.

ÇİDER strives to create services within the framework of economic characteristics of the country. The necessity of the organization's increasing activity as an economic actor is often perceived and represented in terms of national regulations and financial circumstances. Tuzcu thus explains the importance of economic activism:

»[…] Because our country is a country with a low per-capita income; [in contrast] these [treatments] are generally quite expensive in Turkey, and for Turkish people they are [disproportionately] expensive. As the number of our patients is quite large, we can say [to the clinics], so-and-so many patients are coming to you, so lower your profits a bit. They [the members of European patient organizations] have difficulties in understanding this, because their income is large enough to pay for the treatment, and on top of this their countries will pay for up to 3 cycles or up to 2 cycles; our country also pays, but they don't make it easy [›*bin dereden su getirerek*‹].«[46]

The diverse and complex interests and strategies of the actors involved play a central role. These interests and strategies are the basis for the perceptions and needs on the local level – the changing patterns of the multi-dimensional relationships between the diverse actors in the field – but they are also negotiated with discourses beyond the local.

46 The regulation of funding introduced by the Ministry of Health on 09 February 2005 (Official Gazette no. 25722). According to this regulation, eligible couples insured by social security institutions have access to financial aid by the state for two cycles. Eligibility criteria for access to treatment both in private or state clinics are: infertility survey report by a state clinic, marriage for a minimum of three years, no live children of either partner and the age of the women must be 23–29. The couples need a report from a state hospital to get access to financial aid (www.saglik.gov.tr).

Transnational Networking

In this part of the paper I would like to examine ÇİDER's international entanglement with other concerned groups. This entanglement is visible at two levels: First, local concerned groups entertain relationships at a transnational level in order to achieve maximum political impact in their attempt to influence national, political, and social structures. One example of this is the *EIA (European Infertility Alliance)*. This organization brings together European concerned groups under a single banner. The EIA is a sub group of the *International Consumer Support for Infertility (iCSi)*,[47] and ÇİDER cooperates with both.

In 2002, the month of June was declared »World Fertility Awareness Month« (WorldFAM) by the iCSi to increase attention and knowledge regarding issues of fertility and infertility. One of the most important aims of this declaration was to underline the claim that infertility should be recognized as »a treatable disease.«[48] 25 organizations came together from around the world under the initiative of iCSi to organize WorldFAM in their countries under the slogan *Break the Silence*.

ÇİDER was one of the cooperating organizations for WorldFAM. In collaboration with many doctors from both the private and state sector, with politicians, with journalists who made the issue public, and with other professionals from the field of reproductive medicine, such as nurses, or psychologists, ÇİDER organized a number of events under the title *Sessizliğini Kır* (Break the Silence). Important themes were treated at a local level and were reported by Turkish media as the *Tüp Bebek Zirvesi*, »test-tube baby conference.«[49] The *Break the Silence* events were related to national problems, issues, and demands, that is to say, fertility difficulties were examined within the framework of local regulations and locally embedded cultural, socio-economic, and moral-ethical dimensions.

The idea behind this series of events was to make fertility problems visible, to make fertility treatments available for a wider audience, and to

47 iCSi brings together 39 national groups and organizes annual meetings in different countries. EIA attempts to influence politics at a European level by participating in biopolitical debates on regulations, but it also refers to personal and collective experiences.

48 http://www.journalmed.de/newsview.php?id=352.

49 http://www.habervitrini.com.

mobilize the concerned group itself at an administrative and regulative level. ÇİDER attempted to publicize the specific concerns of the involuntarily childless and consumers of ARTs and to actively take part in decision-making. With regard to the definition of infertility, the organization demanded its recognition as a »disease« by local legislation so that infertility »patients« would be eligible for state assistance and couples with insufficient financial resources would gain access to reproductive treatments. On the state level, in negotiating the fertility treatments and access to ARTs, ÇİDER has used statements of transnational norms, standards, and aims to influence the attitude of the public administration and relevant authorities, such as the Ministry of Health and the Ministry for Family Issues. After a long negotiation process they eventually succeeded in securing funding for two cycles of IVF by the Ministry of Health and social security institutions.[50] This demonstrates how transnational and local discourses come into contact and are entangled with one another at a local level in order to push through local demands. The international networking gave the concerned group ÇİDER a basis for its recognition and justification and increased its negotiating power in local power structures.

Conclusion

The purpose of this paper was to discuss some aspects of reproductive technologies in the Turkish context in an attempt to argue that the emergence of the concerned group ÇİDER is embedded in generating and managing diverse forms of knowledge and in operating new knowledge practices. These knowledge practices are directly linked to the dynamics of local social and economic structures. In dealing with personal experiences with IVF and involuntary childlessness and with the social circumstances in which these experiences are made, the concerned group creates a space for itself and becomes a new actor in this field.

ÇİDER operates with notions like *bilinç* (or *bilinçli patient*) and *bilinçlendirmek*, which have a great historical depth reaching back to the Turkish modernization process and beyond. In doing so, it triggers a trans-

50 For the regulation of financial aid through the state see note 46.

formation of existing relationships and constellations and the creation of new categories. On the one hand these notions blur the strict separation of medical experts and laypeople, on the other hand they create a new division between lay experts and ordinary persons who come in contact with ART and with the medical sector. In order to understand the notional shift from patient to consumer and from participant to lay expert in a local context, it is important to look at the encounters between different discourses and the practices of the actors involved. One of the main arguments of the paper is that the relationships enabled by ÇİDER and the mobilization of experience-near narratives and experiential knowledge have a strong influence on the co-production of the reproductive medical sector and local discourses. The growing use of »new« communication and information technologies (such as the Internet) makes it possible to mobilize new forms of knowledge and participation. The example of the *gün* women's group and the narration of »success stories« show that these kinds of relationships and interactions affect the decision-making processes, the motivation to »have a try,« and the creation of personal actor rationalities, logics, and »other« truths. The narrative technologies of hope and success and the performative sharing of them trigger these rationalities, logics, and truths.

In the case of ÇİDER, it is possible to speak of the simultaneous emergence of an economization and mobilization of (personal and/or collective) experience. This is one of the main factors for the proliferation of the concerned groups as »new« actors in the political, private, and economic sphere. The structures of contemporary economic markets and the privatization of the medical sector play a crucial role in the newly emerging forms of concerned group participation. ÇİDER creates its own strategies in managing new services, but it also operates within the structures of networking markets. In a »simultaneous production« of the local and transnational, it develops its own pragmatic way of validating transnational discourses and transferring them into local discourse in an attempt to gain political power, to improve visibility, and to gain access to the local regulative levels.

Tracing Transnational Scapes of Reproductive Technologies: Emergent Forms and Domains of Regulation

Globalization and Gametes: Reproductive »Tourism,« Islamic Bioethics, and Middle Eastern Modernity

Marcia C. Inhorn

Introduction

What motivates the global movements of infertile people searching for new reproductive technologies and human gametes? Inspired by recent developments in globalization theory, medical anthropology, gender studies, and science and technology studies, this chapter focuses on the newly described phenomenon of »reproductive tourism,« also known as »fertility tourism,« »procreative tourism,« and »cross-border reproductive care« (CBRC). Reproductive tourism is defined as »the traveling by candidate service recipients from one institution, jurisdiction or country where treatment is not available to another institution, jurisdiction or country where they can obtain the kind of medically assisted reproduction they desire. As such, it is part of the more general ›medical tourism.‹«[1]

Little is known about the motivations of reproductive tourists in any part of the world. A front-page story in *The New York Times* on January 25, 2005, entitled »Fertility Tourists Go Great Lengths to Conceive,« claimed that infertile Americans were seeking services abroad, »in places like South Africa, Israel, Italy, Germany, and Canada, where the costs can be much lower.«[2] However, economic factors may not be the sole consideration. Scholars who are beginning to theorize the relationship between nation-

1 Guido Pennings, »Reproductive Tourism as Moral Pluralism in Motion«, in: *Journal of Medical Ethics* 28 (2002), pp. 337–341.

2 Felicia R. Lee, »Fertility Tourists Go Great Lengths to Conceive«, in: *The New York Times* [25.1.2005). Lee is mistaken about Germany as a major hub of reproductive »tourism.« Because of a strict law regarding ova donation, embryo transfer, embryo selection and preimplantation genetic diagnosis, few reproductive tourists travel to Germany. Rather, German reproductive tourists travel out of the country, to Spain, Belgium, the Czech Republic, the United States, and India, among others.

states, reproductive tourism, and global reproductive rights suggest that the causes of such transnational tourism may be manifold. Eight discrete, but often interrelated, factors promoting reproductive tourism have been cited in the existing literature: 1) individual countries may prohibit a specific service for religious or ethical reasons; 2) a specific service may be unavailable because of lack of expertise, equipment, or lack of donor gametes (eggs, sperm, or embryos); 3) a service may be unavailable because it is not considered sufficiently safe or its risks are unknown, so that countries exercising safety precautions may prohibit procedures that are available elsewhere; 4) certain categories of individuals may not receive a service, especially at public expense, on the basis of age, marital status, or sexual orientation; 5) services operate on a market or quasi-market basis, particularly in relation to donor gametes, thus affecting both affordability and supply (including shortages and waiting lists); 6) services may simply be cheaper in other countries; 7) patients may have concerns about low-quality medical services; and 8) finally, privacy concerns may lead some patients to travel.[3]

These »causes« of reproductive tourism are still speculative, as little empirical research has yet to be undertaken. Yet even in the absence of empirical data, a policy debate is growing over the desirability of national and international legislation to restrict reproductive tourism. As Penning notes in *The Journal of Medical Ethics*, »The more widespread this phenomenon, the louder the call for international measures to stop these movements.«[4]

Most of the extant literature on reproductive tourism focuses on the West, particularly upon border-crossing between European Union nations.[5] Little is known about reproductive tourism outside of Euro-America, or about the forces that motivate infertile persons to undertake international travel in their »quests for conception«[6]. Only through in-

3 See Eric Blyth & Abigail Farrand, »Reproductive Tourism – A Price Worth Paying for Reproductive Autonomy?«, in: *Critical Social Policy* 25 (2005), pp. 91–114; Ruth Deech, »Reproductive Tourism in Europe: Infertility and Human Rights«, in: *Global Governance* 9 (2003), pp. 425–432; or Pennings, »Reproductive Tourism«, op. cit. (note 1), pp. 337–341.

4 Pennings, »Reproductive Tourism«, op. cit. (note 1), pp. 337.

5 Richard F. Storrow, »Quests for Conception: Fertility Tourists, Globalization, and Feminist Legal Theory«, in: *Hastings Law Journal* 57 (2005), pp. 295–330.

6 Marcia C. Inhorn, *Quest for Conception: Gender, Infertility, and Egyptian Medical Traditions* (Philadelphia: University of Pennsylvania Press, 1994).

depth ethnographic analysis of the actual stories, desires, and migratory pathways of reproductive tourists themselves may scholars begin to shed light on the complex calculus of factors governing this global movement of reproductive actors.

This chapter examines the theoretical interplay between forces of globalization and reproductive tourism in the Middle East.[7] It will begin with Arjun Appadurai's theory of global »scapes,« which is highly relevant and useful in thinking about the global landscape in which assisted reproductive technologies (ARTs) are being rapidly deployed. However, Appadurai's work needs to be »engendered« and expanded to include the complex »reproscape« in which the multiple »flows« of reproductive tourism occur. In the global reproscape, issues of bodily commodification are paramount, given that reproductive tourism may be undertaken explicitly to procure human gametes, both sperm and eggs, which are disassociated from men's and women's bodies and increasingly sold on the open market. Furthermore, the language of reproductive »tourism« itself comes into question when the subjectivities of reproductive travelers themselves are taken into consideration. In short, a whole new vocabulary is needed to represent the global flows and scapes surrounding ARTs in the new millennium.

The second half of the chapter turns to the author's empirical work on reproductive tourism in the Muslim Middle East, based on ethnographic research carried out there over the past 20 years, but particularly since the year 2003.[8]As will be argued, reproductive »tourism« in the Middle East is inflected by local moral attitudes toward science, technology, and

7 This chapter is based on my article, »Globalization and Gametes: Reproductive ›Tourism,‹ Islamic Bioethics, and Middle Eastern Modernity«, part of a special issue on »Healing Holidays? Itinerant Patients, Therapeutic Locales and the Quest for Health«, guest edited by Harish Naraindas & Cristiana Bastos, *Anthropology & Medicine* 17 (2010), 3. Reprinted with minor editorial amendments and with permission of the publisher (Taylor & Francis Ltd, http://www.informaworld.com).

8 This article is based on long-term ethnographic fieldwork conducted in multiple Middle Eastern countries, including Egypt, Lebanon, United Arab Emirates and Iran as well as »Arab Detroit.« It represents nearly 600 Middle Eastern couples (primarily from Egypt, Lebanon, Syria, Palestine, the United Arab Emirates, Iraq, and Yemen). This article is based primarily on my two most recent studies, one on male infertility carried out in Beirut, Lebanon in 2003, and the other on reproductive tourism carried out in the United Arab Emirates in 2007. In addition, fieldwork among infertile Arab Americans took place from 2003 to 2005 and 2007 to 2008.

medicine, as well as varying Islamic bioethical positions on the donation of human gametes. Furthermore, the implications of gamete donation for marriage, kinship, and gender relations are tremendous, perhaps especially for infertile Muslim couples. But first, it is important to situate this topic of reproductive tourism – and the search for human gametes in the Middle East – within the broader theoretical literature on globalization and specifically global flows.

Globalization and Reproductive Tourism: Theorizing Reproscapes

Globalization can be understood, in a most basic sense, »as the ever faster and ever denser streams of people, images, consumer goods, money markets, and communication networks around the world.«[9] Anthropologists have contributed significantly to theorizing the nature of these global flows – and to providing numerous ethnographic examples of the »glocal,« or the reception of things »global« at various »local« levels.[10]

One of the major anthropological theorists of globalization, Arjun Appadurai, has delineated a »global cultural economy« in which global movements operate through five pathways, which he famously calls

9 Birgit Schaebler & Leif Stenberg, *Globalization and the Muslim World: Culture, Religion, and Modernity* (Syracuse, NY: Syracuse University Press, 2004), pp. xv-xvi.

10 For examples see Arjun Appadurai, *Modernity at Large: Cultural Dimensions of Globalization* (Minneapolis: University of Minnesota Press, 1996); Linda Basch, Nina Glick Schiller & Cristina Szanton Blanc, *Nations Unbound: Transnational Projects, Postcolonial Predicaments, and Deterritorialized Nation-States* (Langhorne, PA: Gordon and Breach, 1994); Jonathan Friedman, *Cultural Identity and Global Process* (London: Sage, 1994); Ulf Hannerz, *Transnational Connections: Culture, People, Places* (London: Routledge, 1996); Marcia C. Inhorn, *Local Babies, Global Science: Gender, Religion, and In Vitro Fertilization in Egypt* (New York: Routledge, 2003); Ted C. Lewellen, *The Anthropology of Globalization: Cultural Anthropology Enters the 21st Century* (Westport, CT: Bergin and Garvey, 2002); Aihwa Ong & Stephen J. Collier (Eds.), *Global Assemblages: Technology, Politics, and Ethics as Anthropological Problems* (Malden, MA: Blackwell, 2005); George Ritzer (Ed.), *McDonaldization: The Reader* (Thousand Oaks, CA: Pine Forge Press, 2002); or James Watson (Ed.), *Golden Arches East: McDonald's in East Asia* (Stanford, CA: Stanford University Press, *1997*).

»scapes.«[11] According to Appadurai, globalization is characterized by the movement of people (ethnoscapes), technology (technoscapes), money (financescapes), images (mediascapes), and ideas (ideoscapes), which now follow increasingly complex trajectories, moving at different speeds across the globe. Appadurai reminds us that this transnational movement of people, goods, and ideas is both a deeply historical and inherently localizing process. In other words, globalization is not enacted in a uniform manner around the world, nor is it simply culturally homogenizing in its effects.

The phenomenon of reproductive tourism clearly involves two of Appadurai's five scapes – namely, ethnoscapes and technoscapes. Ethnoscapes, according to Appadurai, involve »the landscape of persons who constitute the shifting world in which we live: tourists, immigrants, refugees, exiles, guest workers, and other moving groups and individuals.« [12] Technoscapes involve »the global configuration, also ever fluid, of technology and the fact that technology, both high and low, both mechanical and informational, now moves at high speeds across various kinds of previously impervious boundaries.«[13]

However, a consideration of reproductive tourism has the potential to expand upon Appadurai's theory of globalization. Despite the heuristic appeal of five discrete global scapes, one scape of significant medical anthropological interest – namely, the *bioscape* of moving biological substances and body parts – might be added to Appadurai's list.[14] Using Appadurai's language of »scapes,« reproductive tourism might be productively thought of as a more complex reproscape – a kind of »meta-scape« combining numerous dimensions of globalization and global flows. To wit, reproductive tourism occurs in a new world order characterized not only by circulating reproductive technologies (technoscapes), but

11 Arjun Appadurai, »Disjuncture and Difference in the Global Cultural Economy«, in: *Global Culture: Nationalism, Globalization and Identity*, ed. by Mike Featherstone (London: Sage, 1990), pp. 296–308; Appadurai, »Modernity at Large«, op. cit. (note 10).

12 Appadurai, »Modernity at Large«, op. cit. (note 10), p. 33.

13 Ibid., p. 34.

14 The term »bioscape« is my own, but bespeaks the strong Foucauldian influences on medical anthropology, where terms such as »biopower,« »biopolitics,« »biocitizenship,« »bioavailability,« and »biocrossings« are becoming common parlance.

also by circulating reproductive actors (ethnoscapes) and their gametes (bioscapes), leading to a large-scale global industry (financescapes), in which images (mediascapes) and ideas (ideoscapes) about making lovely babies while »on holiday« come into play. This reproscape entails a distinct geography traversed by global flows of reproductive actors, technologies, body parts, money, and reproductive imaginaries (e.g., the birth of »miracle« babies).

Furthermore, this reproscape is highly gendered, with technologies enacted on men's and women's bodies in differentiated ways. Gender was never the focus of Appadurai's original work on globalization. Yet the ethnoscape of moving peoples, the technoscape of moving technologies, the bioscape of moving body parts, and the ideoscape of moving procreative scenarios are, indeed, highly gendered, and this is a feature of globalization that must be analyzed. Reproscapes also entail new forms of reproductive labor among reproductive »assistors,« who in many cases are women and who undergo risky forms of hormonal stimulation and oocyte (egg) harvesting. However, reproductive assistance also has the potential to create kin-like female alliances, between actual kin who donate their oocytes to relatives as well as between unrelated women who »share« their oocytes with other women in infertility clinics or donate them for a fee. Oocyte donation in particular invokes the notion of altruistic »gift exchange« between women, even though oocytes are increasingly sold on the reproductive marketplace for up to $50,000, especially for »Ivy League« oocytes of presumed superior intelligence and other ineffable qualities.[15] Indeed, the very language of *reproductive assistance* is called into question when assistance comes at such a high cost.

In addition, using the language of *reproductive tourism* to define this field of global flows is a bit of a misnomer.[16] It is important to note that, in some countries, »clinics that cater to fertility tourists appear to welcome the development of new markets and have undertaken to market their services so as to create a fantasy of conceiving a child during a romantic

15 The term »Ivy League« connotes the most prestigious universities in the United States, including the »triumvirate« of Harvard, Yale, and Princeton. Affluent couples often place advertisements seeking the services of egg donors who are »Ivy League« college students – and thus presumed to be particularly intelligent.

16 Marcia C. Inhorn. & Pasquale Patrizio, »Rethinking Reproductive ›Tourism‹ as Reproductive ›Exile‹«, in: *Fertility and Sterility* 92 (2009), pp. 904–906.

holiday.«[17] But is overseas test-tube baby-making a holiday? In his excellent theoretical analysis of reproductive tourism, legal theorist Richard Storrow (2005) questions the trope of »tourism« as an appropriate gloss for fertility travel. As he notes, tourism is a type of traveling that involves leisure, pleasure, and free time. Fertility tourism, on the other hand, is quite a different story:

»Fertility tourism occurs when infertile individuals or couples travel abroad for the purposes of obtaining medical treatment for their infertility. Fertility tourism may also occur in the reverse, when the infertile import the third parties necessary for their fertility treatment. These definitions of fertility tourism are, on the one hand, difficult to harmonize with the idea of tourism as pleasure travel, particularly given that some infertile individuals describe their condition as devastatingly painful and their effort to relieve it as requiring enormous physical and emotional exertion.«[18]

More neutral terms, such as *reproductive travel* or *cross-border reproductive care* (CBRC), are beginning to enter the clinical lexicon.[19] However, the use of the term *reproductive exile* more accurately captures the feelings and experiences of many infertile couples who feel »forced« to travel to seek ART assistance across borders. Indeed, the term »tourism« must be avoided, for it can never fully capture the stories of travel and hardship experienced by the infertile in their border-crossings. The term »tourism« will be dispensed with for the remainder of this chapter.

Moreover, the notion of *stratified reproduction*, introduced by Shellee Colen in medical anthropologists Faye Ginsburg and Rayna Rapp's seminal volume *Conceiving the New World Order* (1995), comes into play.[20] Stratified reproduction evokes transnational inequalities whereby some well-to-do infertile couples are able to achieve their reproductive desires, including through resort to reproductive technologies and reproductive travel, while others infertile couples of lesser means are disempowered and even despised as reproducers. Only 48 of the 191 member states of the

17 Storrow, »Quests for Conception«, op. cit. (note 5), pp. 326–327.

18 Ibid., p. 300.

19 Inhorn & Patrizio, »Rethinking Reproductive ›Tourism‹«, op. cit. (note 16).

20 Shellee Colen, »›Like a Mother to Them‹: Stratified Reproduction and the West Indian Childcare Workers and Their Employers«, in: *Conceiving the New World Orlder: The Global Politics of Reproduction*, ed. by Faye D. Ginsberg & Rayna Rapp (Berkeley: University of California Press, 1995), pp. 78–102.

World Health Organization offer ARTs to their citizens, with less than one percent of the projected needs for ARTs met in some of the largest countries of the world (China, India, Pakistan, Indonesia). In these countries, the average cost of one cycle of IVF exceeds the average income of half the population, making ARTs easily affordable only for elites.[21] In other words, the global »reproscape« in which reproductive tourism takes place is an uneven terrain in that some individuals, some communities, and some nations have achieved greater access to the fruits of reproductive globalization than others. The term »stratified reproscape« might be added to the lexicon to describe the unevenness of ART access around the world.[22]

In my earlier studies of in vitro fertilization in Egypt, which were characterized as a *quest for conception*,[23] I examined numerous local barriers to ART access, calling these *arenas of constraint*, meaning the structural, ideological, social relational, and practical obstacles and apprehensions that constrain and sometimes prohibit altogether the uses of ARTs.[24] More than a decade later, little is known about the various arenas of constraint that face infertile couples in their *transnational quests for conception.*

However, one of the major prohibitions cited by legal scholars who have written about reproductive tourism are prohibitions on access to human gametes.[25] Several Western nations, including Germany, Italy, Norway, Canada, and Great Britain, have enacted strict legislation prohibiting some or all forms of gamete donation, especially anonymous gamete donation, as well as gestational surrogacy. Such restrictions have triggered European fertility tourism on a massive scale, mostly of infertile Western Europeans to the post-Soviet bloc of Eastern Europe such as Russia, Slovenia, or Romania. There, clinics can »employ the Internet to attract fertility tourists with promises of cut-rate in vitro fertilization, high success rates, liberal reproductive policies and little administrative oversight.«[26]

21 Inhorn, »Local Babies, Global Science«, op. cit. (note 10).

22 Thanks to one of the reviewers for suggesting this composite term.

23 Inhorn, »Quest for Conception«, op. cit. (note 6).

24 Inhorn, »Local Babies, Global Science«, op. cit. (note 10).

25 Blyth & Farrand, »Reproductive Tourism – A Price Worth Paying?«, op. cit. (note 3); Deech, »Reproductive Tourism in Europe«, op. cit. (note 3); Pennings, »Reproductive Tourism«, op. cit. (note 1).

26 Storrow, »Quests for Conception«, op. cit. (note 5), p. 307.

Furthermore, young women in these countries may comprise a vulnerable population of egg donors, who are compelled out of economic necessity to sell their ova in the local reproductive marketplace.[27] Given the newly recognized category of the »traveling foreign egg donor« who seeks economic mobility through the sale of her body parts,[28] Storrow points to the parallels between unregulated fertility tourism and sex tourism, as young women in the economically deteriorated postcommunist societies discover that prostitution and egg donation offer economic rewards. As Storrow argues, »egg donation, like prostitution, will be especially attractive in regions of the world where large numbers of women with few choices want to improve their economic circumstances by any means available.«[29]

Indeed, »bodily commodification« – the selling of gametes and other body parts for the purposes of reproduction and medical research – has become one of the major areas of study in both medical anthropology and science and technology studies.[30] Bodily penetration, fragmentation, and commodification are clearly operative in the world of assisted reproduction, a world that has evolved dramatically since the birth of Louise Brown, the world's first »test-tube baby,« in 1978. Since then, the invention of in vitro fertilization (IVF) to overcome female infertility has paved the way for:

27 Ibid.

28 Boon Chin Heng, »Regulatory Safeguards Needed for the Travelling Foreign Egg Donor«, in: *Human Reproduction* 22 (2007), pp. 2350–2352.

29 Storrow, »Quests for Conception«, op. cit. (note 5), p. 327.

30 For example see Lawrence Cohen, »Where it Hurts: Indian Material for an Ethics of Organ Transplantation«, in: *Daedalus* 128 (1999), pp. 135–164; Lawrence Cohen, »The Other Kidney: Biopolitics beyond Recognition«, in: *Commodifying Bodies*, ed. by Nancy Scheper-Hughes & Loic Wacquant (London: Sage, 2002), pp. 9–29; Margaret Lock, *Twice Dead: Organ Transplants and the Reinvention of Death* (Berkeley: University of California Press, 2002); Nancy Scheper-Hughes, »The Global Traffic in Human Organs«, in: *Current Anthropology* 41 (2000), pp. 191–211; Nancy Scheper-Hughes, »Bodies for Sale – Whole or in Parts«, in: *Commodifying Bodies*, ed. by Nancy Scheper-Hughes & Loic Wacquant (London: Sage, 2002a), pp.1–8; Nancy Scheper-Hughes, »The Ends of the Body: Commodity Fetishism and the Global Traffic in Organs«, in: *SAIS Review* 23 (2002b), pp. 61–80; Lesley A. Sharp, *Strange Harvest: Organ Transplants, Denatured Bodies, and the Transformed Self* (Berkeley: University of California Press, 2006); or Lesley A. Sharp, »The Commodification of the Body and Its Parts«, in: *Annual Review of Anthropology* 29 (2000), pp. 287–328.

1. intracytoplasmic injection (ICSI) to overcome male infertility;
2. third-party gamete donation (of eggs, sperm, embryos, and uteruses, as in surrogacy) to overcome absolute sterility;
3. multifetal pregnancy reduction to selectively abort high-order IVF pregnancies;
4. ooplasm transfer (OT) to improve egg quality in perimenopausal women;
5. cryopreservation, storage, and disposal of unused gametes and embryos;
6. preimplantation genetic diagnosis (PGD) to select »against« embryos with genetic defects and to select »for« embryos of a specific sex;
7. embryonic stem cell research on unused embryos for the purposes of therapeutic intervention; and
8. the future possibility of asexual autonomous reproduction through human cloning.

With virtually all of these technologies, sperm and eggs are retrieved from bodies, embryos are returned to bodies, and sometimes they are donated to other bodies or used for the purposes of stem cell and other forms of medical research.[31] As noted earlier, ARTs exact a significant physical toll on the body, especially for women as both recipients of ARTs and as oocyte donors.[32] Furthermore, despite the existence of national and international statements opposing the commercialization of ART services, significant commodification has occurred as gametes and embryos are increasingly sold on the open market through Internet websites and college newspapers

31 Sarah Franklin, *Embodied Progress: A Cultural Account of Assisted Conception* (London: Routledge, 1996); Susan Martha Kahn, *Reproducing Jews: A Cultural Account of Assisted Conception in Israel* (Durham, NC: Duke University Press, 2000); Maggie Kirkman, »Egg and Embryo Donation and the Meaning of Motherhood«, in: *Women & Health* 38 (2003), pp. 1–18; Monica Konrad, »Ova Donation and Symbols of Substance: Some Variations on the Theme of Sex, Gender and the Partible Body«, in: *The Journal of the Royal Anthropological Institute* 4 (1998), pp. 643–667.

32 Inhorn, »Local Babies, Global Science«, op. cit. (note 10); Kahn, »Reproducing Jews«, op. cit. (note 31); Judith Lorber »Choice, Gift, or Patriarchal Bargain? Women's Consent to In vitro Fertilization in Male Infertility«, in: *Hypatia* 4 (1989), pp. 23–36; Storrow, »Quests for Conception«, op. cit. (note 5); Irma van der Ploeg, »Hermaphrodite Patients: In vitro Fertilization and the Transformation of Male Infertility«, in: *Science, Technology, & Human Values* 20 (1995), 4, pp. 460–481.

(with such advertisements as »Sperm Donors Needed – We Will Pay!«).[33] In her article on »Reproductive Tourism in Europe,« Ruth Deech questions the human rights implications of the documented massive transfer within the European Union of sperm, eggs, and embryos »passed from country to country in search of one that permits the desired treatment or allows the chosen gametes to be used.«[34]

The Middle East is different from the EU countries in terms of its attitudes toward the commodification and bodily transfer of human gametes. In the Middle East, an ART industry is flourishing, with hundreds of IVF clinics in countries ranging from the small Arab Gulf states to the larger but less prosperous nations of North Africa.[35] This florescence of a mostly private Middle Eastern ART industry is not surprising: Islam encourages the use of science and medicine as solutions to human suffering and is a religion that can be described as »pronatalist,« encouraging the growth of an Islamic »multitude.«[36]

33 Robert Blank, »Regulation of Donor Insemination«, in: *Donor Insemination: International Social Science Perspectives*, ed. by Ken Daniels & Erica Haimes (Cambridge, England: Cambridge University Press, 1998), pp. 131–150; Andrea M. Braverman, »Exploring Ovum Donors' Motivations and Needs«, in: *The American Journal of Bioethics* 1 (2001), pp. 16–17; Yoram S. Carmeli & Daphna Birenbaum-Carmeli, »Ritualizing the ›Natural Family‹: Secrecy in Israeli Donor Insemination«, in: *Science As Culture* 9 (2000), pp. 301–324; Anne Pollock, »Complicating Power in High-Tech Reproduction: Narratives of Anonymous Paid Egg Donors«, in: *Journal of Medical Humanities* 24 (2003), pp. 241–263; Mary Lyndon Shanley, »Collaboration and Commodification in Assisted Procreation: Reflections on an Open Market and Anonymous Donation in Human Sperm and Eggs«, in: *Law & Society Review* 36 (2002), pp. 257–283; Charis M. Thompson, *Making Parents: The Ontological Choreography of Reproductive Technologies* (Cambridge, MA: MIT Press, 2005).

34 Deech, »Reproductive Tourism in Europe«, op. cit. (note 3), p. 425.

35 Inhorn, »Local Babies, Global Science«, op. cit. (note 10); Gamal I. Serour, »Islamic Perspectives in Human Reproduction«, in: *Reproductive BioMedicine Online* 17 (2008), Suppl. 3, pp. 34–38; Gamal I. Serour, »Bioethics in Reproductive Health: A Muslim's Perspective«, in: *Middle East Fertility Society Journal* 1 (1996), pp. 30–35; Gamal I. Serour & Bernard M. Dickens, »Assisted Reproduction Developments in the Islamic World«, in: *International Journal of Gynecology & Obstetrics* 74 (2001), pp. 187–193.

36 Jonathan E. Brockopp (Ed.), *Islamic Ethics of Life: Abortion, War, and Euthanasia* (Columbia: University of South Carolina Press, 2003); Inhorn, »Quest for Conception«, op. cit. (note 6); B. F. Musallam, *Sex and Society in Islam: Birth Control before the Nineteenth Century* (Cambridge, UK: Cambridge University Press, 1986).

Yet relatively little is known about Islam and technoscience, if technoscience is defined broadly as the interconnectedness between science and technology through »epistemological, institutional, and cultural discursive practices.«[37] As noted by Lotfalian in his recent monograph on *Islam, Technoscientific Identities, and the Culture of Curiosity*,[38] there is a glaring lacuna in the literature on science and technology in cross-cultural perspective, particularly from the Islamic world, where there are »really only two strains of relevant work« – first, on the Islamic medieval sciences and, second, on philosophical arguments for civilizational differences between Islamic and Western science and technology. This dearth of relevant scholarship clearly applies to the cross-cultural study of ARTs. For example, in the second edition of the seminal volume on *Third Party Assisted Conception Across Cultures: Social, Legal and Ethical Perspectives*,[39] not a single Muslim society is represented among the thirteen country case studies.

Clearly, the time has come to examine the globalization of ARTs in the diverse contexts of the Muslim world, particularly given the rapid development and deployment of these technologies. In addition to examining the ART »technoscape,« it is equally important to examine the »ethnoscape« of reproductive actors as they move across the Middle East. ARTs in the Middle East bespeak a complex reproscape of moving peoples, technologies, gametes, money, images, and ideas involving the pursuit of conception. That infertile couples are willing to participate in this Middle Eastern reproscape bespeaks the love, commitment, and ardent desire for children that characterize most couples in the Middle East, but which are rarely emphasized in Western media discourses about the purported violence, fanaticism, and cruelty of Arab men to women.[40] As will be shown in the story of an infertile Syrian couple that follows, the romantic love and conjugal commitments between many infertile Muslim couples are fueling the

37 Mazyar Lotfalian, *Islam, Technoscientific Identities, and the Culture of Curiosity* (Dallas: University Press of America, 2004), p. 1.

38 Lotfalian, »Islam«, op. cit. (note 37), in particular p. 6.

39 Eric Blyth & Ruth Landau (Eds.), *Third Party Assisted Conception across Cultures: Social, Legal and Ethical Perspectives* (London: Jessica Kingsley, 2004).

40 Marcia C. Inhorn, »Loving Your Infertile Muslim Spouse: Notes on the Globalization of IVF and Its Romantic Commitments in Sunni Egypt and Shia Lebanon«, in: *Love and Globalization: Transformations of Intimacy in the Contemporary World*, eds. Mark B. Padilla, Jennifer S. Hirsch, Miguel Munoz-Laboy, Robert E. Sember, and Richard G. Parker, (Nashville: Vanderbilt U. Press, 2007), pp. 139–160.

IVF industry in the Middle East. Love, commitment, and the desire to become parents are also causing some couples to venture abroad in search of gametes.

The Middle Eastern Reproscape: Understanding Islamic Local Moral Worlds

What motivates infertile Middle Eastern couples to travel overseas in search of ARTs? Although there are a wide variety of motivating factors behind reproductive travel,[41] anthropologists and other scholars studying ARTs in the Middle East have called attention to Islam and the so-called local moral worlds of Middle Eastern Muslim infertile couples. Indeed, nearly a dozen scholars are now participating in this scholarly endeavor.[42]

Arthur Kleinman has called local moral worlds »the commitments of social participants in a local world about what is at stake in everyday experience.«[43] Understanding the rapidly evolving moral-religious climate surrounding ARTs in the Muslim world is imperative. To do so requires examining *fatwa*s, or non-legally binding but authoritative religious decrees, as well as the subsequent ethical and legal rulings that are being issued to enforce or, in some cases, overturn these *fatwa* rulings.[44] However, understanding local moral worlds also involves asking what Muslim ART-seekers think about IVF and specifically donor technologies. When faced with the need for donor gametes to overcome infertility, what do

41 Maria C. Inhorn & Pankaj Shrivastav, »Globalization and Reproductive Tourism in the United Arab Emirates«, in: *Asia-Pacific Journal of Public Health* 22 (2010), 3, pp. 68–74.

42 Marcia C. Inhorn & Soraya Tremayne (Eds.), *Islam and the Biotechnologies of Human Life* (New York: Berghahn Books, in press).

43 Arthur Kleinman, *Writing at the Margin: Discourse between Anthropology and Medicine* (Berkeley: University of California Press, 1995), p. 45.

44 Inhorn & Tremayne, »Islam and the Biotechnologies«, op. cit. (note 42); Ebrahim Moosa, »Human Cloning in Muslim Ethics«, in: *Voices Across Boundaries* (Fall 2003), pp. 23–26; Soraya Tremayne, »Law, Ethics, and Donor Technologies in Shia Iran«, in: *Assisting Reproduction, Testing Genes: Global Encounters with New Biotechnologies*, ed. by Daphna Birenbaum-Carmeli & Marcia C. Inhorn (New York: Berghahn Books, 2009), pp. 144–163.

Muslim IVF patients do? Is the search for human gametes one of the major motivating factors for reproductive tourism in the Middle East, as suggested by the theoretical literature on this phenomenon? At this point, these questions provide compelling material for a study of what might be called »technoscience in practice.«

As explained in the forthcoming volume *Islam and the Biotechnologies of Human Life*,[45] major divergences in Islamic juridical opinion between Sunni and Shia religious authorities have led to striking differences in the practice of ARTs, particularly with regard to the use of donor gametes. These differences in practice have led to new local moral worlds among Muslim IVF patients, as well as new transnational reproflows across Middle Eastern borders. The differences in the dominant Sunni position on ARTs will be briefly described before turning to Shia innovations that have had major moral and practical implications for Muslim couples in their quests for donor gametes.

Sunni Islam and IVF

The Grand Sheikh of Egypt's famed religious university, Al Azhar, issued the first *fatwa* on medically assisted reproduction on March 23, 1980. This initial *fatwa* – issued only two years after Louise Brown's birth in England, but a full six years before the opening of Egypt's first IVF center – has proved to be truly authoritative and enduring in all its main points. In fact, the basic tenets of the original Al-Azhar *fatwa* on IVF have been upheld by other *fatwa*s issued since 1980 in Egypt, Saudi Arabia, Malaysia, and beyond, thereby achieving wide acceptance across the Sunni Muslim world.[46]

The Sunni Islamic position on assisted reproduction clearly permits in vitro fertilization using eggs from the wife with the sperm of her husband and the transfer of the fertilized embryos back to the uterus of the same wife. However, since marriage is a contract between the wife and

45 Inhorn & Tremayne, »Islam and the Biotechnologies«, op. cit. (note 42).

46 Marcia C. Inhorn, Pasquale Patrizio & Gamal I. Serour, »Third-party Reproductive Assistance around the Mediterranean: Comparing Sunni Egypt, Catholic Italy, and Multi-sectarian Lebanon«, in: *Islam and the Biotechnologies of Human Life,* ed. by Marcia C. Inhorn & Soraya Tremayne (New York: Berghahn Books, in press); Serour, »Islamic Perspectives«, op. cit. (note 35).

husband during the span of their marriage, no third party should intrude into the marital functions of sex and procreation. This means that a third party donor is *not* acceptable, whether he or she is providing sperm, eggs, embryos, or a uterus (as in surrogacy). As noted by Islamic legal scholar Ebrahim Moosa,

»In terms of ethics, Muslim authorities consider the transmission of reproductive material between persons who are not legally married to be a major violation of Islamic law. This sensitivity stems from the fact that Islamic law has a strict taboo on sexual relations outside wedlock (*zina*). The taboo is designed to protect paternity (i.e., family), which is designated as one of the five goals of Islamic law, the others being the protection of religion, life, property, and reason.«[47]

As a result, at the ninth Islamic law and medicine conference, held under the auspices of the Kuwait-based Islamic Organization for Medical Sciences (IOMS) in Casablanca, Morocco in 1997, a landmark five-point declaration included recommendations to prevent human cloning and to prohibit all situations in which a third party invades a marital relationship through the donation of reproductive material.[48] Such a ban on third-party gamete donation is effectively in place in the Sunni world, which represents approximately 80–90% of the world's 1.4 billion Muslims.[49]

In interviews conducted by the author with hundreds of Sunni Muslim IVF patients, they agree completely with the religious prohibitions on gamete donation, arguing that gamete donation: 1) is tantamount to adultery, by virtue of introducing a third party into the sacred dyad of husband and wife; 2) creates the potential for future half-sibling incest, if the offspring of the same anonymous donor should happen to meet and marry; and 3) confuses kinship, paternity, descent, and inheritance in the emphatically patrilineal societies of the Muslim Middle East. According to them, preserving the »origins« of each child – meaning its relationship

47 Moosa, »Human Cloning«, op. cit. (note 44), p. 23.

48 Ibid., op. cit. (note 44).

49 Inhorn, »Local Babies, Global Science«, op. cit. (note 10); Marcia C. Inhorn, »*Fatwas* and ARTs: IVF and Gamete Donation in Sunni v. Shi'a Islam«, in: *Journal of Gender, Race & Justice* 9 (2005), pp. 291–317; Dror Meirow & Joseph G. Schenker, »The Current Status of Sperm Donation in Assisted Reproduction Technology: Ethical and Legal Considerations«, in: *Journal of Assisted Reproduction and Genetics* 14 (1997), pp. 133–138; Serour, »Bioethics in Reproductive Health«, op. cit. (note 35); Serour & Dickens, »Assisted Reproductive Developments«, op. cit. (note 35).

to a known biological mother and father – is considered not only an ideal in Islam, but a moral imperative. For Muslim men in particular, ensuring paternity and the »purity« of lineage through »known fathers« is of paramount concern. The problem with third-party donation, therefore, is that it destroys a child's *nasab*, or lineage, which is considered immoral in addition to being psychologically devastating. The child will be deemed illegitimate and stigmatized even in the eyes of its own parents, who will therefore lack the appropriate parental sentiments.[50]

This firm conviction that parenthood of a »donor child« is an impossibility is clearly linked to the legal and cultural prohibitions against adoption throughout the Sunni Muslim world.[51] The original Al-Azhar *fatwa* prohibiting third-party gamete donation also prohibits the legal adoption of orphans, considering both of them to be *haram* (forbidden). As a result, few Sunni Muslim IVF patients will contemplate adopting an orphan, stating with conviction that it is »against the religion.« According to Arab men, an adopted child, like a donor child, »won't be my son.«[52]

Shia Islam and IVF

Having said this, it is very important to point out how things have changed for Shia Muslims since the beginning of the new millennium. Shia is the minority branch of Islam with its epicenter in Iran. The countries of Iraq, Lebanon, and Bahrain are thought to have Shia majorities, and Shia minority populations are also found in Syria and the eastern coast of Saudi Arabia, which is an otherwise ardently Sunni Muslim country. Shia populations can also be found in the South Asian countries of Afghanistan, Pakistan, and India, where the Ismaili and Bora Shia communities form distinct subgroups.

50 Inhorn, »›He Won't Be My Son‹«, op. cit. (note 40).

51 Marcia Inhorn, *Infertility and Patriarchy: The Cultural Politics of Gender and Family Life in Egypt* (Philadelphia: University of Pennsylvania Press, 1996); Amira el Azhary Sonbol, »Adoption in Islamic Society: A Historical Survey«, in: *Children in the Muslim Middle East*, ed. by Elizabeth Warnock Fernea (Austin: University of Texas Press, 1995), pp. 45–67; Sherifa Zuhur, »Of Milk-Mothers and Sacred Bonds: Islam, Patriarchy, and New Reproductive Technologies«, in: *Creighton Law Review* 25 (1992), pp.1725–1738.

52 Inhorn, »›He Won't Be My Son‹«, op. cit. (note 40).

Many Shia religious authorities support the majority Sunni view: namely, they agree that third-party donation should be strictly prohibited. Iraq's Ayatollah al-Sistani, for example, opposes any form of third-party donation.[53] However, in the late 1990s, the Supreme Leader of the Islamic Republic of Iran, Ayatollah Ali Hussein Khamene'i, the chosen successor to Iran's Ayatollah Khomeini, issued a *fatwa* effectively permitting donor technologies to be used under certain conditions.[54] With regard to both egg and sperm donation, Ayatollah Khamene'i stated that *both* the donor and the infertile parents must abide by the religious codes regarding parenting. However, the donor child can only inherit from the sperm or egg donor, as the infertile parents are considered to be like »adoptive« parents.

However, the situation for Shia Muslims is actually much more complicated than this. The Shia valorize a form of intellectual reasoning known as *ijtihad*, in which individual Shia religious leaders make judgments and issue opinions (*fatwas*) for their followers. Although Sunni Muslims also practice *ijtihad*, it is especially prominent among the Shia. As a result, various Shia religious authorities have come to different conclusions about sperm and egg donation.[55] As a result, there are now major disagreements about:

1. whether third-party donation truly constitutes *zina,* or adultery, if no actual gaze or touch takes place with the gamete donor;
2. whether the child should receive the name of the infertile father or the sperm donor in cases of male infertility;
3. whether donation is permissible at all if the donors are anonymous;
4. whether the husband of an infertile woman needs to do a temporary *mut'a* marriage with the egg donor, then release her from the marriage

53 Morgan Clarke, *Islam and New Kinship: Reproductive Technology and the Shariah in Lebanon* (New York: Berghahn Books, 2009).

54 Morgan Clarke, »Shiite Perspectives on Kinship and New Reproductive Technologies«, in: *ISIM Newsletter* 17 (2006), pp. 26–27; Clark, »Islam and New Kinship«, op. cit. (note 53); Inhorn & Tremayne, »Islam and the Biotechnologies«, op. cit. (note 42); Tremayne, »Law, Ethics, and Donor Technologies«, op. cit. (note 44).

55 Farouk Mahmoud, »Controversies in Islamic Evaluation of Assisted Reproductive Technologies«, in: *Islam and the Biotechnologies of Human Life,* ed. by Marcia C. Inhorn & Soraya Tremayne (New York: Berghahn Books, in press); Tremayne, »Law, Ethics, and Donor Technologies«, op. cit. (note 44).

immediately after the embryo transfer, in order to avoid *zina*, or adultery. Such *mut'a* marriages are condoned in Shia, but condemned in Sunni Islam;

5. and whether a Shia Muslim woman married to an infertile man can do a *mut'a* marriage with a sperm donor, which would constitute an illegal state of polyandry.

In theory, only widowed or otherwise single women – who are not currently married – should be able to accept donor sperm, in order to avoid the implications of *zina*, or adultery. However, in the Muslim countries, single motherhood of a donor child is unlikely to become socially acceptable. Indeed, Iran has made sperm donation officially illegal, although surrogacy has been permitted and is now widely practiced.[56] To get around this problem, some Iranian Shia women are temporarily divorcing their infertile husbands, temporarily marrying the sperm donors, ending the temporary marriage once the pregnancy is firmly established, and then remarrying their infertile husbands.[57] As Tremayne notes, such sperm donation in Iran does not necessarily make »happy families,« suggesting the need to think through the future well-being of both women and the children conceived in this manner.

Given these moral ambiguities and uncertainties, those married infertile Shia couples who are *truly* concerned about carrying out third-party donation according to religious guidelines find it difficult to meet these various requirements, particularly regarding sperm donation. Yet, having said that, in Iran and Lebanon at least some Shia couples *are* beginning to receive donor gametes, as well as donating their gametes to other infertile couples. In Iranian clinics that follow Ayatollah Khamene'i's lead, all manner of egg, sperm, and embryo donation, as well as surrogacy, continue to take place, with his *fatwa* prominently displayed as moral justification.[58] Indeed, since the new millennium donor gametes are now being donated, shared, and even purchased by infertile couples in IVF clinics in Shia-

56 Shirin Naef Garmaroudi, »Gestational Surrogacy in Iran: Uterine Kinship and the Notion of Reproduction in Shia Thought and Practice«, in: *Islam and the Biotechnologies of Human Life*, ed. by Marcia C. Inhorn & Soraya Tremayne (New York: Berghahn Books, in press).

57 Tremayne, »Law, Ethics, and Donor Technologies«, op. cit. (note 44).

58 Garmaroudi, »Gestational Surrogacy in Iran«, op. cit. (note 56).

majority Iran and Lebanon, the only two countries in the Muslim world to allow this practice.[59] For infertile Shia couples who accept the idea of donation, the introduction of donor technologies has been described as a »marriage savior,« helping to avoid the »marital and psychological disputes« that may arise if the couple's case is otherwise untreatable.

Who is the source of these donor gametes? In the Lebanese IVF clinics in this study, some of the donors were other IVF patients (mostly Shia Muslims who accept the idea of donation), some were friends or relatives (including egg-donor sisters), and some were anonymous donors who provided their oocytes for a fee. In at least one clinic catering to a largely Shia clientele, some of these donors were young non-Muslim American women who travel from the Midwest to Lebanon for extra payment in order to anonymously donate their eggs to infertile Lebanese couples.[60] Ironically, those most likely to receive these »American eggs« are »conservative« Shia couples, who accept the idea of donation because they follow the teachings of Ayatollah Khamene'i in Iran. In Lebanon, it least, such Shia recipients of American eggs are likely to be members of or sympathizers with Lebanon's Hizbullah political party, which is officially described by the U.S. administration as a terrorist organization!

Furthermore, quite interestingly, in multi-sectarian Lebanon the recipients of these donor eggs are not necessarily only Shia Muslim couples. Some Sunni Muslim patients from Lebanon and from other Middle Eastern Muslim countries such as Egypt and Syria are quietly slipping across transnational borders to »save their marriages« through the use of donor gametes, thereby secretly »going against« the dictates of Sunni Muslim orthodoxy. That such reproductive travel is done in secrecy – usually under the guise of a »holiday in Beirut« – is quite important, given the moral condemnation of gamete donation in the Sunni Muslim countries. Although such Sunni Muslim gamete seekers may have made peace with their own

59 Inhorn, Patrizio & Serour, »Third-party Reproductive Assistance around the Mediterranean«, op. cit. (note 46).

60 This Shia-serving clinic was run by a transnational Lebanese Shia Muslim physician, who operated several clinics in the US and the Middle East and was able to recruit egg donors from the US to travel to Lebanon. Because of the difficulty of recruiting egg donors within Lebanon, there is a »demand« there for »American eggs.« American donors are also presumed to be »white,« and most Lebanese infertile couples do not want to bear a »black« donor child that will not resemble them.

moral decisions to use donor technologies, they often remain extremely concerned about maintaining anonymity and confidentiality, in order to avoid moral censure of themselves and their future donor offspring. The story of Hatem and Huda, a long-term infertile Muslim couple, bespeaks the complexities within the Middle Eastern reproscape.

The Story of Hatem and Huda's Secret Egg Quest

Hatem and Huda were patients in a hospital-based IVF clinic in Beirut, which catered to all of the religious sects found in multi-sectarian Lebanon. However, Hatem and Huda were not Lebanese, having traveled from rural Syria to Beirut in order to undergo a cycle of IVF. Like most Syrian reproductive travelers to Lebanon Hatem was convinced that Lebanese IVF clinics were superior to the fledgling clinics in neighboring Syria, a Middle Eastern nation-state that has long been isolated from, and even sanctioned by, the West. Thus, he had been bringing his wife to Beirut for IVF since 1997. Hatem had another reason for bringing Huda to Lebanon: There, they could access donor eggs, which were unavailable in the Sunni-dominant country of Syria, where third-party gamete donation is strictly prohibited.

Double first cousins married for 17 years,[61] Hatem and Huda clearly loved each other, despite the perplexing dilemma of her premature ovarian failure. Although Huda was only 36 at the time, she had entered menopause in her twenties and required hormonal stimulation followed by IVF in order to achieve a pregnancy. After five unsuccessful trials of IVF, the IVF physicians in Beirut recommended egg donation as the most likely successful option. As Sunni Muslims, Hatem and Huda knew that egg donation was forbidden in the religion. Yet, as Hatem explained, they rationalized their use of donor eggs in a previous IVF cycle in the following way,

»As long as the donor agrees, then this would reduce the *haram* [forbiddenness] based on our religion. Because she, the donor, is in need of money, she gave

61 They are first cousins on both their mothers' and fathers' sides, because their parents are also closely related.

nine to ten eggs, and the doctor divided the eggs between that couple and us. We took five, and that couple, who were recently married, took five. And I personally entered into the lab to make sure that *my* sperm were being used. It's okay because it's *my* sperm.«

Indeed, Huda became pregnant with donor twins, a male and a female, in 1999. At six months and seventeen days of pregnancy, she began to miscarry, and Hatem rushed her to a hospital in Syria. As Hatem recounts,

»They opened her stomach [by cesarean], and there were twins, who still lived for 48 hours. They had lung deficiency because they were little and not fully developed. The girl died twelve hours before the boy.«

After this traumatic experience, Huda could no longer accept the idea of egg donation, although Hatem persisted in his search. According to Hatem, who spoke for Huda as she sat quietly in the room,

»She was tortured [during the pregnancy]. She stayed four months vomiting whatever she ate, and she lost weight – from 88 kilograms to 55 kilograms. And she was under a lot of stress because of our social environment in Syria. In our [farming] community, they stare at babies and see if they resemble the mother and father. We are not living in a city of 4–5 million. We are in a closed community of 15,000 people. And so, the first time, when we had twins, they [the hospital] did a blood test and everyone [in the family] was surprised. Their blood group was AB, and it didn't match ours.[62] Now everyone will *really* examine the personal traits of this [donor] baby if we do it again. They will look at us suspiciously. Not the doctors; they keep everything confidential. But people in the community who might come to visit and look at us curiously.«

For his part, Hatem is willing to accept donor eggs again and has already made inquiries about finding a willing Shia Muslim egg donor in Syria. On the day of his interview, he also spoke about the possibility of finding a willing donor within the Beirut IVF clinic. Hatem saw no other way to achieve parenthood, given that he loves his wife and refuses to divorce her. Although Hatem is an affluent farmer from a large family of twenty children (by one father and three co-wives), he continues to resist all forms of social pressure to divorce or marry polygynously. His commitment, he says, is based on his deep love for Huda. As he said,

62 The twins needed a blood transfusion, which is why a blood test was performed and a familial blood donor was sought.

»Had I not loved her, I wouldn't have waited for seventeen years. I would have married another. By religious law, I can remarry, but I don't want to. She told me I should marry another woman, and she even offered or suggested that she would get me engaged, because we're already old. We've reached middle age without kids. We're living in a large family with six of my brothers, and they all have children. That's why she's feeling very depressed and very angry that she's alone without children, although she's always surrounded by children. But, of course, she keeps these feelings to herself.
The love between us – I love her *a lot*. I was the one who considered going for IVF, for her sake. But we must keep it secret, because if my parents knew about us having an IVF child, the child would be marginalized and living a lonely life. So we keep everything secret, and we just mention to our families that she's receiving treatment.«[63]

As in so many IVF stories, Huda and Hatem were ultimately unsuccessful in their seventh attempted IVF cycle. Huda's own eggs failed to mature under hormonal stimulation, and no egg donors were currently available at the clinic. Thus, Hatem and Huda returned home quietly to Syria, with little remaining hope of achieving parenthood, but with the love that had kept them together for nearly twenty years.

Conclusion

The arrival of donor technologies in both Lebanon and Iran – the only two Middle Eastern countries to offer these services at the present time – has led to a brave new world of reproductive possibility never imagined when ARTs were first introduced there nearly 25 years ago. These technologies have engendered significant medical transnationalism and reproductive tourism; the mixing of gametes across national, ethnic, racial, and religious

63 At the time of the study, IVF was relatively new to Syria compared to Lebanon. As I have shown for Egypt, IVF was very stigmatizing when it was first introduced to Egypt. Egyptians did not understand how »test-tube babies« were being made, and so they assumed that donor gametes were being used to produce »mixed« offspring. Infertile Egyptian couples were extremely secretive about undertaking IVF, which had a »technological stigma.« Over time, there has been some degree of normalization in parts of the Middle East where IVF has become better known to the public. See Inhorn, »Local Babies, Global Science«, op. cit. (note 10).

lines; and the birth of hundreds of donor babies to devout infertile Muslim couples. For their part, at least some infertile Muslim couples, both Shia and Sunni, have begun to reconsider traditional notions of *nasab,* or the meaning of biological lineage, even if »social parenthood« of a donor child is still not widely embraced in the Middle Eastern Muslim world.[64] Nonetheless, because donor technologies are now widely available in both Iran and Lebanon, the power of the Sunni Muslim ban on third-party donation is being weakened across the region, with some infertile Sunni Muslim couples such as Hatem and Huda reconsidering their own anti-donation moral stances. As a result of these social processes, Shia gametes are finding their ways into Sunni bodies, despite the current regional tensions between these branches of Islam. Indeed, in the new millennium, hundreds – perhaps even thousands – of infertile Sunni Muslim couples are traveling abroad in search of such Shia donor gametes.

As suggested by the Middle Eastern reproscape, reproductive travel is a growing global phenomenon,[65] one that is taking place well beyond the boundaries of the Euro-American nations. In the Middle East as elsewhere, anthropologists are exceptionally well positioned to gather important ethnographic information from reproductive travelers themselves, thereby understanding the motivations that compel them to seek ARTs outside their own countries. In doing so, our discipline can serve to humanize the legal and policy discourses on this subject, and to shed light on both the macro-and micro-level dynamics of the global reproscape, which is still shrouded in mystery.

The author's own multi-sited ethnographic investigation of the Middle Eastern reproscape has begun to uncover the motivations of a diverse set of infertile men and women as they travel to and from ART sites within the region and beyond. Indeed, global travel is part and parcel of the modern-day quest for conception among Middle Eastern Muslim couples. The deployment of the most high-tech forms of assisted reproduction is a facet of Middle Eastern modernity that is rarely emphasized in either the sparse literature on Islamic technoscience[66] or in Western polemics on the »back-

64 Inhorn, »›He Won't Be My Son‹«, op. cit. (note 40).

65 Blyth & Farrand, »Reproductive Tourism – A Price Worth Paying?«, op. cit. (note 3); Deech, »Reproductive Tourism in Europe«, op. cit. (note 3); Pennings, »Reproductive Tourism«, op. cit. (note 1).

66 Lotfalian, »Islam«, op. cit. (note 37).

wardness« of the region.[67] Moreover, such modernity is being supported by Islamic juridical and bioethical discourses, which are being used to justify some forms of technological assistance while limiting others.[68] Islamic bioethics have caught the attention of a new generation of Middle Eastern Studies scholars, who in recent years have compiled four edited volumes on this subject.[69] In short, although the Middle East is rarely regarded in this way, it is a key site for understanding the intersection of technoscience, religious morality, and modernity, all of which are deeply implicated in the Middle Eastern reproscape.

Acknowledgments

I would like to thank Michi Knecht, Maren Klotz, and Stefan Beck for inviting me to be part of this volume and the conference in Berlin upon which it is based. They also made very useful editorial suggestions. I am also extremely grateful to two particularly perceptive and creative reviewers, who engaged seriously with this paper, its wish for a new and better vocabulary to describe reproductive »tourism,« and its exploration of Islamic discourses on ARTs. One reviewer provided particularly helpful feedback on the expansion of Arjun Appadurai's work. The other provided useful cautionary advice to avoid essentializing Islam and its Sunni and Shia variants, as well as the notion of romantic love. The author has attempted to answer most of the reviewers' suggestions, and has referenced a new and growing body of work on Islamic bioethics and Islam and ARTs, which deals with many of the nuances beyond those contained in this brief chapter. Mostly, I want to thank the many gracious and candid women and men who have participated in my ethnographic research on infertility and

67 For more see Lara Deeb, *An Enchanted Modern: Gender and Public Piety in Shi'i Lebanon* (Princeton, NJ: Princeton University Press, 2006).

68 Inhorn & Tremayne, »Islam and the Biotechnologies«, op. cit. (note 42).

69 See: Brockopp, »Islamic Ethics of Life«, op. cit. (note 36); Jonathan E. Brockopp & Thomas Eich (Eds.), *Muslim Medical Ethics: From Theory to Practice* (Columbia: University of South Carolina Press, 2008); Hamada Hamid & Zareena Grewal, *Treating Muslims* (Thousand Oaks, CA: Sage, in press); and Inhorn & Tremayne, »Islam and the Biotechnologies«, op. cit. (note 42).

ARTs in the Middle East. This research was approved by the Behavioral Science Institutional Review Boards (IRB) at the University of Michigan and Yale University's Human Subjects Committee (HSC). Final thanks go to the U.S. Department of Education Fulbright-Hays Faculty Research Abroad Program and the National Science Foundation's Cultural Anthropology Program for generous funding of this research.

Reproducing Hungarians: Reflections on Fuzzy Boundaries in Reproductive Border Crossing

Eva-Maria Knoll

In June 2004 – the year of the most extensive eastern enlargement of the European Union – BBC News in a lurid headline announced »EU faces fertility tourism threat.« The baleful scenario foresaw a massive migration of patients and a corresponding loss of patient fees. This vision was based on a warning by fertility physicians from the United Kingdom, according to whom the »EU enlargement could encourage ›fertility tourists‹ to travel to Eastern Europe for cheap IVF.« Data from a comparative survey across Europe, presented at the annual ESHRE[1] congress on fertility in Berlin in 2004, had shown that in the field of assisted conception the joining member states of Eastern Europe were by no means behind. Already in 2001 Hungary had carried through roughly the same amount of IVF cycles per million of the population as the UK, and Slovenia had even managed twice as many. As a consequence, Slovenia and Hungary were ranked as the most likely destinations for UK fertility travelers. The future scenario of frequent border crossing along IVF routes was based on two additional facts: First, that »IVF success rates are as good in Eastern Europe as elsewhere,« as media coverage claimed. Second, that treatment costs in these countries were roughly fifty percent cheaper than in the UK. Reflecting on these facts, Suzi Leather, chairwoman of the UK's Human Fertilisation and Embryology Authority (HFEA), said she »can understand why people could be tempted to go abroad.« The best combination

1 ESHRE (European Society for Human Reproduction and Embryology) was founded in 1985 to stimulate research in the field of reproductive medicine and embryology, to disseminate respective results to the wider public, and to improve clinical practice on a European level. Around ESHRE's annual fertility conference in June 2004, media coverage predicting an increase in reproductive travel activities towards the East hit its peak (see e.g. BBC News 30.6.2004, Times Online 1.7.2004, Medical News Today 1.7.2004, and BioNews 5.7.2004).

of low »Eastern prices« and »Western standards« in IVF, of local costs and global quality, was offered in Slovenia and Hungary. These two countries therefore might turn out to be the most attractive Eastern destinations for fertility travelers from the West. It remained rather vague, however, what the alleged »threat« of prosperous transnational flows of patients towards fertility clinics in former Eastern Europe was actually about. Discrepancies in prices, in quality, and in efficacy of treatment, an overburdened UK health system, and the restrictions on IVF procedures were mentioned as pull and push factors. Additional worries referred to uncontrollable patient mobility linked to the freedom of movement within the EU, and to a lack of patients' safety in countries where treatment was not regulated and where counseling could be missing. This connection between an expanding political sphere of influence and a (potential) expansion of the realm of medical services can be read as the need of diverse actors to reflect, reassess, and demarcate standards, quality, costs, patients' rights and safety, and ethical considerations regarding fertility treatment within a new transnational competition.

Changes of political, economic and ideological borders, boundaries, and frontiers such as the fall of the Iron Curtain and the subsequent eastward enlargement of the European Union create opportunities and transformations while simultaneously producing uncertainty and fear. Hence pessimistic prophecies mushroomed in newspapers at the time of EU enlargement in 2004. Differences in labor cost and wages were the source of repeatedly raised concerns about change for the worse in Western labor markets. IVF and related biotechnologies, in turn, produce their own kind of uncertainty and fear, precisely because they are perceived to engender other, morally related forms of boundary crossing. The vision of IVF tourism along a West-East axis thus combines and multiplies several fears. No wonder that the turning East of fertility travel as a combination of geopolitical and moral transgression raised such strong concerns as voiced in the headlines and statements around the ESHRE conference 2004.

However, as a resident of Vienna, situated close to the Hungarian border, the evocation of a »fertility tourism threat« in the course of eastern EU enlargement came as no big surprise to me. Austria's south-eastern neighbor enjoys the well-established reputation of a dynamic medical tourism destination. In my childhood memories Hungary figures as a poor but close country and a cheap shopping destination. In the 70s and 80s my parents and relatives used to undertake the one-hour car ride to Hungary every once in a while in order to buy groceries, get a decent haircut, or enjoy an opulent meal at an extremely bargain price. In my current perception, this south-eastern neighbor is a country of low-cost dentistry.[2] Cross-border treatment in dental care is driven first of all by cost, while the short distance as well as entrepreneurial behavior and the development of a service cluster for this specific sector in the border region also play significant roles. Dental tourism towards Hungary is well developed, organized, and intensively advertised these days.[3] Austrian citizens regularly cross the border both for dental work offered in a myriad of surgeries in the border region, as well as for the relaxing and healing powers of the thermal waters in countless spas all over Hungary. The conceptual link between *health* and *tourism* therefore is widely taken for granted on both sides of this border.

2 Austria once directly faced the Iron Curtain, which nevertheless remained permeable to some extent for cross-border activities, especially after Hungary opted for a soft form of economic liberalization as a third way between communism and capitalism from the 1970s onwards, the so-called »Goulash Communism.« Today, Austria shares borders from the north-east to the south-west with four »new« EU member states of the 2004 extension. Since the country is so small, the border to the Czech Republic, to Slovakia, to Hungary, and to Slovenia is never far, especially for citizens in the eastern part of the country. Thus eastern Austria can basically be seen as a border region with corresponding incentives, possibilities, and potentials for cross-border activities such as health care mobility. A research project on the external frontiers of the European Community therefore has explicitly dubbed this intensified border region »health region«; cf. August Österle, »Health Care across Borders: Austria and its New EU Neighbors«, in: *Journal of European Social Policy* 17 (2007), 2, pp. 112–124; August Österle & José Delgado, »Dental Care Migration in Central Europe«, in: *Economic and Sociopolitical Perspectives for Health Services in Central Europe. Healthregio Report*, ed. by Renate Burger & Martin Wieland (Vienna: Gesundheitsmanagement OEG, 2006); see also http://www.healthregio.net.

3 The promotion of dental tourism to Hungary includes advertisements in Austrian newspapers, specific travel guides, and web pages. A dental surgery called »Dental Tourism Hungary,« for example, is located 15 km from the Austrian border and offers a web page in four languages (but not in Hungarian) with subtitles such as »Holiday and Dental Treatment« or »Travel for Health at Bargain-Price.« See http://www.dental-tourism-hungary.com, retrieved 14.8.2007.

The sensational media coverage on a »threat of fertility tourism flowing towards the East« and my personal experiences with border traffic with the neighboring country encouraged me to explore whether Hungary might be an attractive destination in the global market for fertility medicine. I traveled there in 2006 for a short-term visit as part of a broader multi-sited research project on reproductive tourism.[4] Ironically, I shared my compartment on the train to Budapest with a dental tourist from Vienna.

What I would like to address and discuss in my contribution to this volume is the existence of conceptual and legal grey zones and the forms of personal agency involved in dealing with transnational fertility treatment.[5] By comparing the comments and opinions on reproductive tourism voiced by representatives of different fertility clinics in Hungary's capital, I will show that key categories regarding personal identity and body substances become easily blurred when IVF is investigated within a transnational perspective. I went to Hungary with the intention of tracing reproductive border traffic, i.e. close-range reproductive traveling along a west/east trail.[6] My findings and insights made it inevitable, however, to conceive of boundaries as blurred along more than just one axis: Consulting a private IVF facility, a university clinic, and an IVF center located in a public

4 This research project explores the mobility of IVF patients under premises that conceptualize reproductive technologies in global and transnational terms, e.g. Arjun Appaduai's notion of »technoscapes« and Ulf Hannerz's »transnational connections.« Cf. Arjun Appadurai, *Modernity at Large: Cultural Dimensions of Globalization* (Minneapolis: University of Minnesota Press, 1996); Ulf Hannerz, *Transnational Connections. Culture People Places* (London/New York: Routledge 2003 [1996]). The ensuing methodological procedures have included multi-sited and comparative analyses in various European contexts with necessarily shorter ethnographic investigations on the local level. Since 2004 I have thus collected and analyzed various ethnographic vignettes which derive from visits to fertility clinics and interviews with IVF providers and users. This was carried out with a particular interest in some of the EU's more peripheral and less well-known arenas of IVF mobility such as Ljubljana, Lisbon, and Budapest.

5 I am grateful to Michi Knecht for inviting me to the workshop »IVF as a Global Form.« I would like to give my thanks to the workshop participants, to the editors of this volume, and to Andre Gingrich for inspiring contributions, remarks, and thoughts. The Theodor Körner Award 2006 of Austria's Chamber of Labor encouraged my research project and helped me realize my stay in Budapest.

6 For insights into reproductive treatment abroad involving long distance travel see the contributions of Marcia Inhorn, Michal Nahman, and Sven Bergmann in this volume.

hospital, my inquiries about fertility tourism into Hungary revealed fuzzy boundaries of belonging and knowledge, both related to transnational and interpersonal flows of people and bodily substances. These multidimensional, shifting, and blurred boundaries are due to interactions between national regulation and personal agency, i.e. the options and strategies of local actors in transnational IVF. As one group of actors involved, medical experts will be discussed in more detail in the second part. A particular example will demonstrate the scope of medics' options in defining who does and who does not count as a foreign patient and, thus, to whom IVF treatment is offered and to whom it is not. In the end, I will reflect on the tension between altruistic acts of egg cell donation and their commodification, as well as on known versus unknown donors for these contexts. However, let me first offer some reflections on terminology regarding tourism.

On Terminology: Health Tourism versus Reproductive Tourism

Health-related border crossing, such as the case of Austrians seeking cheap dentistry in Hungary discussed here, has brought about a corresponding terminology. Terms addressing tourist- and health-related aspects are established for some, but contested for other health service segments. I therefore will discuss the merging of tourist and health care practices in the following, providing some arguments for the appropriateness of the term »reproductive tourism.«

Border traffic for dental care and for health spa visits belongs to the booming economic sphere of *health tourism*. The Hungarian Tourist Authority has declared health tourism as a major goal in its National Tourism Development Strategy 2005–2013. According to the Hungarian Tourist Authority, health tourism comprises the two key sub-sectors of *medical tourism* and *wellness tourism*. Both these forms of cross-border health care »will be the priority product of the next planning period,« as the relevant strategy paper declares.[7] Dental tourism has played a significant role in the medical tourism boom in Hungary and has become even more attractive since Hungary joined the EU in 2004. According to estimates by the European Consumer Centre, 160.000 dental tourists go on such a medical pilgrimage to Hungary every year. For this reason, the Centre offers a specific collection of reports and some safety warnings.[8]

In contrast to the well-established and flourishing dental border traffic, reproductive travel has not yet been incorporated into official Hungarian tourism development strategies and has not yet concerned European Consumer Associations.[9] Nevertheless, this medical or health tourism segment has a significant growth potential:[10] EU enlargement has had a marked impact upon neighboring regions of »old« and »new« EU member states.

7 Hungarian Tourist Authority, *National Tourism Development Strategy 2005–2013* (Budapest: 2005), in particular p. 41, http://www.ungarn.dk/main.php?folderID=1657, [last accessed: 14.8.2007].

8 The handout »Zahnbehandlung in Ungarn« (dental treatment in Hungary) by the European Consumer Centre Vienna is a collection of reports on dental treatment (see http://www.evz.de/UNIQ118710538125735 [last accessed: 14.8.2007]. No lesser an institution than the Hungarian Tourist Authority offers another handout in German to those interested in Hungarian dental treatment (see http://www.ungarn-tourismus.de/wegzahn.pdf [last accessed: 14.8.2007]. The fact that a tourist authority comments and evaluates medical treatment options represents another surprising instance of fuzziness.

9 Although official consumer associations in Europe so far have not concerned themselves with reproductive travel, there is a patient organization advocating consumer rights in cross-border fertility treatment. The *International Consumer Support for Infertility*, in short *iCSi* (the pun with ICSI, short for »intracytoplasmic sperm injection,« seems to be intended), was initiated in 1999 by an Australian patient group. The goal of iCSi is to empower patients to become full partners in transnational fertility healthcare and public policy. The coordinators of iCSi are from three different parts of the world, Australia, Argentina, and Germany. iCSi organized a section at the ESHRE conference in 2008 where implications of reproductive traveling were discussed on the basis of case studies from Italy, Germany, Spain, and Eastern Europe (Petra Thorn, German iCSi coordinator, personal communication 11.9.2008; see also http://www.icsi.ws, and ESHRE 2008, *Abstract Book of the 24th Annual Meeting of the ESHRE, Barcelona, Spain, 7–9 July, 2008*).

10 Eric Blyth and Abigail Farrand have argued that although »reproductive tourism has its own idiosyncratic manifestations, it may be seen as part of the wider phenomenon of globalization and health tourism« (2005:96). Eric Blyth & Abigail Farrand, »Reproductive Tourism – A Price Worth Paying for Reproductive Autonomy?«, in: *Critical Social Policy* 25 (2005), 1, pp. 91–114, in particular p. 96.

Medical tourism has increased, driven by price differences between East and West (and reproductive tourism might follow suit, as indicated by the vision of a »fertility tourism threat« mentioned at the beginning).[11] A second reason is the existence of a well-beaten track of health tourism to Hungary, as I have argued above. Third, legal aspects can be an important incentive for reproductive travelers: Egg donation ranks as one of the most frequent motives among German-speakers in Europe for seeking fertility treatment abroad, and Hungary is occasionally mentioned as a promising new fertility destination in respective Internet exchange forums. Egg donation is lawful in Hungary whereas it is outlawed in Austria and Germany. Precisely these two countries have generated the strongest flow of health and medical tourists towards Hungary so far.[12]

11 Philipa Mladovsky, research officer in Health Policy at the London School of Economics, stresses that such price discrepancies are a first important incentive for people to seek treatment abroad. Personal expenses usually include two dimensions: price differences for treatment and travel costs. Philipa Mladovsky, »IVF and Reproductive Tourism«, in: *Euro Observer. The Health Policy Bulletin of the European Observatory on Health Systems and Policies* 8 (2006), 4, p. 5.

12 In my home country Austria, IVF is offered to the so-called stable heterosexual couple with or without marriage up to the age of 40 (woman) and 50 (man) while access is denied for homosexual couples and single women. Under specific conditions (blocked tubes and other forms of diagnosable forms of infertility) about 70% of IVF costs are covered by social insurance for four cycles per desired pregnancy. Illegal techniques include surrogacy and the donation of eggs or embryos. Donor insemination is lawful, but IVF is restricted to the homologous system (only sperm from the husband or partner can be used in IVF cycles). Preimplantation Genetic Diagnosis (PGD) is restricted to polar body biopsy procedures. The polar body is cell material of the egg cell, left over during the process of fertilization. Since the polar body is not part of the developing embryo but sticks to the outside of the egg membrane (while the embryo is developing inside), it can be extracted and used for genetic testing even in a country like Austria, where »regular« PGD (of one cell removed from an embryo) is outlawed. PGD of the polar body has been carried out since 2005 as a creative way for IVF providers and researchers to circumvent the law. Austrian patients travel abroad seeking donor eggs and the more comprehensive forms of PGD performed on an one-cell biopsy of the embryo, to circumvent the age limit, or simply for cheaper IVF. However, Austria is also an attractive IVF tourism destination for German and Swiss patients seeking blastocyst transfer and other legislative advantages. Blastocyst transfer is said to increase the chance of successful implantation because the embryo is under scrutiny in vitro for about 5 days and only »the best« developing embryos get transferred. A further motivation for German and Swiss IVF tourists is the so-called ›rule of three‹ (Dreierregelung) of their home countries, according to which only a maximum

Such regional legal diversity intersects with the emergence of new elements in the power relations of reproduction, which Shellee Colen has called »stratified reproduction.«[13] In principle, the process of egg donation is distributing the IVF procedure together with the risks and burdens of treatment across different female bodies. This includes the healthy bodies of young donor women.[14] However, the spreading of IVF burdens and risks and the flow of human eggs show a counter-directional movement. On one hand, human eggs move, as human organs do, along existing disparities from East to West, »from South to North, from poorer to more affluent bodies.«[15] In Europe, young Eastern European women and their bodily substances more and more often produce »miracle babies« for older, affluent women in the West. On the other hand, my current research indicates that an increasing number of people from Western Europe, desperate

of three embryos can be produced within one IVF cycle. In Austria the amount of produced embryos is left to the discretion of the medic (in accordance with medical standard of knowledge says the law). Surplus embryos can be frozen in Austria and can be used for another cycle in the future (which is also outlawed in Germany and Switzerland).

13 Faye D. Ginsburg & Rayna Rapp, »Introduction: Conceiving the New World Order«, pp. 1–17, in particular p. 3. Cf., Shellee Colen, »»Like a Mother to Them«: Stratified Reproduction and West Indian Childcare Workers and Employers in New York«, in: *Conceiving the New World Order: The Global Politics of Reproduction,* ed. by Faye D. Ginsburg & Rayna Rapp (Berkeley: University of California Press. 1995), pp. 78–102.

14 Cf. Marta Kirejczyk, »Enculturation through Script Selection: Political Discourse and Practice of In Vitro Fertilization in the Netherlands«, in: *Bodies of Technology. Women's Involvement with Reproductive Medicine*, ed. by Ann Rubinow Saetnan, Nelly Oudshoorn & Marta Kirejczyk (Ohio: Columbus, 2000) pp. 183–206, in particular p. 185.

15 Cf. Nancy Scheper-Hughes, »The Last Commodity: Post-Human Ethics and the Global Traffic in »Fresh« Organs«, in: *Global Assemblages. Technology, Politics, and Ethics as Anthropological Problems,* ed. by Aihwa Ong & Stephen Collier (Malden/Oxford/Victoria: Blackwell Publishing, 2005), pp. 145–167, in particular p. 150. In sharp contrast to organs, however, eggs (and sperm) do not move from black and brown bodies to white ones because of what Charis Thompson describes as »identity properties,« i.e. phenotypical and cultural characteristics are of no significance to a liver or a kidney recipient, but of central concern for the egg recipient and her desired offspring. Donors from Eastern European countries thus display two advantages: they are fair-skinned and fair-haired, and their body substances are low-priced. Cf. Charis Thompson, *Making Parents. The Ontological Choreography of Reproductive Technologies* (Cambridge/London: MIT Press, 2005), in particular p. 10. In her contribution in this volume, Michal Nahman discusses egg cells imported to Israel from Romania.

to conceive, are heading towards the cost-saving East. How can we conceptualize these IVF travelers and their activities?

When it comes to travel activities for procreative matters, terminology is a sensitive and contested terrain. Terms linking the medical and the tourist segments, such as health tourism, medical tourism, dental tourism, patient tourism, or abortion tourism seem to represent an academically well established and respected terminology.[16] Strong objections are raised, however, against terms like *reproductive tourism* or *fertility tourism* to describe cross-border traveling activities of fertility patients. These objections often argue that undergoing a physically and emotionally demanding fertility treatment should not be equated with a holiday and has nothing in common with recreation, leisure time, and therefore by implication with tourism. The insistence upon a clear-cut terminological separation between the two economic segments of tourism and reproductive medicine is upheld by both some patients and some providers. Some scholars tend to share this view, thus the appropriateness of tourism terminology for the description of the transnationalization of IVF treatment was also subject to a lively debate in the course of the international workshop that forms the basis of this volume. In order to present the scope of the controversy and to get a better understanding of the points of contention, I shall now briefly discuss tourism-related concepts and terminology and cast some light on their contradictory connotations.

Since the 1970s the anthropology of tourism has theorized interactions between host and guest communities and the touristic experience with its ritual-like structure that raises it above the everyday. Tourism thus is a complex phenomenon, a system rather, which cannot be limited to human travel activities. The most comprehensive and generally accepted definition of tourism is offered by the World Tourism Organization (WTO) and covers the elements of space, time, and diverse motives: „Tourism comprises the activities of persons travelling to and staying in places outside their usual environment […] for leisure, business and other purposes».[17]

16 See for example Milica Z. Bookman & Karla R. Bookman, *Medical Tourism in Developing Countries*, (New York: Palgrave, 2007), in particular the introduction, pp.1–19.

17 World Tourism Organization – WTO, as cited in Monika Rulle, *Der Gesundheitstourismus in Europa – Entwicklungstendenzen und Diversifikationsstrategien* (München/Wien: Profil 2004), in particular p.19. Another conception of tourism broadly quoted in anthropology comes from Valene Smith, who sees tourism as a

Following this definition, there is more to tourism than merely holiday and leisure time. It also includes the burdens of business traveling and »other purposes« as motivating mobility.

Anthropologists have considered different terms and metaphors in analyzing tourist activities. The notion of *traveling* is linked to the Grand Tour of European aristocrats, who traveled for educational purposes between the sixteenth and eighteenth centuries.[18] The term travel thus is rooted in a Western and class-oriented discourse and genre, being intertwined with travel writing.[19] Travel refers to the older and more cumbersome ways of movement, while the term *tourism* is related to modern transportation.[20]

The term *reproductive tourism* is used or rejected by scholars of diverse academic disciplines. Economist Debora Spar describes reproductive medicine as a growing international market due to regulatory and price differences that attract affluent and mobile customers.[21] Bioethicist Guido Pennings in his earlier work also wrote about reproductive tourism, which he positively characterized as »moral pluralism in motion«

---

social practice that comprises the three elements of temporary leisure (non-working time), disposable income, and travel ethic. Cf. Valene Smith, response to Dennison Nash »Tourism as an Anthropological Subject« in: *Current Anthropology* 22 (1981), 5, pp. 461–481, in particular p. 475, as cited in Peter M. Burns, *An Introduction to Tourism and Anthropology* (London/New York: Routledge, 2002 [1999]), in particular p. 26.

18 Cf. »Tourism«, in: *Encyclopedia of Cultural Anthropology*, ed. by David Levinson & Melvin Ember (New York: Holt, 1996) pp. 1316–1320, in particular p. 1318.

19 James Clifford, »Traveling Cultures«, in: *Routes. Travel and Translation in the Late Twentieth Century* (Cambridge/Massachusetts/London: Harvard University Press, 1997) pp. 17–46, in particular p. 34.

20 According to James Clifford, the term »pilgrimage« would be »a nice way of subverting the constitutive modern opposition between traveler and tourist. But its ›sacred‹ meanings tend to predominate – even though people go on pilgrimages for secular as well as religious reasons.« Clifford, »Traveling Cultures«, op. cit. (note 19), p. 39. A more detailed discussion on the subject of terminology will be offered in Eva-Maria Knoll, *Managing Distances and Navigating Moral Landscapes: Reproductive Tourism in Europe* (forthcoming).

21 As mobile customers, reproductive tourists »will go where prices are lowest and quality highest, and where regulations are most conducive on their own needs and interests.« Debora L. Spar, *The Baby Business. How Money, Science, and Politics Drive the Commerce on Conception* (Boston: Harvard Business School Press, 2006), in particular p. 216; see also Debora L. Spar, »Reproductive Tourism and the Regulatory Map«, in: *New England Journal of Medicine* 352 (2005), 6, pp. 531–33.

– a »safety valve that avoids moral conflict« by making available outside a country's border what a majority has determined as morally unacceptable inside. Pennings was criticized for using the terms reproductive tourism or (in)fertility tourism because the word tourism is linked to travel for pleasure and thus trivializes fertility problems. As a consequence he renamed the phenomenon as *cross-border reproductive care.*[22] Marcia Inhorn, who has provided the most comprehensive anthropological contribution to reproductive travel activities in the Muslim world,[23] takes her informants' objection against the term tourism seriously. She suggests »reproductive traveling« instead, a term used by one of her informants meant to emphasize the exhaustion and burden of traveling instead of projecting images of a holiday. Sven Bergmann offers the term cross-border treatment as an alternative to tourism vocabulary.[24]

Although these various objections, doubts, and reservations with regard to tourism-related terminology are perfectly understandable, I am not entirely convinced, neither by the critics' arguments nor by the terminological alternatives. To my mind they offer an »emic« terminology that is not necessarily *more accurate* for analytical purposes. From my anthropological perspective, tourism is an analytical term that captures the complexities of various kinds of peaceful movements across borders – even though some members of the special interest groups involved may not

22 Currently IVF providers prefer and promote the notion of cross-border reproductive care. Cf. Guido Pennings, »Reproductive tourism as Moral Pluralism in Motion«, in: *Journal of Medical Ethics* 28 (2002), pp. 337–341; Guido Pennings, »Legal Harmonization and Reproductive Tourism in Europe«, in: *Human Reproduction* 19 (2004), 12, pp. 2689–2594; Guido Pennings, Reply: »Reproductive Exile versus Reproductive Tourism, Letters to the Editor«, in: *Human Reproduction* 20 (2005), 12, pp. 3571–3572; Guido Pennings et al., »ESHRE Task Force on Ethics and Law 15: Cross-Border Reproductive Care«, in: *Human Reproduction* 23 (10) (2008), pp. 2812–2184; Roberto Matorras, »Reproductive Exile versus Reproductive Tourism, Letters to the Editor«, in: *Human Reproduction* 20 (2005), 12, p. 3571.

23 Marcia C. Inhorn, »Making Muslim Babies: IVF and Gamete Donation in Sunni versus Shi'a Islam«, in: *Culture, Medicine and Psychiatry* 30 (2006), 4, pp. 427–450; Marcia C. Inhorn, »Religion and Reproductive Technologies: IVF and Gamete donation in the Muslim World«, in: *Anthropology News* 46 (2005), 2, pp. 10–14; Marcia C. Inhorn, »Middle Eastern Masculinities in the Age of New Reproductive Technologies: Male Infertility and Stigma in Egypt and Lebanon«, in: *Medical Anthropology Quarterly* 18 (2004), 2, pp.162–182.

24 See the contributions of Marcia Inhorn and Sven Bergmann in this volume.

share this perspective. Tourism is a complex phenomenon encompassing the mobile person of the tourist, the facilities supplied by a tourist industry, and a society of destination. Accordingly, reproductive tourism comprises the border crossing patient; the supply industry in the form of fertility clinics, travel agencies, and infrastructure; and the norms and values of a destination society, articulated in laws, rules, regulations, and policies. It may even include bodily substances from the destination society such as egg cells. Tourism is a complex ethnographic field that includes front-stage and backstage dealings, as will become evident in the following case study on egg donation in Hungary.

Tourism, as I have argued, is not inherently linked to fun and leisure; travel and stay may be motivated by »other purposes« like the visit of a spa, a dentist, or a fertility clinic. Consequently, the objections against too broad a meaning of the term tourism are not well substantiated. On the one hand, cross-border tourism for medical purposes like dentistry, which may include implants after root treatment, has little in common with a great holiday. Fertility treatment, on the other hand, has intentionally been carried out in a holiday setting by several of my informants. They were more or less forced to combine fertility treatment with leisure, or else they would have spent their whole annual holiday entitlement on IVF treatment. The majority of my informants had actively and deliberately worked out a creative combination of IVF treatment with a tourist interest.[25]

25 One of my informants was an Austrian manager in her forties searching for donor eggs. As she and her husband were forced to travel abroad to obtain egg cells (the donation of which is outlawed in Austria), they wanted at least to see the world. She decided to continue her IVF treatment as long as it would take, but to strategically change the country after each failure. For further examples of how fertility travelers combine medical treatment with tourist interests, see Eva-Maria Knoll, »Fortpflanzungsmedizin ohne Sexualität als gesellschaftliche Irritation: Diskurse über ‚Jungfrauen-Geburten«, in: *Sexualität als Experiment. Identität, Lust und Reproduktion zwischen Science und Fiction*, ed. by Nicolas Pethes & Silke Schicktanz (Frankfurt/New York: Campus, 2008), pp. 331–348; Eva-Maria Knoll, »Transnationale AkteurInnen im Geschäft mit der Hoffnung. Österreichische Momente globaler Verflechtungen der In-Vitro-Fertilisation«, in: *Kulturelle Dynamik der Globalisierung. Ost- und Westeuropäische Transformationsprozesse aus sozialanthropologischer Perspektive*, ed. by Johanna Riegler (Wien: Verlag der Österreichischen Akademie der Wissenschaften, 2005), pp. 203–232; Eva-Maria Knoll, »Globale Assemblagen«, in: *Lexikon der Globalisierung*. ed. by Fernand Kreff, Eva-Maria Knoll & Andre Gingrich (Bielefeld: transkript, 2011).

In addition to these patients' activities, there have also been the first attempts at an IVF-specific tourist service and an IVF-related tourist infrastructure in the field of reproductive medicine, as I have outlined elsewhere.[26] Evidently the two socio-economic segments of tourism and reproductive medicine increasingly overlap. Using a specific academic term to refer to this new form of mobility that blurs the distinctions or boundaries between tourism and medical treatment is but a logical consequence.[27]

With regard to cross-border activities in fertility treatment, the term *tourism* – in contrast to *traveling* – does not exclusively focus on moving patients, i.e. on transnational users of reproductive technologies and their travel and treatment. Rather, I would like to understand the term in a broader and more general sense as comprising demand and supply in global IVF. The notion of reproductive tourism therefore captures new forms of choice and consumerism in health care that tend to undermine the distinction between tourism and health care. I see IVF-based tourism as a relatively new therapeutic culture emerging in the context of tourism. Tourism terminology also points to negative effects (e.g. the exploitation of egg donors), and it includes the supply activities of technology providers, i.e. fertility physicians and their agency. The following example from Hungary will demonstrate that technology providers play a crucial role in shaping global/local forms of IVF.

26 Eva-Maria Knoll, »So weit gehen für ein Kind: Reproduktionstourismus als grenzüberschreitender Umweg«, in: *Umwege zum eigenen Kind. Ethische und rechtliche Herausforderungen an die Reproduktionsmedizin 30 Jahre nach Louise Brown*, ed. by Gisela Bockenheimer-Lucius, Petra Thorn & Christiane Wendehorst, Göttinger Schriften zum Medizinrecht, Band 3, (Göttingen: Universitätsverlag, 2008), pp. 63–79.

27 Development economists and attornies Milica and Karla Bookman have convincingly argued that medical tourism entails what they call »the splicing« (namely the merging and intersecting) of the two biggest industries across the globe, medicine and tourism. Cf. Bookman & Bookman, »*Medical Tourism in Developing Countries*«, op. cit. (note 16).

Additional Terminological Boundaries: Who Counts as Foreign Patient?

As in many other parts of Europe, the fertility market in Hungary is dominated by private clinic activities.[28] One private facility, which I will call *Prospect IVF*, performs up to 70 percent of the approximately 6000 annual cycles in Hungary.[29] The first Prospect IVF Centre was established in 1991 in Budapest with the help and expertise of a prominent Austrian IVF specialist.[30] It was soon followed by additional centers in other parts of the country and within a few years a nation-wide network had been established. In 2006, Prospect IVF network announced in a press release that it was the sixth largest fertility institution worldwide. It was claimed that two percent of annual births in Hungary were due to this institution. »We are very proud,« explained Hungarian-American clinic owner Ákos Raćz, who is a prominent figure in the Hungarian fertility landscape, »this is a little bit of a Guinness Book Record that *one* institute, Prospect IVF institute, provides two percent of the entire nation's population per year.«[31]

28 According to Hungary's Hospital Act, health care can be offered in public institutions, private institutions, and health care institutions that belong to a religious organization. University clinics, however, are organizational units of universities with differing ownership status. They provide theoretical and practical training for medical students within the broader framework of general health care. Cf. Judit Sándor (s.n.), »Hungary«, in: *Kluwer International Encyclopaedia of Laws. Medical Law Vol. 2*, ed. by Herman Nys (London/New York: The Hague, 2003), pp. 1–148, in particular p. 29.

29 If not otherwise marked, all information is derived from interviews with representatives of three fertility clinics in Budapest in 2006. Both the clinics' names and the identity of the clinic representatives have been anonymised.

30 The very first IVF unit in Hungary was established in a public hospital and Hungary's first IVF baby was born there in the summer of 1989. Private clinics started business in the early nineties and soon outnumbered public facilities. In 2006, only three of the eleven existing fertility centers in Hungary were run publicly, as the head of a university-based public fertility unit explained.

31 Considering the dominating position of the Prospect IVF clinic conglomerate on the Hungarian market, this claim of producing two percent of annual Hungarian births does not seem unrealistic. By comparison, ESHRE results for 2005 show that 1,3 percent of births in Germany were induced by assisted conception; Slovenia was leading with 3,9 percent, followed by Denmark und Belgium with 3,5 percent each. Cf. The European IVF Monitoring Program (EIM) for the European Society of Human Reproduction and Embryology (ESHRE), »Assisted Reproductive Technology and In-

On a national Hungarian level, Ákos Raćz's ambitious activities of reproducing Hungarians have received a number of official honors.[32] These official honors indicate that Hungarian domestic policy displays a marked interest in the process of producing Hungarians under laboratory conditions.[33] The Hungarian health care system also contributes extensive financial support to IVF. It is based on a national health insurance system which theoretically provides almost complete coverage for nearly all citizens.[34] Political interest and health care traditions thus shape public financial support for assisted conception in Hungary, and this support is among the highest within the European Union. Fertility patients can expect reimbursement for five cycles per desired pregnancy.[35]

trauterine Inseminations in Europe, 2005: Results Generated from European Registers by ESHRE«, in: *Human Reproduction* 1 (2009) 1, pp. 1–21.

32 He has been awarded several medals, which can be viewed on the clinic's homepage, and even the above-mentioned Austrian physician who supported him was honored for his activities with the Officer's Cross of the Order of Merit of the Republic of Hungary in April 2006.

33 The entanglement of reproductive medicine with national economies has a long history that goes back to the incipience of artificial insemination in the late 19th century. At the beginning of the 20th century there was an increasing interest in artificial insemination due to a growing awareness for demographic developments and the fear of a declining population; cf. Christine Schreiber, *Natürlich künstliche Befruchtung? Eine Geschichte der In-vitro-Fertilisation von 1878 bis 1950*, Kritische Studien zur Geschichtswissenschaft, Bd. 178 (Göttingen: Vandenhoeck & Ruprecht, 2007), in particular p. 108. In the 1980s and 90s, public funding for IVF was frequently argued for with the visionary promise of an increase in citizens and tax payers against the background of an allegedly dramatic decline of birthrates, especially in small European countries like Hungary or Austria; cf. Eva-Maria Knoll, *Reproduktionsmedizinische Imaginationen. Überlegungen zum österreichischen IVF-Diskurs aus ethnologisch-feministischer Perspektive* (University Vienna: unpublished Master Thesis, 2001), in particular pp. 58–59.

34 In reality, however, health care demands a growing proportion of direct out-of-pocket payments, of co-payments (on pharmaceutical and on some dental treatments), and of under-the-table payments (the so-called »gratitude money«) in Hungary, as jurist Judit Sándor explains (see »Hungary«, op. cit. [note 28], p. 21).

35 This reimbursement policy is only surpassed by Belgium, where six IVF cycles are funded. Cf. Corinna Sorenson, »ART in the European Union«, in: *Euro Observer. The Health Policy Bulletin of the European Observatory on Health Systems and Policies* 8 (2006), 4, pp. 1–4. In some other European countries (e.g. Portugal or Spain) reimbursement is theoretically unlimited if treatment is carried out in public facilities.

In line with the claim that the Prospect IVF conglomerate performs the majority of IVF circles in Hungary, Ákos Raćz declares that it is mostly Hungarians who receive fertility treatment in his clinics.[36] Egg donation is carried out, but, as Raćz emphasizes, »[…] only between Hungarians. We do not treat foreigners with egg donation. Hungarian eggs are staying in the country and are reserved for Hungarians. Usually, somebody brings a sister along.« Nevertheless, after persistent questioning from my side, Ákos Raćz eventually admitted that Hungary and Prospect IVF *do* play some role as a destination for reproductive tourists:

»Unfortunately, like anything else, IVF tourism is already there. IVF tourism will be more widespread in the future, but since we have such a large national program and it is supported generously by the government, this is very, very secondary to us. We *do* perform some IVF cycles on quote, foreigners, unquote – *because they are Hungarians* living abroad. Because Hungary was, you know … the territory of Hungary was reduced to half, as you know. So, half of the Hungarians are living outside of its borders. I consider them as Hungarians. I live in the US, I am Hungarian – once Hungarian, always Hungarian, so we treat them.« (emphasis Ákos Raćz)

The fact that the speaker explicitly inserts a phrase from written language, namely »quote/unquote,« into his argument is a very clear marker and statement: He would not call Hungarians living abroad »foreigners.«

In the immediacy of this interview situation I did not pursue this evident conflation between Hungarians as citizens of a nation-state and Hungarians as an ethnic group any further. Hence it was left to the present analysis to reconsider and interpret this rather elastic boundary regarding

36 All interviews discussed here were scheduled in advance and conducted in the offices of the respective clinics during regular opening hours. Squeezed in between patient's appointments, they lasted between 20 and 45 minutes, were semi-structured and recorded. Two interviews were conducted in English, one interviewee preferred to speak German. I talked to the directors of the respective clinic alone, except at the Prospect IVF clinic. There a third person, the scientific director, was also present during the interview. Among other topics, I straightforwardly asked whether patients from abroad were entitled to fertility treatment in Hungary both generally and at their respective clinic. It became quite obvious during these interviews that, at least in 2006 when this research was carried out, there was no sign of a beaten path of Western IVF patients seeking cheap egg cells in Budapest as evoked by the media. However, the clinics' representatives were reluctant to speak about flows of foreign patients and flows of bodily substances.

national and transnational identities within the field of IVF. Inspired by Aihwa Ong, we might call this tricky subject a specific and creative variant of flexible reproductive citizenship:[37] What does it mean if Prospect IVF *treats no foreigners in Hungary except for those considered Hungarians living abroad?* Does Ákos Raćz's classification of »Hungarian patients living abroad« refer to labor migration? Does it merely reflect a nostalgic attitude towards a perished empire? Or does it concern questions of ethnicity? I shall briefly discuss these three possibilities in the following three sections. Although the third option will turn out to be the most accurate one, discussing all three of them will illustrate the rich potential of transnational confusions in patient mobility and how they are co-determined by the observers' perspective.

A first possible interpretation of Ákos Raćz's reference to the clinic's treatment of »quote, foreigners, unquote« as long as they are Hungarians would relate it to labor migration. For labor migrants, »going home« for procreative matters is often a question of language proficiency in the face of considerable bureaucratic obstacles, of differences in income and treatment costs, or of experiences of discrimination in the health care sector of their host country. Thus reproductive border crossing frequently does not lead abroad into foreign and unknown countries, but paradoxically turns back home. Albania, for example, is a country that offers low-cost IVF. Although assisted conception is hardly developed in Albania, with not even 300 cycles carried out in the only existing IVF clinic in 2006, the country nevertheless was chosen as a fertility destination by patients from Kosovo, Macedonia, and Italy, as biologist Rezarta Reimann from the University of Tirana reported at the European Biopolitics Conference in 2006.[38] These fertility travelers were Albanian emigrants, living and working in these and other parts of the world. For matters of assisted procreation, however,

37 Cf. Aihwa Ong, *Flexible Citizenship: The Cultural Logics of Transnationality* (Durham: Duke University Press, 1999); Aihwa Ong (s.n.), »Flexible Staatsbürgerschaft« in: Kreff, Knoll & Gingrich (eds.), *Lexikon der Globalisierung*, op. cit. (note 25).

38 Cf. Rezarta Reimann, »Workshop IVF Trafficking and Egg Cell Donation«, in: European Biopolitics Conference. Connecting Civil Society – Implementing Basic Values, by Heinrich Boell Foundation 17.-19.03.2006 Berlin, Conference Documentation, http://www.boell.de/en/04_thema/4202.html, retrieved 24.08.2007; Rezarta Reimann, »Bioethik in Albanien«, GID – Gen-ethischer Informationsdienst 175 (April 2006), pp. 50–52, http://www.gen-ethisches-netzwerk.de/GID175_Reimann [last accessed: 28.10.2008].

they traveled to their home country. Like all reproductive travelers, they traveled across international borders – but in contrast to most other (Western, middle-class) repro-tourists, they were traveling from a host country back to their place of origin. Quite often these people would face considerable bureaucratic and financial obstacles in their host countries, barring them from fertility treatment with their migrant workers' salaries. We can thus observe a two-fold migration movement: Many migrants move towards a foreign country that seems to promise a better economic future, while moving back to their home country or the country of ethnic origin for medical assistance in procreation. This counter-directional migratory mobility might point to modes of Arjun Appadurai's disjunctive entanglement of distinctive global flows.[39] In this case, these are the disjunctive flows of manpower and purchasing power, of technological options and (socio-economically determined) practical access.

In the case of Slovenia, anthropologist Dorijan Keržan highlights an additional component in »labor migrants returning home for fertility treatment.« In his research on public debates on kinship and reproductive technology, he shows the importance of avoiding fuzzy ethnic boundaries in procreation. When in need of donor semen, Slovenian emigrants travel to their home country for fertility treatment to ensure »certified ethnicity,« as I am tempted to call it: When it is necessary to use the semen of a stranger, for many Slovenians it should at least be »ethnically appropriate semen,« namely semen from Slovenian donors.[40]

Concerns regarding language skills, income, and ethnicity were the motivating forces discussed so far regarding emigrant technology users choosing a reproductive travel route that brings them home to their »country of origin.« The technology providers' side offers additional insights into the phenomenon of »going home for procreative matters«: Stefan Beck has shown that the transnational arena of reproductive medicine is also structured by different business models. One of these business models is exemplified by the foundation of an IVF center in Izmir. This IVF clinic

39 Appadurai, »*Modernity at Large*«, op. cit. (note 4).

40 Dorijan Keržan, »Kinship and Family in Public Debate on Assisted Conception in Slovenia«, in: *MESS – Mediterranean Ethnological Summer School Piran, Slovenia 2001 and 2002,* ed. by Rajko Muršič & Irena Weber (Ljubljana: Županjčeva knjižnica, 2003), pp. 211–228, in particular pp. 215–218, and personal communication 20.05.2004, Ljubljana.

was established by Turkish siblings. After their education and graduation in reproductive medicine in Germany, sister and brother had re-migrated to their hometown Izmir where they now run the fertility clinic together.[41] Ákos Raćz from Prospect IVF in Hungary can also be seen as a re-migrant who put his medical skills into the service of his home country. These two examples of re-migrating IVF professionals thus represent a specific form of »returning home for procreative matters.« They are part of a process of technology and knowledge transfer and dissemination in the field of reproductive medicine. These two examples furthermore show that the phenomenon of reproductive traveling does not only consist of transnational flows of patients: knowledge, technology, human substances, and IVF providers like Ákos Raćz himself are highly mobile as well.

Hungarian emigrants traveling home for procreative matters is but one possible interpretation for Ákos Raćz's identification of »Hungarians living abroad,« the category that makes them eligible for IVF treatment in Prospect IVF clinics. My own national identity as an Austrian, however, leads me to the alternative interpretation that Raćz may be mourning the territorial losses of Hungary, which have led to parts of the former population living outside today's nation-state. Talking about the loss of territorial sovereignty brings the former Austro-Hungarian Empire to *my* mind. Following this interpretation, could one refer to today's citizens of successor states to the former multiethnic empire as »Hungarians living abroad«? The dual monarchy harbored over 50 million people in 1914 and included the state territories of today's Austria, Hungary, Czech Republic, Slovakia, Slovenia, Croatia, Bosnia and Herzegovina, and parts of what today are Romania, Montenegro, Poland, Ukraine, Italy, and Serbia. If the category of »Hungarians living abroad« means »former Austro-Hungarians,« there would be a very large pool of potential border crossing patients to Hungarian Prospect IVF clinics. Unlike other foreigners, these patients would be accepted by the clinics since they would not be classified as foreign. Despite a certain proportion of returning labor migrants among the patients in Prospect IVF clinics and despite my admittedly provocative train of

41 Stefan Beck, »Globalisierte Reproduktionsregimes: Anmerkungen zur Emergenz biopolitischer Handlungsräume«, in: *Berliner Blätter. Ethnographische und ethnologische Beiträge* 42 (2007), pp. 124–151, in particular pp. 136–143.

thoughts about the Austro-Hungarian Empire, yet another interpretation seems much more plausible than these two.

Pan-Nationalism and Ethnic Identity in Reproductive Tourism

Ákos Raćz's description of »Hungarians living abroad« revealed indications for a third interpretation. In our conversation, Raćz emphasized that he and his clinics were not profiting from reproductive tourism because he was treating exclusively Hungarians – including those living abroad. To my mind, what is at stake here is a distinctive form of language-based pan-nationalism. This kind of nationalism promotes and enhances members of one's own language group and often receives its first impulses from the implosion of empires, as anthropologist Andre Gingrich has exemplified.[42] Pan-Slavism and Pan-Turkism are examples for comparable nationalist attitudes and movements. By contrast to the multi-ethnic Austro-Hungarian Empire discussed before, this alignment not only has nostalgic and royalist connotations, but also points to an ethnic reference. The taped interview section quoted above made this dimension evident. When a speaker explicitly puts the term »foreigners« between quotation marks, he indicates that he actually regards these so-called foreigners as nationals. On the basis of such a pan-nationalist point of view, Ákos Raćz refers to the changeful history of the Kingdom of Hungary and the »Magyars,« the ethnic group of Hungarians.[43] 10 million Magyars live within the borders of today's Hungary, while approximately 3 million live as substantial ethnic and linguistic minorities in Romania, Slovakia, Serbia, and Ukraine, with smaller minorities in Austria, Slovenia, and Croatia. As migrants, ethnic Hungar-

42 Cf. Andre Gingrich, »Pan-Nationalismus«, in: Kreff, Knoll & Gingrich (eds.), *Lexikon der Globalisierung*, op. cit. (note 25).

43 The Magyars originated from an Asian nomadic horse-people who spoke Hungarian, an Ugric language unrelated to most other languages spoken in Europe. Around 1000 A.D. Stephen I founded the Kingdom of the Hungarians. In the modern era their main settlement areas formed part of the Austro-Hungarian Dual Monarchy from 1867 until 1918. With the Treaty of Trianon at the end of World War I, Hungary lost about two-thirds of its former territory and a large part of its population to the other successor states of the Austro-Hungarian Empire.

ians and their descendants are scattered all over Western Europe, Canada, the Americas, and Israel.[44] If even some of them were to travel home for IVF treatment, they would constitute a significant additional clientele for a private clinic conglomerate like Prospect IVF.

The 2004 EU enlargement did not only affect flows of fertility patients from Western countries, as mentioned at the beginning of this article. It also had a strong effect on the Hungarian minorities in Serbia, Ukraine, and Romania. As non-EU citizens, members of these ethnic Hungarian minorities have since 2004 had to deal with visa and immigration procedures at an external EU border whenever they interact with their ethnic home country and with relatives living there.[45] Ákos Raćz's pan-nationalist attitude and practice of privileging ethnic Hungarian patients from abroad is neither unique nor is it a strictly private matter; rather, it stands for the broader political tendency of pan-nationalism.[46] Reproductive border crossing is related to this attitude.

Relatives outside EU borders have such an importance on private and political levels that their status is discussed and challenged both within and outside the Hungarian border. Such discussions include topics like

---

44 See http://www.hhrf.org. In contrast to the term *ethnic Hungarian* (or *Magyar*), which denotes a feeling of ethnic belonging regardless of the actual place of birth or residence, the term *Hungarian* refers to citizens of the present Hungarian nation-state, including all people with a Hungarian passport – i.e. a majority of Magyars as well as Roma, Slovaks, and people with other ethnic roots.

45 Petra Szavics argued that the EU accession has reinforced the awareness of the existence of state borders, which after the fall of communism had become more permeable. This was noted among Hungarian minorities as the creation of a second Iron Curtain. Cf. Petra Szavics, *The Boundaries of European Union Citizenship. The Problem of Third Country Nationals* (MA Theses, Central European University, Nationalism Studies Program, 2004), http://www.mtaki.hu/docs/petra_szavics_boundaries_of_-eu_citizenship.pdf, in particular p. 15. See also the Government Office for Hungarian Minorities Abroad, http://www.hhrf.org/htmh/en/index.php.

46 The pan-nationalist political ideology of a Great Hungary, which unites all ethnic Hungarians within the nation's historic borders preceding the treaty of Trianon following the end of World War I, has a strong impact on religious and linguistic minorities *within* Hungary. Anthropologist Donna Meryl Goldstein shows this by the example of the contested (and denied) belonging of Jews throughout Hungarian history. Cf. Donna Meryl Goldstein, »Re-imagining the Jew in Hungary: the Reconstruction of Ethnicity through Political Affiliation«, in: *Rethinking Nationalism and Ethnicity. The Struggle for Meaning and Order in Europe*, ed. by Hans-Rudolf Wicker (Oxford/New York: Berg, 1997), pp. 193–210.

extraterritorial, non-resident, and dual forms of citizenship, questions of territorial autonomy and territorial sovereignty; minority rights and privileges; the minority policy of the EU; and the possibility of recognizing a nation that is not defined by territorial boundaries.[47] The case of treatment for ethnic Hungarians (but not for other patients) from abroad in Prospect IVF clinics can thus be seen as an example of the complex entanglements and interactions of IVF as a global form with contested politicised boundaries and with a national and transnational identity politics that turns IVF technology and practice into a »politics by other means.«[48] Yet these ideologies of belonging and of solidarity were not the only themes with blurred contours that I encountered in Hungary. After dealing with potential flows of foreign patients in the previous section, I shall now discuss the potential flows of egg cells.

On the Fuzzy Boundaries of Two-directional Flows: Substances and Compensations

Egg donation in Hungary is an ambiguous and complicated field, as the head of a fertility section at one of Budapest's universities explained to me. I call him József Baltaś. He founded the clinic in 1992 after a five-year IVF training at a small university town in Germany. József Baltaś refers to egg donation as an ambiguous field because, until recently, the procedure in Hungary was regulated in a contradictory and even paradoxical way. Due to this former regulation he describes egg donation in Hungary as lawful, but »practically not feasible.« A law from 1997, the Parliamentary Act CLIV on Health Care Chapter IX, ruled that egg donation

47 Cf. Stephen Deets, »Reimagining the Boundaries of the Nation: Politics and the Development of Ideas on Minority Rights«, in: *East European Politics and Societies* 20 (2006), 3, pp. 419–446; Mária Kóvacs, »The Politics of Dual Citizenship in Hungary«, in: *Citizenship Studies* 10 (2006), 4, pp. 431–451; Myra A. Waterbury, »Internal Exclusion, External Inclusion: Diaspora Politics and Party-Building Strategies in Post-Communist Hungary«, in: *East European Politics and Societies* 20 (2006), 3, pp. 483–515.

48 Cf. Simone Abram, »Introduction: Science/Technology as Politics by Other Means«, in: *Focaal – European Journal of Anthropology* 46 (2005), pp. 3–20.

must not be connected to financial interests and at the same time must be anonymous. The crux of the matter was that without payment, hardly any woman would be willing to endure the painful and time-consuming procedure, explains József Baltaś. If, on the other hand, the donor was a sister or a friend, she no longer satisfied the requirement of an anonymous or »nameless relation«[49] set by the law. However, this contradiction in the 1997 Health Care Act was resolved by an amendment, which repealed the requirement of anonymity for egg donors from the 1st of July 2006, a few months before my sojourn in Hungary.

On the basis of this new law, foreign patients are now allowed to receive donor eggs in Hungary. According to József Baltaś, however, this requires that they bring along their own donors. Since July 2006, when donor anonymity was revoked, IVF treatment with donor eggs may also be offered to foreign patients; to a German patient with her sister, for example. However, a transnational flow of egg cells from Hungarian donors to Western recipients is, according to Baltaś, »virtually not working,« because without pay there simply aren't any donors. Nevertheless, he remarks with a whiff of sarcasm, he had »indeed received some phone calls from Germans searching for egg cells.« Occasionally there are foreign patients at this university fertility center. They come from Romania, Slovakia, Serbia, and some also come from Germany. However, according to Baltaś they live or have lived in Hungary, or his former colleagues in Germany, with whom he has collaborated for several years, have recommended them.

István Zoltai is my third interlocutor in Budapest. He runs an IVF clinic located in a public hospital, which I have called Péter Hospital IVF. He explains to me the complexity of the flow of organic matter, or, to paraphrase Nancy Scheper-Hughes and Margaret Lock, of »mindful body« substance:[50]

»The tricky thing in egg donation – the difficult thing is the financial situation [...]. Officially there is no money, which could move before or after. So we do not

49 Cf. Monica Konrad, *Nameless Relations. Anonymity, Melanesia and Reproductive Gift Exchange Between British Ova Donors and Recipients* (New York/Oxford: Berghahn, 2005).

50 Nancy Scheper-Hughes and Margaret Lock coined the notion of the »mindful body« to remind us of individual, social, and political aspects when analyzing and theorizing the human body. Cf. »The Mindful Body: A Prolegomenon to Future Work in Medical Anthropology«, in: *Medical Anthropology Quarterly* 1 (1987), 1, pp. 6–41.

sell eggs. This would be completely impossible and illegal. [...] From now on it is not anonymous, so they [donor and recipient; EMK] can talk to each other. I do not mind what they discuss [...]. Whether it is traveling, or money, or a present, or whatsoever just a handshake, or a ›thank you.‹ I do not mind. We do *not* take care of *this* part. We are very careful because it could be very, very difficult if we were [implicated] in that. But we are definitely not! We assume that there is also some kind of financial movement behind it, but this is between the donor and the recipient.«

There are two ways by which Péter Hospital IVF center recruits egg donors and deals with the moral and legal dilemma of altruism versus payment. Either the recipient brings a donor along or there are donors themselves »who approach this institute and want to give eggs for someone.« In both cases, the clinic's activities are limited to matching procedures, as István Zoltai once again stresses:

»If we find out that they [...] match [...] we enable them to meet. *We* are discussing the medical part, and the other part *they* discuss. I know of course that there is something behind [i.e. going on behind the scenes; EMK], but officially this is not done. There is no price. [...] of course we know that maybe there is something behind. But this is completely outside of this institute.«

He also points out that the majority of these unrelated donors, who are neither anonymous nor entirely altruistic, are lower class people from Hungary's periphery.

»They [...] do not come from the cities but from the villages. A [...] poor mother who is raising kids and who needs that money for the kids. This is 80 per cent of our donors, nice village women who need a little support. At least this is what I think; this is what I see with most of our donors. But [...] we do not have the donor who is *really* needy, not *very* poor, not *very* low class. They have a normal family life, they are normal people, but of course they would like to have something. In other countries you could *see* a price: how much the donor gets [as compensation; EMK]. Here, it is not clear.«

Conclusion

In my attempt to trace activities and grey zones related to reproductive tourism in Hungary I have followed a comparative approach. The interviewed representatives of a private fertility clinic, a university center, and a public IVF facility provided insights into remarkably divergent practices and differing interpretations.[51]

The image of Western IVF travelers following a traditional trajectory towards the East for cheap egg cells seems to contradict with Ákos Raćz's public image as a state-honored producer of Hungarians. Raćz denies reproductive patient border traffic and stresses that Hungarian eggs stay with Hungarian patients in Prospect IVF clinics. However, the concept of national belonging in his perspective has attained considerable flexibility, and thus some of the private clinic's »Hungarian« patients may in fact come from abroad.

Ever since anonymity is no longer legally required, a German patient can bring her sister or her friend as an egg donor to the university's fertility center. There, the German fertility traveler will get an IVF cycle far cheaper than in Germany, and she may undergo IVF treatment with donated eggs, a procedure which is outlawed in Germany. However, the German fertility tourist is still not able to use Hungarian egg cells because she is not allowed to acquire female gametes by purchase. Since the number of altruistic Hungarian egg donors is very limited, the German patient would need to bring a donor to the university's fertility clinic, and this would have to be a known donor from within her family or from the circle of her friends. In Péter Hospital IVF, by contrast, egg donation is also arranged with donors unrelated to the recipient. In Prospect IVF clinics,

51 The divergent interpretations of both the legal framework for egg donation and the assumed grey areas of unofficial flows of money and other forms of compensation for egg donations, as well as the personal pan-nationalistic attitude of one informant can be seen as information belonging to the »para-ethnographic« sphere. Douglas Holmes and George Marcus have discussed the relevance of such »para-ethnographic« strategies for gaining access to emergent policy formations by making use of anecdotal remarks, marginal or even illicit thoughts of professional subjects Cf. Douglas Holmes & George Marcus, »Cultures of Expertise and the Management of Globalization: Toward the Re-Functioning of Ethnography«, in: *Global Assemblages. Technology, Politics, and Ethics as Anthropological Problems,* ed. by Aihwa Ong & Stephen Collier (Malden, Oxford and Victoria: Blackwell Publishing, 2005), pp. 235–252.

treatment for patients from abroad first of all depends on their belonging: being ethnic Hungarian defines them as equal to national patients.

These divergent practices are based on different interpretations and assessments of the legal situation in Hungary and of the ways in which this situation shapes the fuzzy intermingling of flows of human body substances (egg cells) with flows of knowledge (the non-anonymity of the donor), and flows of money or other benefits (compensation). The private fertility clinic, the university center, and the public IVF facility all showed heterogeneous clinic policies in their attempt to keep these flows apart and to provide clear boundaries for them.

According to the self-portrayal by the clinic representatives, only Péter Hospital IVF is explicitly a meeting place for the supply and demand of donor eggs, potentially including Eastern supply and Western demand. Here, clinic policy with the help of a »matching procedure in two stages« draws a clear line. A genetic-biological matching process inside the clinic's laboratory is flanked by (an assumed) financial one, which is strictly banished from the clinic. The genetic-biological matching procedure is based on scientific knowledge and mediated through medical professionals and technology. By contrast, the assumed financial matching is a non-mediated procedure. It is neither mediated through the clinic nor through legal regulations. It is instead a kind of backdoor dealing between donor and recipient.

For an ethnography of reproductive tourism in a broader sense, the Hungarian example clearly demonstrates that national laws themselves neither primarily, exclusively, nor distinctively shape »glocal«[52] practices of IVF. The relevant laws always combine with manifold interpretations and with diverse clinic policies. They all have to be taken into consideration as additional powerful factors, forces, and actors. While two fertility professionals have argued that the ban on financial compensation for egg donors limits or even prevents Western egg tourism to Hungary, for the third physician the legal frame leaves enough room to tolerate a shady kind

52 Cf. Roland Robertson, »Glocalization: Time-Space and Homogeneity-Heterogeneity«, in: *Global Modernity*, ed. by Mike Featherstone, Scott Lash & Robert Robertson (London: Sage Publications, 1995), pp. 25–44; Marta Kirejczyk, *Bodies of Technology. Women's Involvement with Reproductive Medicine*, ed. by Ann Rubinow Saetnan, Nelly Oudshoorn & Marta Kirejczyk (Ohio: Columbus, 2000) pp. 183–206, in particular p. 185.

of »expense allowance,« as long as this secret commercial sphere of conception[53] occurs exclusively outside the clinic as a purely personal affair between donor and recipient. Of course, what is *actually* going on between donors and recipients remains hidden, unclear and behind the scenes – at least within the limited scope of this inquiry.

Researching reproductive tourism as one manifestation of IVF as a global form means exploring fuzzy and blurring grey zones of legality: Is it illegal, or illicit, or informal to look for egg cells abroad (e.g. in Eastern Europe) when egg donation and egg transfer is outlawed in one's (Western European) home country? It is a delicate, often confusing, and sometimes even discouraging matter to do ethnographic research on the shifting and blurred boundaries between legality and illegality. Anthropologist Carolyn Nordstrom discusses the difficulties of this kind of ethnographic research and employs the useful term *il/legal* to »designate the intersections of legality and illegality.«[54]

The exploration of transnational egg donation in Hungary as both a new and traditional medical tourism segment in-the-making revealed a number of fuzzy boundaries. Performing or not performing donor egg procedures, the definition of who counts as a foreign patient and therefore what counts as reproductive tourism, donor recruitment and compensation, and the resulting hierarchies (between East and West and between urban center and rural periphery within Hungary) are highly dependent on socio-economic, geographical, and legal structures as well as on the individual agency of the actors involved.

The Hungarian case shows, furthermore, that the nation-state and its borders have not become obsolete in transnational medical travel activities. Exploring IVF as a global form, we should also pay attention to connections and proximities between assisted conception, nationalisms, and pan-nationalisms, as I have argued in the present case. We should not take »given« borders for granted and we should try to avoid the episte-

53 Spar, »The Baby Business«, op. cit. (note 21).

54 Cf. Carolyn Nordstrom, *Global Outlaws. Crime, Money, and Power in the Contemporary World* (Berkeley, Los Angeles and London: University of California Press, 2007), in particular p. XVIII. For a more detailed discussion of the il/legal spheres in reproductive tourism see Eva-Maria Knoll, »*Managing Distances and Navigating Moral Landscapes*«, op. cit. (note 20).

mological trap of methodological nationalism,[55] which seems all the more tempting since national laws have such a high impact on the opportunities and exclusions in the *reproscape.*[56] Technological zones like the *reproscape*, which has emerged around IVF as a global form, may have more or less clear-cut borders, as Andrew Barry argues, but he also stresses that these borders increasingly *depart* from the borders of nation-states.[57] IVF as a global form and reproductive traveling as one part of medical tourism does not necessarily reproduce the state's own account of territorial boundaries and sovereignty. Ákos Raćz's imaginary mapping of Magyar settlement has little in common with the official political and geographical images of the actual borders of Hungary and its neighboring countries today. Rather, it is a complex and fuzzy relation between mobility and immobility; between an imaginary community and its shared imaginary territorial space.

In my contribution to this volume I have reflected on the complexity of terminology and borders in reproductive medicine. By applying some ideas and thoughts from international migration studies and the anthropology of borders and by comparing the practices of different clinics, I have tried to look beyond the border-as-line and to shed some light on social space instead, i.e. on borders as a »messy [...] conjunction of barriers and passages.«[58] The legal and moral sovereignty of an EU state over its territory is materialized in a variety of (partially arbitrary) legal and moral interpretations that corresponds to distinctive or even contrary treatment practices in different clinics.

55 With »methodological nationalism« Andreas Wimmer and Nina Glick Schiller refer to a topic which was introduced by Ulrich Beck and has been discussed since the 1970s. In a nutshell, methodological nationalism means that »nationally bounded societies are taken to be the naturally given entities to study.« Andreas Wimmer & Nina Glick Schiller, »Methodological Nationalism and Beyond: Nation-State Building, Migration and the Social Sciences«, in: *Global Networks* 2 (2002), 4, pp. 301–334, in particular p. 304–308.

56 The term »reproscape« was independently developed by several scholars as quite an obvious derivation from Arjun Appadurai's concept of scapes (e.g. mediascape, ideoscape, technoscape) into the sphere of global-local interaction of IVF. Cf. Appadurai, »*Modernity at Large*«, op. cit. (note 4).

57 Andrew Barry, »Technological Zones«, in: *European Journal of Social Theory* 9 (2006), 2, pp. 239–253.

58 Madeleine Reeves, »Materializing Borders«, in: *Anthropology News* 49 (2008), 5, pp. 12–13, in particular p. 13; Hastings Donnan & Thomas M. Wilson, *Borders. Frontiers of Identity, Nation and State* (Oxford/New York: Berg, 2001 [1999]).

What is Europeanization in the Field of Assisted Reproductive Technologies?

Maren Klotz & Michi Knecht

Recently, the Grand Chamber of the European Court of Human Rights (ECHR) decided that the Austrian ban on sperm and ova donation for heterologous forms of in vitro fertilization is not in breach of the European Convention on Human Rights and in particular does not conflict with Article 8 providing the »right to respect for one's private and family life.« With this judgment the ECHR revoked a prior decision issued by the First Section of the Court on 1 April 2010 and granted the member states of the European Union considerable room for maneuver in legislating reproductive technologies. While the judges observed a »clear trend [...] towards allowing gamete donation for the purpose of in vitro fertilization, which reflects an emerging European consensus,« this consensus according to the Chamber's assessment is not »based on settled and long-standing principles established in the laws of the member states.« Rather, it simply »reflects a stage of development within a particularly dynamic field of law.« The Court therefore argued that Austria should be given a wide margin of appreciation in legislating sperm and ova donation and that local or national »moral considerations and social acceptability« had to be taken seriously. The Court additionally mentioned »there is no prohibition in Austrian law on going abroad to seek treatment of infertility that uses artificial procreation techniques not allowed in Austria.«[1]

What makes this decision so interesting is that, in a nutshell, it captures three simultaneous and at least partly contradictory developments within the European regulation of assisted reproductive technologies: *First* a trend toward increasing coordination and »consensus,« brought about not only by general social and cultural dynamics, but also by European regulations

1 Grand Chamber of the European Court of Human Rights (ECHR), *Case of S.H. and Others v. Austria (Application no. 57813/00) Judgement*, Strasbourg, 3 November 2011.

directed towards the harmonization and standardization of practices and procedures within the field of reproductive medicine. *Second* the tendency toward the persistence of a patchwork of widely diverging national laws and even a proliferation of new differences in the legislation of reproductive technologies.[2] And *third*, an increase in reproductive mobility across national borders within the European Union as well as beyond. In explicitly mentioning the possibility of women and couples to travel abroad in search of treatments legally banned or for other reasons unavailable in their own nation states the Court seemed to imply that while individuals and bodily substances such as gametes (ova and sperm) can and should be mobile, »moral considerations and social acceptability« are not. The judgment is formulated as if to officially confirm what Norwegian anthropologist Marit Melhuus has described as a double capacity of national law not exclusively but pronouncedly playing out in the field of reproductive technologies: At once a »localizing strategy« in itself that reflects and defines cultural values, territorial boundaries and a characteristic stance vis-à-vis other forms of legislation, such law in practice also »opens up a world, setting persons and things in motion and thereby laying the basis for new social relations.«[3]

For anthropologists the legislation and regulation of reproductive technologies in the European Union affords a unique possibility to grasp the complexities involved in such a transnational constellation and to rethink the process of Europeanization not only in terms of changing practices of identification and the circulation of political ideas, images and ideals, but also with respect to more mundane aspects such as laws, safety directives and standards. In this article, we will zoom in on one small and fairly specific piece of European regulation within the legislation of assisted reproductive technologies: the EU Tissue and Cells Directive of

2 Important legal differences among European nations exist for example in banning, approving or not regulating specific procedures such as surrogacy arrangements, ova donation or heterologous insemination; with regard to the status and storage of fertilized ova, fetuses and embryos, and with respect to preimplantation genetic testing. Together with Austria, Ireland, Italy, and Portugal (and Switzerland as a non-EU country), Germany belongs to those nations within the European Union that are more restrictive about ARTs.

3 Marit Melhuus, »Exchange Matters: Issues of Law and the Flow of Human Substances«, in: *Globalisation – Studies in Anthropology*, ed. by Thomas Hylland Erikson (London: Pluto Press, 2003), pp. 170–197, in particular p. 171.

2004, which got implemented into German national law in 2007. We will look into one moment of its translation into actual practice when the EU Tissue Directive arrives at two Berlin sperm banks and fertility clinics and leads the actors there to pass through a number of transformations. By ethnographically focusing on the effects and ramifications of the EU Tissue Directive from a local perspective and by way of a single case study, we want to show how the threefold process of »increasing similarities,« »increasing differences,« and »increasing reproductive mobilities« engendered by the local articulation of transnational regulation is playing out within a specific assemblage. We want to illustrate the role of seemingly »unspectacular« or, as Leigh Star would probably have argued, »boring«[4] aspects of transnationalization in structuring our research field and making the discursive and material space called Europe. While the explicit aim of the EU Tissue Directive is rather narrowly formulated as providing »a safe and stable supply of human tissue and cells for therapeutic treatment,«[5] we trace unintended social, material, and political implications that clearly reach farther than the officially declared intention. We show how, within the Berlin sperm bank, the Tissue Directive has effects on emerging legal and social forms of kinship, on new medical actors, on changing institutional hierarchies and work routines. Simultaneously, in the local process of translating the new directive into the everyday routines and procedures of a Berlin sperm bank, Europe emerges as a specific space for the different actors involved

In what follows, we first locate our attempt toward an ethnography of transnational regulation within a more general anthropological perspective on Europeanization processes. We then contextualize the implementation of the EU Tissue Directive in Germany and ethnographically describe some of the implications and articulations it has had in our field of research, detailing one moment of its installment at two Berlin sperm banks and briefly pointing to some of the implications it has had beyond these institutions. In summing up we discuss research approaches and tools for

4 Susan Leigh Star, »Infrastructure and Ethnographic Practice. Working on the Fringes«, in: *Scandinavian Journal of Information Systems* 14 (2002), 2, pp. 107–122, in particular p. 110.

5 Klaus Hoyer, »An anthropological analysis of European Union (EU) health governance as biopolitics: The use of the EU Tissue and Cells Directive«, in: *Social Science & Medicine* 70 (2010), pp. 1867–1873, in particular p. 1867.

an ethnography of transnational regulation that may contribute to a better understanding of Europeanization processes in the field of reproductive technologies.

Anthropological Perspectives on Europeanization in the Field of Reproductive Technologies

Europeanization is an open, unfinished and contested process. With John Borneman and Nick Fowler[6] we point to the difference between on the one hand the political process of European integration and the establishment, enlargements and crisis of the European Union and on the other hand a more encompassing, fuzzy cultural and social process transforming everyday routines, processes, and practices of diverse actors and institutions, often without much notice.[7] Both dimensions of Europeanization are closely interlinked; however, they are neither congruent with regard to territory and space nor synchronized with regard to temporalities and time.

Europeanization can be viewed both as an example of a supranational integration process and of the emergence of a transnational regional unity. On both levels, tensions between the established structures of European nation states and transnational or supranational politics, practices, laws, and procedures persist – in our case study it is the tension between national regulation and legislation of sperm banks and a transnational directive aimed at raising safety standards and harmonizing European cooperation and transfer. Far from gradually decreasing, such tensions rather seem to form an enduring and characteristic feature of Europeanization.[8]

6 John Borneman & Nick Fowler, »Europeanization«, in: *Annual Review of Anthropology* 26 (1997), pp. 487–514.

7 Cf. Gisela Welz & Annina Lottermann, »Projekte der Europäisierung – Einleitung«, in: *Projekte der Europäisierung. Kulturanthropologische Forschungsperspektiven*, ed. by Gisela Welz & Annina Lottermann. Kulturanthropologische Notizen no. 78, (Frankfurt: Johann Wolfgang Goethe-Universität Frankfurt, Institut für Kulturanthropologie, 2009), pp. 11–16.

8 Cf. Aihwa Ong, *Flexible Citizenship. The Cultural Logics of Transnationality* (Durham: Duke University Press, 1999).

From the perspective of social and cultural anthropology, Europeanization is more than the top-down implementation of formal and informal rules, the installation of political and economic institutions and procedures, and the negotiation of shared political and economic objectives. Ethnographers have experimented with different approaches in order to investigate Europeanization as a vision and process[9] from the perspective of local situations and positioned actors. Early paradigmatic studies of Europeanization within anthropology have accessed their field both from the center – e.g. by studying bureaucrats and lobbyists in Brussels and Strasbourg – and by taking fringe perspectives.[10] Other studies have taken their inspiration from the anthropology of policy and tried to »research through« different interlinked levels and hierarchies.[11] At first ethnographic research mainly focused on the means of political and cultural management like ideas, images, symbols and identifications. During the past decade more recent studies have also highlighted the importance of regulation, standardization, knowledge practices and infrastructural. To better understand Europeanization within the field of reproductive medicine, we suggest to develop an ethnography of regulation that focuses on the interplay of knowledge practices, standardization, and normativity as formulated through law and policies. The more general observations on Europeanization by Andrew Barry bear instant plausibility for our field of research:

9 Borneman & Fowler, »Europeanization«, op. cit. (note 6), p. 487.

10 For a useful overview cf. Welz & Lottermann, »Projekte der Europäisierung«, op. cit. (note 7), pp. 11–12; for an exemplary case study Chris Shore, *Building Europe. The Cultural Politics of European Integration* (London and New York: Routledge, 2000); also Iréne Bellier & Thomas M. Wilson (Eds.), *An Anthropology of the European Union. Imagining and Experiencing the New Europe* (Oxford: Berg, 2001); Maryon McDonald, »Unity in Diversity. Some Tensions in the Construction of Europe«, in: *Social Anthropology* 3 (1996), pp. 47–60; and Gisela Welz, »Ethnografie Europäischer Modernen«, in: *Ort. Arbeit. Körper. Ethnografie europäischer Modernen,* ed. by Beate Binder, Silke Göttsch, Wolfgang Kaschuba & Konrad Vanja (Münster: Waxmann, 2005), pp. 19–32.

11 Cf. Kerstin Poehls & Asta Vonderau (Eds.), »Turn to Europe. Kulturanthropologische Europaforschungen«, in: *Berliner Blätter. Ethnographische und ethnologische Beiträge* 41 (2006), pp. 11–26; Chris Shore & Susan Wright, *Anthropology of Policy. Critical Perspectives on Government and Power* (London: Taylor & Francis, 1997); Chris Shore, Susan Wright & Davide Però (Eds.), *Policy Worlds. Anthropology and the Analysis of Contemporary Power* (Oxford: Berghahn, 2011).

»For what has developed across Europe is a whole range of regulations and devices, governing and monitoring everything from the cleanliness of beaches to the design of electrical equipment and the safety of toys. The European Union has surprisingly few bureaucrats, no teachers, no prisons, and no doctors. It has few human representatives with which it is possible to identify. But it does possess an array of procedures, regulations, and standards that govern the behavior of human and nonhuman devices throughout its territory and, indeed, beyond.«[12]

In this article we are particularly interested in the work done with and by standards defined through EU-regulation. Standards are an important element of transnational orders.[13] They construct »uniformities across time and space through the generation of agreed-upon rules.«[14] At the same time, however, these standards are altered in the process of integration into local structures like the daily routines of a sperm bank. All the protagonists of our research – laboratory staff, doctors, donors, patient-consumers – are permanently concerned with comparing, translating, questioning and modifying standards. In our understanding these practices all contribute in their own specific way to a provisional and fragile stabilization of a »Europeanized« space in reproductive technology. While standardizations require the development of partly relaxing routines and make more and more things fit the same pattern by aligning and subjecting elements to norms, »translations« in Michael Callon's sense[15] contribute to the tentative stabilization of emerging transnational – in our example, European – spaces of reproductive medicine precisely by creating diversity. »Translation« here means all those appropriations, reinterpretations and representations that emerge in dealing with, for instance, the stan-

12 Andrew Barry, »In the Middle of the Network«, in: *Social Studies of Knowledge Practices*, ed. by Annemarie Mol & John Law (Durham, London: Duke University Press, 2002), pp. 142–165, in particular p. 143.

13 Cf. Elizabeth C. Dunn, »Standards and Person-Making in East Central Europe«, in: Global Assemblages. Technology, Politics, and Ethics as Anthropological Problems, ed. by. Aihwa Ong & Stephen J. Collier (Malden, MA and Oxford: Blackwell, 2005), pp. 173–193.

14 Stefan Timmermans & Steven Epstein, »A World of Standards but not a Standard World: Toward a Sociology of Standards and Standardization«, in: *Annual Review of Sociology* 36 (2010), pp. 69–89, in particular p. 71.

15 Michel Callon, »Some Elements of a Sociology of Translation. Domestication of the Scallops and the Fishermen of St. Brieuc Bay«, in: *The Science Studies Reader*, ed. by Mario Biogioli (New York and London: Routledge 1999), pp. 67–83.

dards introduced by an EU Directive in German sperm banks, creating a broad field of variations that leads to an ever widening interplay and more extensive alliances.[16]

Focusing not only on the work done by standards but also on what actors do with them connects our perspective on Europeanization with knowledge practices. We hark back here to the broader understanding of knowledge developed in social and cultural anthropology that sees knowledge not only as a pool of information, but also as performative and relational, in short: as a social practice.[17] In everyday life knowledge appears as bricolage, as a way of making sense.[18] Analytically we can distinguish between the validated content, the medium and genres of its transmission, and the social organization of knowledge[19], in practice, however, these registers always coincide. Standards are worked into the fabric of daily life by knowledgeable actors and only by taking their everyday acts and experiences seriously can we discern those spaces that in spite of thick regulation remain open to configuration. Only the analysis of *practices* of knowledge may lead to an understanding of the interactive dynamics, social struggles, multi-faceted processes of negotiation and diverse networking activities that are the basis both for translating regulation into everyday life and also for legal change. Only in view of these practices can we perceive the difference between regulations and their execution, can variations in the implementation of regulative guidelines and subjective, even oppositional appropriations be discerned.

16 Michel Callon, »Techno-economic networks and irreversibility«, in: *A Sociology of Monsters. Essays on Power, Technology, and Domination*, ed. by John Law (London: Routledge, 1991), pp. 132–162, in particular p. 143.

17 Kirsten Hastrup, »Getting it right: Knowledge and evidence in anthropology«, in: *Anthropological Theory* 4 (2004), 4, pp. 455–472, in particular p. 458.

18 Bernd Jürgen Warneken, *Die Ethnographie popularer Kulturen. Eine Einführung* (Basel, Köln, Weimar and Wien: Böhlau/UTB, 2006), pp. 109–114.

19 Cf. Fredrik Barth, »An Anthropology of Knowledge«, in: *Current Anthropology* 43 (2002), pp. 1–18.

Contextualizing the EU Directive on Human Tissue and Cells in Germany

During our various research endeavors into reproductive technologies in Germany, almost all professional actors we came into contact with since 2005 mentioned the EU Tissues and Cells Directive in some context or other. Particularly sperm donation has been realigned within the German legal landscape by the specific regulatory power the Directive has unfolded in Germany. To begin our analysis of a specific assemblage engendered through the implementation of the Tissue Direction it is necessary to give a rough introductory sketch of German policies on reproductive technologies and, in particular, sperm donation: Artificial insemination in Germany has never been affected by the regulatory initiatives on reproductive technologies and biotechnologies that developed in Europe at the beginning of the 1990s. While the British Human Fertilisation and Embryology Act, the most elaborated piece of regulation on NRTs worldwide installed in 1990, comprehensively discusses sperm donation, there is no mention of it in the German law regulating reproductive medicine, the so called »Embryo Protection Law« (Embryonenschutzgesetz), which was equally enacted in 1990. There is a complicated genealogy to this obvious omission. Firstly, German discourse on reproductive and genetic technologies pronouncedly centered on the status of the embryo. As a result of the development of German abortion laws in the 1980s and 1990s and, more generally, as a way of dealing with the experience and memory of the Holocaust and with the use and abuse of medical experiment and genetic classification during Nazism, »a strong moral protection of fetus and embryo« had become a »distinguishing feature of German law« in general and of German legislation on reproductive technologies in particular.[20] Secondly, as soon as general questions entered the policy discussions, they quickly became subject to so-called slippery slope arguments leaving little

20 John A. Robertson, »Reproductive Technology in Germany and the United States: An Essay in Comparative Law and Bioethics«, in: *Columbia Journal of Transnational Law* 2004 (43), pp. 187–226, in particular p. 195. For a comparative view on the legal status of the embryo in British and German law see Nicole Richardt, »A Comparative Analysis of the Embryological Research Debate in Great Britain and Germany«, in: *Social Politics: International Studies in Gender, State and Society* 10 (2003), 1, pp. 86–128.

or no room for – in the words of many of our medical interview partners – »low-tech« and »primitive« reproductive technologies such as donor insemination. Thirdly, although it is hard to assess how much this influenced policy discourse on important levels, sperm donation has had a somewhat dingy public image in Germany for a long time, because of pervasive myths that the Nazis had used artificial insemination for their *Lebensborn* »human breeding« programs during World War II.[21] As a result of this lack of political interest and legislative attention, sperm donation in Germany has long been, and in many instances still is, an underregulated grey area compared to many other European countries.

Before the integration of the EU Directive into German national law in 2007, sperm donor anonymity – or non-anonymity – was not mentioned in any regulatory statement. This is particularly interesting since there is a German Federal Constitutional Court ruling from 1989 which is unrelated to reproductive technologies, but which nevertheless declares »knowledge about ones parentage«[22] to be a basic constitutional right. However, the ruling was not applied to sperm donation until the implementation of the EU Directive. The full extent of the legal uncertainties and entanglements surrounding sperm donation in Germany cannot be unfolded in detail within the scope of this article.[23] Suffice it to give one additional impression: To date, a German donor conceived child could – in theory – contest his social and legal father's paternity and try to instead

21 For a short discussion of the – falsely attributed – connection between DI and the *Lebensborn* program see Thomas Katzorke, »Entstehung und Entwicklung der Spendersamenbehandlung in Deutschland«, in: *Umwege zum eigenen Kind. Ethische und rechtliche Herausforderungen an die Reproduktionsmedizin 30 Jahre nach Louise Brown* [Göttinger Schriften zum Medizinrecht no. 3], ed. by Gisela Bockenheimer-Lucius, Petra Thorn & Christiane Wendehorst (Göttingen: Universitäts-Verlag Göttingen, 2008), pp. 80–103, in particular pp. 92–93.

22 Our translation. German: »Kenntnis der eigenen Abstammung,« BVerfGE 79, 256.

23 For more detailed juridical discussions see Eva Maria K. Rütz, *Heterologe Insemination – Die rechtliche Stellung des Samenspenders«* (Berlin: Springer, 2008); Christiane Wendehorst, »Die rechtliche Regulierung donogener ART in Deutschland und Österreich«, in: *Umwege zum eigenen Kind. Ethische und rechtliche Herausforderungen an die Reproduktionsmedizin 30 Jahre nach Louise Brown* [Göttinger Schriften zum Medizinrecht no. 3], ed. by Gisela Bockenheimer-Lucius, Petra Thorn & Christiane Wendehorst (Göttingen: Universitäts-Verlag Göttingen, 2008), pp. 103–133.

have the sperm donor recognized as his or her father, thereby transferring legal and financial obligations.[24]

How did the Directive on Human Tissue and Cells figure within this gray area? Before we can answer this question from a localized ethnographic point of view, we need some further contextualization. The Directive, aimed at »setting standards of quality and safety for the donation, procurement, testing, processing, preservation, and distribution of human tissues and cells,« was put into force on EU level in 2004. Mainly directed at safety standards for new high-tech varieties of medical therapies with organic materials such as tissue transplants the Directive still came to affect fertility clinics and low-tech treatments such as artificial insemination. Gametes and their medical-commercial handling obviously fell under the label of »human tissues and cells« and were thus just as much subject to the Directive's regulations as other medical and biotechnical procedures involving, for example, the culturing of skin or tissue and bone banking. It was presumably due to what Hoyer[25] calls the »›technical nature‹ of safety standards« and to the complex, lengthy and divergent national implementations, that the Directive has engendered neither public attention nor much interest from the social sciences, with the notable exception Hoyer, who ethnographically analyzes the implementation of the Directive with regard to bone banking in Denmark and interprets its biopolitical implications.

The Directive was implemented as the German »Tissue Law« in 2007, which actually amounted to a complex and concerted change of various existing German laws on organ transplantation, pharmaceuticals, and blood transfusion. During the implementation process, the German Federal Chamber of Physicians campaigned against the inclusion of gametes under the new law, essentially giving them the status of pharmaceuticals, but to no avail.[26] Again, fully mapping the maze of legal requirements, clinical protocols, and lobbying activities, the implementation of the EU Directive has engendered in Germany would be beyond the scope of this article. However, before we leave the juridical birds-eye perspective in or-

24 Rütz, »Heterologe Insemination«, op. cit. (note 23), p. 217.

25 Hoyer, »An anthropological analysis«, op. cit. (note 5), p. 1867.

26 Bundesärztekammer, »Erweiterte und aktualisierte Stellungnahme zum Regierungsentwurf für ein Gewebegesetz«, (2007), http://baek.de/downloads/ZRegStell20070124.pdf [last accessed 13.4.2012].

der to address our ethnographic material it is important to keep in mind that the German implementation of the Directive has, in our view, had a tremendous impact and has worked to eliminate at least some of the legal gray areas surrounding the anonymous – or non-anonymous – status of sperm donors. We would argue it has essentially been the Tissue and Cells Directive with its somewhat surprising application to fertility clinics and sperm banks that has tipped the scales in Germany from a de facto anonymity in sperm donation practices to a still fragile and not very clearly defined form of non-anonymity. One important detail in this context is that, in the past, medical records (including donor records) have often been destroyed after the minimum storage period of ten years, leading to an »untraceability« of donors for grown-up children. The concurrence of the Federal Court ruling on the right to know ones genetic parentage (which had not been applied to sperm donation in earlier years) and the general extension of the storage period of all medical records (which has made the legal scenario of a grown-up child *successfully* suing for access to donor files much more likely) has essentially made it necessary expressly to deal with the anonymity status of donors in German regulations. The 2007 law for the first time in German legal history stated that a grown-up child has the right to look at the files. While the relevant paragraph (§14(3)) generally states that organ donations should always be managed anonymously, it specifically declares that »with sperm donation the right of the child to information on its parentage« has to prevail.[27] The paragraph does not give any detailed guidelines on how this right is to be safeguarded in practice. Whether it has been the question of record storage periods or not, it has clearly been the implementation of the EU Tissue Directive that has lead to the first explicit reference to donor *non*-anonymity in a German legal text. To our knowledge, there were no other policy endeavors discernible at the time that might have put the issue on the agenda, had not the Directive pushed questions surrounding gamete donation from relative obscurity into the glaring light of Federal politics.

27 Our translation. In German: »Von diesen Vorschriften unberührt bleibt im Falle der Samenspende das Recht des Kindes auf Kenntnis der eigenen Abstammung.«

The EU Tissue Directive in two Berlin Sperm Banks: Remaking Kinship, Work Routines and Authority within a »European Assemblage«

After we and our colleagues of the »Kinship Cultures and Reproductive Technologies« project«[28] had focused quite extensively on reproductive cross-border mobility (of patient-consumers in search of particular treatments as well as of practitioners) within a previous phase of research, during our ethnographic research at two Berlin sperm banks we began to see the ubiquitous EU Tissue Directive as a sort of traveler itself: Now the traveling regulation rather than the travelling patients or medical professionals became a transnational, in this case »Europeanizing« actor of sorts. Starting interviews and further fieldwork only shortly after the implementation of the Directive in Germany in 2007, the laboratory personnel kept rolling their eyes at us about their changed routines, doctors mused how it might further influence their work, medical consultants came and went to advise and train staff on the Directives' requirements, often combining the »shop-floor« implementation of the Directive with the installment of the ISO 9001 quality management system. [29]

Donor recruitment at the North Berlin Sperm Bank[30], a clinic located in a rather working class neighborhood of Berlin with many Turkish cafés and betting shops around, has hardly changed despite the significant change that the 2007 law introduced by officially guaranteeing non-anonymity. Since its establishment through andrologist and owner Dr. Dettmaringen in 2000 the North Berlin Sperm Bank has always opted for very openly informing their donors about the fragmentary state of German legislation regarding anonymity and legal relations between donor and child. Interestingly, the sperm bank has never had problems finding donors to come forward, even though it only occasionally advertises donor requests in two Berlin city magazines comparable to the Time-Out series. Sperm donors in Germany receive a recompense of roughly 400–600 Euro

28 For further information about this research project see [http://www.sfb-repraesentationen.de /teilprojekte/c4/english].

29 The Directive asks for a quality management system to be put in place, without specifying a particular typ. Many clinical institutions within the IVF sector in Germany and in wider Europe opt for the ISO system.

30 The name of the sperm bank and all personal names have been changed.

for one donation cycle of about eight weeks, within which the donor has to donate at least once weekly.

Dr. Dettmaringen quite passionately claims he always thought that knowledge about genetic ancestry was a »constitutional right since its establishment in 1949« (here he in fact seems to predate the much younger ruling by the Federal Constitutional Court). He never destroyed donor information and feels that the EU tissue Directive, now arriving in its national »translation« at his Berlin sperm bank, »proves him right.« One has to grant, however, that he has actually never faced the decision whether to destroy records after ten years or not since the Tissue Law came into force before his sperm bank's records were this old. Sitting in the reception area of the practice, white tiled, the desk partially decorated with »cuddly sperm« – colorful stuffed animals in the iconic shape of a sperm cell – physician's assistant Ruth Tolmin shows us the new donor consent forms they have started to use after the Directive was implemented: Complete anonymity is impossible, the paper informs possible donors, it cannot be entirely ruled out that a child resulting from a sperm donation one day might contact its donor. The clinic may have to comply and hand over data to the child, donors are warned on the document. Tolmin, a young woman who takes the sometimes metaphorical and always literal »seediness« of her job with mild humor, says that only very rarely are donors so concerned about this uncertainty that they do not return. On the new consent form they now have to sign the page informing them of their rights – and the uncertainties surrounding these – not just once, but twice:

»We always ask whether something is unclear. And in the donor consent form the paragraph about children having the right from the age of 18 to ask the gynecologist whom the donation came from now has a special bar around it. The donor has to specially sign this excerpt.«

These new routines did *not*, however, originate from new and detailed instructions on how to deal with sperm donor identity. While consultants are making a living out of training laboratory and administrative medical staff in new safety standards and other quality management measures, the very specific questions facing the relatively small amount of sperm banks in Germany have remained largely unattended and unsolved. Neither Ruth Tolmin nor her boss Dr. Dettmaringen has received any further description or explanation on how exactly the request for information from a donor-child should be dealt with: Whether Dr. Dettmaringen is in charge or rather the inseminating gynecologist and what would be considered a legitimate ground for disclosure – notwithstanding the legal uncertainties surrounding the juridical relation between donor-child and donor-father.

In this situation Dr. Dettmaringen excels in what seems to be the identifying marker of his trade – networking and interpreting the regulatory situation to his own end, displaying what we would characterize as a marked »pioneer spirit.« Legal consultants have been contacted by mail and phone to produce all the documents and contracts used within his practice; ISO experts, patient, and other interest groups have been asked for their opinion of the situation. As member in a professional medical organization concerned with donor insemination he is also in close contact with other sperm bank owners and IVF practitioners throughout Germany. However, many of the very mundane problems regarding forms, contracts, routines and standards connected to the EU Tissue Directive somehow fall »below« the level of responsibility of this association.

When looked upon ethnographically on the »shop floor« Europeanization in the field of reproductive technologies presents itself as a global – or one might say European assemblage[31]: a field of heterogeneous con-

31 Collier defines the term global assemblage as follows: »Global assemblages are the actual configurations through which global forms of techno-science, economic rationalism, and other expert systems gain significance. (…) The relationship among the elements in an assemblage is not stable; nor is their configuration reducible to a single logic. Rather, an assemblage is structured through critical reflection, debate, and contest,« (Stephen J. Collier, »Global Assemblages«, in: *Theory, Culture & Society* 23 (2006), 2/3, pp. 399–401, in particular 400). The somewhat elusive concept has been used by Rabinow (Paul Rabinow, *Anthropos today: reflections on modern equipment* (Princeton, N.J: Princeton University Press, 2003)) and has been first introduced, at least as a descriptive term, by Deleuze and Guattari (Gilles Deleuze & Félix Guattari, *A thousand plateaus: capitalism and schizophrenia* (London, New York: Continuum, 2004) and has also been followed up within art and architectural theory by Marcus and Saka (George E. Marcus & Erkan Saka, »Assemblage«, in: *Theory, Culture & Society*, 23 (2006), 2/3, pp. 101–109). More recently, it has been applied, in a less complex theoretical fashion, to anthropological studies of globalization by Aihwa Ong and Stephen J. Collier (Eds.), *Global Assemblages. Technology, Politics, and Ethics as Anthropological Problems* (Malden, MA: Blackwell 2006). Marcus and Saka have been quite critical of the elusiveness of the concept, but underline its potential for »an evocation of emergence and heterogeneity amid the data of inquiry (…) without rigidifying into the thingness of final or stable states that besets the working terms of classic social theory« (Marcus & Saka »Assemblage«, op. cit. (this note), p. 106.).

nections between state and EU regulation, transnational standards for quality management, professional and activist, the anticipation of future events, and miniscule interpretations and perspectives of local actors – in the ethnographic vignette presented above notably by Dr. Dettmaringen. We shall continue to look at this assemblage from a variety of angles throughout the course of this article, pointing to new forms of kinship, working routines, institutional hierarchies, and specific »manifestations« of the contested space called Europe.

By making sperm donation non-anonymous, or at least *less* anonymous, kinship is being reconstituted as part of a process of Europeanization of reproductive medicine in Germany. In affected families, new kinship practices may emerge, for instance regarding openness about the donation, donor or half-sibling contacts etc. These tendencies are observable in other countries,[32] but so far are more or less unheard of in Germany (also see Klotz in this volume). Following Strathern[33] and also Carsten[34] we believe that, ultimately, kinship in current Western society produces – constitutes – itself in knowledge practices. And it is knowledge practices which the EU Tissue Directive, as an unintended Germany-specific side-effect one could argue, surely changes. Even if emerging new kinship practices do not include the setting up of social relationships, they will still have effects on children-by-donation concerned. Strathern argues that kinship knowledge (in its »Western version« mostly knowledge on biological relatedness) has immediate consequences for our sense of self and does not allow for acceptance or dismissal on the basis of personal »usability.« To quote Marilyn Strathern: »It's social effects are immediate, built-in.«[35]

The traveling regulation – or rather the assemblage which was formed through the various interfaces the Directive has enacted – has also greatly affected the daily work routines in the two sperm banks that where part

32 E.g. Tabitha Freeman, Vasanti Jadva, Wendy Kramer & Susan Golombok, »Gamete Donation: Parents' Experiences of Searching for Their Child's Donor Siblings and Donor«, in: *Human Reproduction* 24 (2009), 3, pp. 505–516.

33 Marilyn Strathern, »Refusing Information«, in: *Property, Substance, and Effect: Anthropological Essays on Persons and Things* (London: Athlone Press, 1999), pp. 64–88.

34 Janet Carsten, »Constitutive Knowledge: Tracing Trajectories of Information in New Contexts of Relatedness«, in: *Anthropological Quarterly* 80 (2007), 2, pp. 403–426.

35 Strathern, »Refusing Information«, op. cit. (note 33), p. 77.

of the research field. This is a second unintended, but socially important, implication we want to trace in the process of translation of a piece of regulation into a specific »local« practice. At the much posher Charlottenburg Fertility Clinic and Sperm Bank, located in an affluent business and tourist area, head biologist Dr. Hagedorn explains some of the changes to us. She is still slightly baffled by the amount of work entailed by re-training all her laboratory personnel on those routines:

»Those new regulations prescribe a form of traceability. That means we have to be able to prove for every patient with which materials the gametes came into contact. That is an extreme effort, every test tube, every pipette tip, every Petri dish has a batch number, which gets documented. The batch number stands for a certificate that certain tests have been done with the materials. All of this we have to be able to document and account for, and all of this needs to be administrated. So, changes are mostly about administration, documentation and about the materials used and to a much lesser extent about the actual workflow in the laboratory.«

Her colleagues had to be shown how to fill out the new documentation papers and to administer the large amounts of additional information. This has also been the case in the North Berlin Sperm Bank, where young lab technician Maria Reusch additionally underlines that changes in laboratory materials do have a severe impact on her daily routines. She shows us how as part of the changed routines she now has to weld shut the straws within which the sperm is then frozen and stored in liquid nitrogen containers. Before, the straws were corked by sterile metal balls and Reusch still finds the welding process which is performed with a newly acquired welder, much more time-consuming.

For the employees in the North Berlin Sperm Bank, the new work flows make new demands on their internal communication and with their boss Dr. Dettmaringen. Lab technician Reusch explains to us – with her colleague, the administrator Tolmin sitting next to us:

»We don't really have the time to talk to each other, and yesterday I thought that maybe we should use a notebook and then you [her colleague Tolmin] could write what is new with the paperwork and how you do it correctly. I can't remember everything at first try and my colleague also doesn't remember to tell me everything at once... Maybe it is not the whole routine, but it is the small things that have changed... But I can't always go to the doctor and say ›Doctor, I don't know what I should do.‹«

Interestingly, as we talk further about the new work flows, it becomes clear that her statement about the impossibility of always asking the doctor what to do, does not only refer to not wanting to interrupt the boss, but also to the fact that at the moment of our research, Dr. Dettmaringen indeed did not have the final word on work routines. In fact, he hardly knew them himself. Instead he deferred research questions to the consultant sent by the medical consulting firm he had hired, Claire Herrmann, who conducts external trainings and internal consultations. Similarly, head biologist Dr. Hagedorn from the other sperm bank in Charlottenburg – who is in an analogous position of weight regarding the lab procedures as Dr. Dettmaringen who does not employ an additional head biologist to run his lab – actually mentions feelings of relief for being able to cede some of her authority to a consultant:

»When I read these regulatory guidelines, I keep thinking: ›My god, I am never going to be able to do this.‹ And then you are told that it is actually quite banal a thing. However, the language in these documents is so fundamentally different.«

Back at the North Berlin Sperm Bank, Reusch and Tolmin explain to us how their patience has often been taxed and how a certain disbelief about the new procedures started to mount during their work with consultant Frau Hermann:

»There always seems to be something. You think ›Great, now you're done.‹ And then« – Reusch completes Tolmins sentence with a glint in her eyes »then Frau Herrmann says that you actually cannot do this [...] and then you think that it cannot actually go on like this [...].«

Moreover it is not only new medical experts from »outside« sperm banks that are bestowed with authority within the assemblage engendered through the implementation of the European Directive but also the professional associations of the actors involved in reproductive medicine in Germany who gain additional significance. Biologist Dr. Hagedorn, for instance, expresses relief about the lobbying and policy watching initiatives of the German association of health professionals in reproductive medicine. She has experienced their work like a »shield« against some highly problematic aspects lurking in the implementation process. At some point she says she has been threatened by the scenario of a mandatory »class A cleanroom status« for her lab (a complicated standard on the amount of particles per cubic meter allowed), which would have essentially required to build a new one and change all lab procedures. As Hagedorn says:

»So I was looking at these potential regulations to come and actually got a bit shaky. We all started to hope that through the work of the association it would not get as horrible as we all thought it might. And I actually think that in certain areas it has worked out well.«

In the end, Dr. Hagedorn did not need to rebuild the Charlottenburg Sperm Bank's complete lab in order to conform to the EU Tissue Directive. In hindsight she expressed relief to have been spared by some of the seemingly grotesque implications the application of the European cleanroom standard would have had for her lab. As our analysis of micro interactions and vernacular talk during the incorporation of European standards into the everyday practices of two Berlin sperm banks has shown, the influence of such standards and regulations is not merely a technical matter:[36] Without intent and largely unnoticed by the public – »below the level of social visibility« – the EU Tissue Directive in very contingent ways massively modifies how kinship can be done with donated sperm in Germany. It has tipped the scales to a fragile donor non-anonymity, changed the uneven distribution of authority, knowledge and competencies within the sperm bank's labs, it has promoted the emergence of a new type of EU health consultant and has itself been modified by a myriad of small practices of everyday appropriation, transformation or avoidance.

We would also like to argue that the assemblage described here is co-producing the contested physical and imaginary space of »Europe.« The narratives of our interview partners time and again stress the perceived absurdity of the new regulations and the near impossibility of actually »living« them as lab personnel, doctors, and administrators. Sometimes these regulations are simply evaded, e.g. by not wearing the new face masks that are now officially required or by using up old lab materials instead of complying with the new standard. And they are reflected on with disbelief – and humor. Reusch and Tolmin for example laugh at the procedures for sending out sperm samples to other gynecologists:

36 Cf. Hoyer, »An anthropological analysis«, op. cit. (note 5).

»We now have to fill out extra transport papers. These papers state that, although it is a human tissue sample, on the basis of its properties it does *not* fall under the regulations for identifying hazardous goods. Before the EU Directive, we didn't do anything of this kind. It simply wasn't hazardous and there was no notice specifically stating that no special security measures were needed because – obviously – sperm is not a hazardous object.«

Here, Europe becomes a pronounced locus for the apparent absurdities of an increasingly overregulated late modernity – *Europe as Absurdistan*. In other situations, shop floor talk in the sperm bank labs figures *Europe as a repository of comparative knowledge*. Everyday comparison, we might say, pervades our transcripts and field notes. Lab staff, donors, consumer-patients and medical practitioners not only juxtapose the times »before« and »after« the implementation of the EU Tissue Directive, but also display a pronounced comparative consciousness about the wide spectrum of different regimes of reproductive governance installed in various European countries and beyond, evaluating, amongst other dimensions, access, cost, quality, and availability and by such acts of comparison creating new linkages and complexities.

Toward an ethnography of transnational regulation

By focusing on the effects of standardization and on knowledge practices involved in the implementation of the EU Directive on Human Tissue and Cells in two Berlin sperm banks it has become apparent that such standards in many ways not only produce »more sameness,« but also »more difference.« Regulation such as the EU Tissue Directive at the same time harmonizes and diversifies, depending on level and concrete situation. For an emerging ethnography of transnational regulation it is mandatory to capture this simultaneity and to develop analytical tools that adequately grasp this new complexity.

To better understand the development of reproductive technologies and reproductive medicine as a transnational or even global form in the future it will be important to pay attention not only to the scientific and medical developments but also to the regulation and legislation accompanying new technologies. An emergent ethnography of regulation will want to know more about the interaction of regulation and law, standards and norms, material and discursive dimensions. It is in this interplay of standards, norms and social practices that the obscure notion of an »implementation« of directives and standards can be unpacked in order to make visible the huge amount of work, negotiation, and the creative range of agency of the actors in the field.

Transnational Reproductive Mobilities, Materialities, and Agencies

Making Interferences: The Cultural Politics of Transnational Ova »Donation«

Michal Nahman

Introduction: Interferences

It is an aim of all good ethnographers to represent and interpret what they have seen »out there« in the world as faithfully as possible. But the question remains of what and to whom must one be faithful? Strands of anthropology have developed dedicated to examining anthropological modes of production – how we write; how or whether we intervene. It is clear from the last few decades of work in this discipline that there is always a kind of intervention when we enter a place and attempt to extract a »story« out of it.[1] Writing, itself, is a kind of intervention. Feminist science studies and philosophy have added the possibility of doing fiction and/or »figuration« as a way of not only acknowledging the role of the ethnographer/author, but also of doing something about the problems that we confront.[2] This

1 It may also be a kind of self-promotion of the ethnographer to write about what we have seen. Hence there is an inherent tension in the practise of ethnographic representation to do with being »good« at what we do (a moral obligation to those we study) and being »good« for our career. I discuss this later on in the paper when I think about the problems arising from my »intervention« in the ethnographic space in which I conducted research.

2 Haraway's idea of feminist cyborg revisionings is precisely a call to pay attention to the ways in which writing is always fiction, but also to use that truism to promote feminist critique and politically invested writing that accounts for historical and global effects on the women's bodies as they are mediated by technoscience. In the introduction to her book *Nomadic Subjects* (1994), Braidotti states that, »A figuration is a politically informed account of an alternative subjectivity« (Braidotti 1994: p. 1). Both Braidotti and Haraway call for a proliferation of feminist figurations which subvert »old ways« of viewing what is happening to/in /through women's bodies. Haraway draws her notion of »figuration« from Auerbach 1957. For more on this approach see Donna Haraway, *Simians, Cyborgs and Women: The Reinvention of Nature* (New York: Routledge, 1991); Claudia Castañeda, *Figurations: Child, Bodies, Worlds* (Durham and

is a resolutely political project that takes questions of power seriously; not just the power of the author to objectify, but the power of the academic-as-activist to make interferences.

This paper is an experiment in doing political feminist anthropology, and it is part of a larger project of seeing what kinds of connections can be made through writing, which will also have repercussions for social scientific and socio-cultural practice. It is tentatively prescriptive, and inevitably a product of my own situatedness in a time of persistent »war on terror,« global financial crisis, and, closer to home, the massive privatization of UK universities, which is affecting academic and scholarly work in unprecedented ways. Such times reflect the »absurdity of capitalist modernity«[3] and may generate fantastical responses. The »fantastical response« revives anthropological attempts at bringing fiction into ethnography. By this I do not revert to the »all ethnography is fiction position,« a postmodern interpretation of ethnography that makes a potentially nihilistic claim about the possibility of doing or saying anything. Rather, after providing an ethnographic account of Israeli-Romanian transnational egg or ova »donation,« what this paper brings in at the very end is a fictitious but possible ending. In an attempt to think through feminist and anthropological »interferences« in research and writing, the role of the researcher and writer in *making culture* is pursued. This is a topic that has been examined extensively, to say the least. Here, in presenting face-to-face research I conducted with young Romanian ova »donors« in an Israeli clinic in Bucharest,[4] I am trying to see what such »interference« can do for thinking about the politics of inequality or global »stratified reproduction.«[5]

London: Duke University Press, 2002); Rosi Braidotti, *Nomadic Subjects: Embodiment and Sexual Difference in Contemporary Feminist Theory* (New York: Columbia University Press, 1994).

3 China Miéville, »Introduction to Marxism and Fantasy«, in: *Fantastic Literature: A Critical Reader*, ed. by David Sandner (Westport, CT: Praeger, 2004), pp.334–344, in particular p. 337.

4 The idea of an »Israeli clinic in Bucharest« is explained below.

5 See Shellee Colen, »'Like a Mother to Them': Stratified Reproduction and West Indian Childcare Workers and Employers in New York«, in: *Conceiving the New World Order: The Global Politics of Reproduction*, ed. by Faye Ginsburg and Rayna Rapp (Columbia: University of California Press, 1995), pp. 78–102.

If, as Nancy Scheper-Hughes[6] argues, anthropology has the opportunity to contribute to emancipatory change, how do we do this in our writing and/or actions? Rather than simply *having awareness* and *responsibility* towards our subjects/objects of study, what if we sought to make allegories and myths that helped to convey what we have witnessed? *What if what we have seen cannot be adequately explored and explained without myth, allegory, and invention?* This approach is not simply about reflexivity in research, but rather in remaking epistemology and ontology – we are making society by writing it. The question then remains: what kind of society are we making? One approach is to make it as we would like it to be. Sociologists John Law and Kevin Hetherington, borrowing from the work of Haraway, have indicated that interference is about representational strategies and practice.[7] They are drawing on a feminist technoscience representational practice known as diffraction: »[d]iffraction is a mapping of interference, not of replication, reflection or reproduction.«[8] Diffraction is the way light waves are changed when put through a prism – the light wave is changed or interfered with. We know already through anthropological and feminist critique of representational practices that we always affect those we are studying and that the author creates as much as she describes. *Making interferences* is about writing in a way that does not merely describe, replicate, or reflect. It is about placing politics and power at the center of the social scientific practice of writing. When we go out there to study something, we are not merely representing it – we are interfering with it.

Making an interference indicates that there is a tension between *intervention* and *interference*. The former is more about practice – writing and acting on a moral question or problem (in the field), for example: writing to challenge a particular point of view or acting to bring about change in the particular area one is researching. An instance of this can be found ahead, when I discuss my »intervention« in an egg donation clinic. Interference, on the other hand, may involve writing as a vehicle for tran-

6 Nancy Scheper-Hughes, »Making Anthropology Public«, in: *Anthropology Today* 25 (2009), pp. 1–3.

7 John Law & Kevin Hetherington, *Allegory and Interference: Representation in Sociology*, (1998) http://www.lancs.ac.uk/fass/sociology/papers/law-hetherington-allegory-interference.pdf [last accessed: 12.11.2010].

8 Donna Haraway, *The Haraway Reader* (New York: Routledge, 2004), in particular p. 70.

scending the problems which present themselves in the field. In my case, the way in which I »intervened« in an egg donation clinic seemed to be a dead end that only posed the potential for ending my access to the research site. Hence »interference« in the form of writing a different story seemed another useful route for anthropological critique. This will, I hope, become clearer below.

Anthropology has a history of being uncomfortable with intervening in the cultures we study. And with good reason. Part of our disciplinary history comes from assisting in colonial administration. Anthropology's legacy of cultural relativism, from Franz Boas to Ruth Benedict onward, represents a strong disciplinary bias against intervening in other cultures. The ethos is that cultures should be taken in their own terms and not judged. To intervene on the basis of one's own ethics or cultural precepts would be to presume those to be superior. Also, to intervene on behalf of others can be seen as patronizing. Yet there are times when intervention seems necessary despite the potential of being seen to be culturally imperialist. Indeed it has been argued that there is a long-history of value-laden work in anthropology, which histories of anthropology have only partially represented, and that understanding the world must not be a substitute for being committed to improving it.[9]

The Research

This paper draws on observational and interview research I conducted into Romanian-Israeli ova donation.[10] This research, begun in 2002, involved following discursive-practices[11] of ova extractions, exchanges, and implantations to the various sites of their enactment: in clinics, in people's homes,

9 Barbara Rylko-Bauer, Merrill Singer & John Van Willigen (Eds.), »Reclaiming Applied Anthropology: Its Past, Present and Future«, in: *American Anthropologist* 108 (2006), 1, pp.178–190.

10 This research was fully funded by the Wenner Gren Foundation for Anthropological Research and by the Social Science and Humanities Research Council of Canada.

11 Here I am referencing Butler's notion of discursive-practice, in which it is not possible to separate discourses from practices or vice versa. See Judith Butler, *Bodies That Matter: On the Discursive Limits of Sex* (London, New York: Routledge, 1994).

in labs, and in waiting rooms in Israel and Romania. I will not refer much to the research in Israel here[12] but will focus on the research in Romania. The research in Romania was a fortunate opportunity that arose while I was conducting participant observation at a private IVF clinic south of Tel Aviv, Israel. The head of this clinic was keen for me to observe all the steps of their IVF »brand« known as the »embryo method.«[13]

But why do Israelis turn to Romania for ova? In 2001 there was a »crisis« in Israeli ova donation, where ova were stolen from women in public clinics and sold to women in private clinics.[14] A woman became unwell in the course of receiving hormonal treatment for IVF and was diagnosed

12 See Michal Nahman, »Materialising Israeliness: Difference and Mixture in Transnational Ova Donation«, in *Science as Culture* 15 (2006), 3, pp.199–213; Michal Nahman, »Making More Disposable People. Reflections on Biosociality in Israeli Egg Donation«, in: *Genetics, Biosociality and the Social Sciences. Making Biologies and Identities*, ed. by Sahra Gibbon and Carlos Novas (London: Routledge, 2007); Michal Nahman, »Embryos Are Our Babies: Condensing the Body in Israeli Ova Donation«, in: *Technologized Images, Technologized Bodies: Anthropological Approaches to a New Politics of Vision*, ed. by Jeanette Edwards, Penny Harvey and Peter Wade (Oxford and New York: Berghahn Books, 2010).

13 In another paper I argue that the approach to doing transnational egg donation that this clinic takes can be seen as a »brand.« The clinic itself names it the »embryo method« and uses a logo and other branding conventions to make this happen. The »embryo method« is the label given by the clinic in its glossy brochures and website to the entire set of practices and techniques involved in ova donation. For more on this practice, see Nahman »Embryos Are Our Babies«, op. cit. (note 12).

14 The women had agreed to donate one or two ova and instead were »hyperovulated« to produce many more ova, and large numbers of eggs were sold to other women. Hence, this was known in the media as the »theft« of eggs. See Ran Reznick, »The Lives of Women Patients Were Put at Risk«, in: *Ha'aretz Newspaper* (in Hebrew), 2000; Ran Reznick, »Ministry Demands Medical Records in Human Egg Trading Investigation«, in: *Ha'aretz Newspaper* (in Hebrew), 2000; Ran Reznick & Nicole Kraw, »House Arrest for Two Doctors: Suspected of Fraud and Endangerment of Lives«, in: *Ha'aretz Newspaper* (in Hebrew), 2000; Ran Reznick & H. Shadmi, »Professor Raphael to be Suspended from Administration of the Women's Wing of Beilinson Hospital«, in: *Ha'aretz Newspaper* (in Hebrew), 2001; Ran Reznick & H. Shadmi, »The Solicitor General Will Soon Decide Whether to Rule against the Doctors in the Episode of the Eggs«, in: *Ha'aretz Newspaper* (in Hebrew), 2001; S.Rozenblum, »The Suspicion: Doctors Extracted Eggs and Sold Them to Other Women«, in: *Yediot Aharonot Newspaper* (in Hebrew), 2000; S. Rozenblum, »Women Fear Commerce in Eggs: Thousands of Couples Wait in Vain for a Donation«, in: *Yediot Aharonot Newspaper* (in Hebrew), 2000; Judith Siegel-Itzkovich, »Health Ministry Investigating Claims of Illegal Ova Sales«, in: *The Jerusalem Post*,

with ovarian hyperstimulation syndrome. It was subsequently revealed that she had been asked to donate some of her ova to other women in IVF in return for cheap or free IVF. After this was reported in the media, other women brought up similar allegations against two doctors who were subsequently arrested and charged with theft of ova. They had been asking women to »donate« eggs in a state-run clinic and then selling these eggs to women in privately run IVF clinics for significant personal profit.

Due to the wide publicity this received, the laws tightened up and ova donation virtually came to a halt in Israel, with doctors afraid to ask women to donate eggs for fear of being implicated in trafficking.[15] In order to alleviate this perceived shortage[16], some physicians looked outside Israel's borders to Cyprus or Central and Eastern Europe for ova, in places where regulation of these practices was light and where there was greater »bioavailability.«[17] The donors were perceived to be good ones because they were seen to »ethnically« or »phenotypically« match Israeli Jews (Israel has a very large population that originated in Romania and Eastern Europe); but also, and crucially, the donors were seen to be available in large numbers due to their own relative poverty and perceived willingness to participate in selling their ova. One Israeli doctor, himself raised in Romania until his family immigrated to Israel, had set up a clinic with an Israeli business partner who was already based in Romania. That was in 2002. Today this research would look very different, as ova donation is currently voluntary and unpaid in Romania. Yet, despite being criminalized in Romania as in the rest of Europe payment of donors did not completely stop. In July 2009 the Israeli newspaper *Ha'aretz* reported that two doctors with both Israeli and Romanian citizenship who had set up a clinic in Bucharest had been arrested and charged with unlawful practices. It should be noted that their clinic did not have the approval of the Israeli

2000. www.jpost.com/Editions/2000/02/10/Health/Health.443.html [last accessed 23.1.2001].

15 See Michal Nahman, 2005. *Israeli Extraction: An Ethnographic Study of Egg Donation and National Imaginaries,* unpublished PhD thesis, Lancaster University.

16 Much of the feminist literature on the topic of egg donation stresses that these are produced and perceived shortages, which relate to the pressure on women to reproduce and cultural perceptions that all women should/must have babies.

17 Lawrence Cohen, »Operability, Bioavailability, and Exception«, in: *Global Assemblages: Technology, Politics, and Ethics as Anthropological Problems,* ed. by Aihwa Ong & Stephen J. Collier (Malden, MA: Blackwell Publishing, 2005).

Ministry of Health, while the one whose practices I am describing in this article did.[18]

Reverse Traffic Ova Donation

Whilst most transnational ova donation practices involve the travel of women who wish to buy eggs across borders into other states, the practices I am describing involve a »reverse traffic.« Instead of prospective recipients traveling, what travels here are the gametes, machines for fertilizing ova, hormones, embryologist and doctor. At the time of conducting the observation this was the only clinic known to practice in this fashion, but currently this model has been taken up by others in different places around the world.

Each month the head physician and embryologist traveled from Israel with canisters of cryopreserved sperm from commissioning couples or donated sperm. They went to their clinic abroad, where they extracted ova, fertilized them with the thawed sperm, cryopreserved these fertilized ova,[19] and transported them to Israel in canisters.[20] Ova were extracted by a local doctor, who was assisted by several nurses. The embryologists (in my observations the Israeli embryologist Nachum[21] was joined by a young female Romanian embryologist) sat in the adjoining laboratory to perform the *in vitro* procedure of inserting sperm into ovum. Consent was obtained by the clinic through forms, but there were some issues with them. For instance, the forms were not explicit about the potential risks involved in the treatment; the women also signed that they consented not to seek treatment from another medical institution should complications

18 Representatives of the Israeli Ministry of Health actually visited the clinic and approval was given in order to facilitate the support for treatments by the national health system. This is discussed further in Nahman, »Israeli Extraction«, op. cit. (note 15).

19 It is crucial that these are not embryos but fertilized ova, as they have a different legal status in Israel.

20 This is a greatly condensed description that does not capture the socio-technical dimensions of the practices. I analyze these elsewhere, see Nahman, »Making More Disposable People«, op. cit. (note 12).

21 All names have been changed.

arise; finally, the forms stipulated that a woman who had an unplanned pregnancy during the course of hormonal injections or who simply decided that she was no longer interested in selling her eggs was obliged to repay the clinic for the hormones given to her.[22]

The women who sold their ova at this clinic were paid 200 US dollar per »batch« of 20–30[23] eggs. This, I was told by several of the women sellers, equaled three months' of their salary. The clinic sold the fertilized ova to Israeli couples for $3000 US dollar. Clearly the profit-margin is high. The business worked so well that they expanded to other countries around the world where they are still practicing this »reverse traffic« ova donation.

Intersecting »Aspirations«

»Aspiration« is both literally and figuratively a reproductive technology that reproduces a particular global order of things.

Aspiration refers to several aspects of ova donation in Romania. First, »aspiration« is the medical term used to designate the series of medical techniques for extracting ova from women's bodies (with the aid of a machine called an »aspirator«) that I observed in the Bucharest clinic.[24]

---

22 The pitfalls of consent forms are widely known and critiqued by anthropology and the social sciences more broadly (see for instance Oonagh Corrigan, »Empty Ethics: The Problem with Informed Consent«, in: *Sociology of Health and Illness* 25 (2005), pp. 768–92, and are further discussed in a previous paper Nahman, »Making More Disposable People«, op. cit. (note 12). During my research I found out that a few years prior there had not even been a consent form. This form was introduced because some young women had unprotected sex and became pregnant as a result of the hormones making them hyperfertile. The clinic became concerned that they were losing money and introduced the consent form.

23 This is a very high number of ova to obtain in one cycle. The women were hyperstimulated with hormones to produce such a large number of eggs.

24 The process of extracting ova from women's bodies is called different things in different contexts. For instance in Israel it is often termed »dikkur,« Hebrew for »poking.« See Nahman, «Israeli Extraction», op. cit. (note 15), and Nahman, »Making More Disposable People«, op. cit. (note 12), for a discussion of the local significance of »dikkur.«

»Aspiration« also refers to the complex desires[25] of ova donors and of clinic staff I encountered during the week I spent at this clinic. Finally, »aspiration« could be associated with my own desire to conduct »critical« research and to intervene both through writing and actions in situations I find morally troubling. In all three dimensions of »aspiration« examined here, there is some sense of transcendence, crossing a boundary of bodies, borders, or intellectual disciplines, as well as a sense of becoming »stuck« or immobile. In these various sites and forms, aspirations are technologies that embody dynamic processes – both social and biological. I thus see these intersecting sites of aspiration as technologies that reproduce[26] aspects of inequality in the world order.

I came to ask questions about the entangled aspirations of ova donors and recipients because of the particularly complicated practices and processes of choosing and selecting eggs that I had observed in Israel.[27] I wondered about the implications of these selections and choices for donors, and of the concerns of Israelis about what »Romanian eggs« might offer. As my research in Israel progressed, I realized it would be impossible to tell a story about what is allowed and disallowed into the Jewish Israeli body or nation without considering the discursive practices of ova procurement. The story of Israeli ova donation would be incomplete without an examination of this key aspect of its enactment.

The research I conducted in the ova donation clinic in Romania was the most deeply troubling experience of my research on Israeli ova donation. I struggled with how to represent it while I was still in Romania, and subsequently I found that I could not write about my experiences without conveying shock and anger. Yet that would be self-serving and not analytically interesting. What is interesting is how to deal with the complex intersections of aspirations and reactions that come out in research.

---

25 I am aware that there is an extensive body of psychoanalytic literature on the notion of »desire.« However, in this paper I use the term in its more colloquial sense of »want.« Nevertheless, it is interesting and worthy of note that the psychoanalytic aspect of desire involves both a »pull« and a »push« aspect (attraction and repulsion).

26 I want to emphasise that they reproduce the global order, but always in shifting, unexpected, and variable ways.

27 Michal Nahman. »Materialising Israeliness: Difference and Mixture in Transnational Ova Donation«, in: *Science as Culture* 15 (2006), 3, pp. 199–213.

I came to Bucharest primarily as a researcher. Yet my experiences and observations there were so complex because of other factors. I went to Bucharest not only as a researcher but also as a feminist and a middle-class woman. I also went as someone with close ties to Israel and as a woman who had herself been asked to donate eggs. These positionings help me to »make sense« of the questions with which I was preoccupied during my research in Bucharest. I came to Bucharest to speak to women who had chosen to donate their eggs, or who felt they had no choice but to donate eggs. Hence, it seems likely that our differential positioning affected how we related to each other. I hope to convey that the intersection of my positioning with those of the donors and the clinic is a complicated one, in order to foreground the idea that ethnographic research can evoke many emotions in the researcher. It was also done in order to suggest that a culturally relativistic approach to practices like transnational ova donation is neither possible nor desirable. The proximity and entanglement of the responses of the researcher with the aspirations of those who participated in this research project are centrally important.

The following story provides an ethnographic representation that helps to further explore the questions of intervention and intersecting aspirations.

Anna

In the round of ova extractions I observed there were 20 egg donors. Over a period of one month the women were injected with ovarian stimulating hormones. They arrived at the clinic for three nights in a row to receive this injection, which was administered by a nurse. Six or seven women came to the clinic each night, and each morning six or seven came for extraction. Thus, monthly 20 women were involved, and the ovum extraction divided up over three days.

At around 10:30 p.m.[28] the nurse arrived, tired and dressed in clothing that seemed too large and ill fitting. She had spent the day working at another hospital and was now about to administer hormone injections to seven egg donors. The first woman, Anna, arrived and sat looking a bit nervous. I chatted with her and told her about my research. She appeared to be interested in this and told me about some of her experiences with ova donation. As the others arrived they joined in the conversation. Three women could understand and speak English relatively well, so they acted as translators. It seemed as if the young women knew one another, but they told me they had met only at the clinic.

Anna was the first egg donor I interviewed. Through her broken English and my broken Romanian, I learned in my first conversation with her that she was nineteen years old and scared of doctors. She was a student and wanted to become a police officer. Anna told me she would use the money she received from the clinic to take courses for her university entrance exams. A friend had told her that she could donate eggs for money at this clinic. So she had decided to come and try it out. The trip to the clinic took her half an hour by bus and the buses usually stopped running by the time her injection was over. Anna made it clear that she was afraid to come to this part of town, and told me »it's not safe.« A second-time donor, she had not told her parents that she was going to the clinic and donating eggs. She lived with them and when she went to the clinic late at night, she told them that she was going to a friend's house. If her parents had known, they would not have let her do this.

When I arrived at the clinic that day, I was still largely ignorant of how things worked in Romania. Orit, the clinic manager in Israel, had told me »donors« were paid a »fair amount,« but he would not provide me with details. I had decided to wait until I met the ova sellers themselves to find out. In both Israel and North America, stories about high-earning donors from the United States and elsewhere abound: from models, to high IQ scorers, to Jewish donors, all of whom are paid a premium for their eggs.

28 The nurse explained that the final pre-aspiration injection had to be given exactly 36 hours prior to ovum extraction and so this final shot had to happen late at night for the extraction to happen in the morning 36 hours later. If the hormones were given too early and ovulation happened, there would be no ova to extract and the whole month's preparation would be wasted.

I was therefore interested to see how much the donors at this Bucharest clinic would be paid.

In our first conversation in the waiting room, I asked Anna about the amount of money she received for her eggs. Taking charge of the conversation, Anna turned the tables around and asked me how much women make for selling their eggs in North America. I had worried that this question would arise, and despite my concern that it would be a lot more money than she would be receiving from this clinic, and that that might upset her, I had decided to simply tell the truth. I told her it can be in the range of several hundred to 20,000 US dollar, although I knew donors can even be paid much more. I myself had been offered the equivalent of four years' doctoral tuition plus living expenses from an academic who had wanted to buy my ova a few years earlier. The information about how much donors were paid abroad obviously had an effect on Anna. I discovered this the next day after her »aspiration.«

Anna's Aspiration

After we met in the waiting room on my first night in Bucharest, Anna asked me to accompany her during her ovum extraction procedure the following day. I agreed. Prior to this she had prepared for »aspiration« by showering and taking a painkiller in the form of a suppository. She had waited with five other women in the small recovery room. The recovery room had three beds for after the operation . The atmosphere in the recovery room was jovial, with much nervous chatter about what was going on in the surgery room. Medical assistants came and went. Staff and patients are all women in their twenties or early thirties. The donors all acted as if they had known one another for a long time. They advised, cajoled, and tried to make each other comfortable by providing food and coffee.

On the morning of Anna's »aspiration« I had been observing ovum extractions, moving between the recovery room and the surgery room with the consent of the ova sellers. So I was already in the surgery room when a clean bed was wheeled in and Anna entered. Anna was brought in wearing a light blue hospital gown bearing the company logo. She lay down on the bed and her legs were placed in stirrups. She was prepared for surgery with iodine and a saline solution. The lights in the room were bright and cold

As she lay on the bed I tried to make casual conversation in order to take her mind off of her fear of doctors. We talked about mundane things: food, how nice it is to sleep, how good the doctor was. Ioanna, the Romanian doctor, was making jokes with her, as was the anesthetist. Anna asked me to hold her hand as the anesthetist injected a white liquid into her arm. This was meant to induce a light gentle sleep. So light, in fact, that several of the women had woken up during surgery and had more of the liquid injected. Within minutes, Anna was asleep and the lights were dimmed, except for a large light used by the clinicians. I noted that there was no heart monitor here, as I had seen used in clinics in Israel when a general anesthetic was employed.

Stephania, one of the nurses, entered to assist with the extraction. Nachum, the embryologist, could be seen in the lab getting mediums and utensils ready for separation of eggs from fluid, insertion of sperm into ova, and cryopreservation.

Back in the surgery room, the ultrasound stick (transducer) was ready and covered with a large disposable cover. A long aspirator needle was attached to the transducer and inserted vaginally. Dr. Ioana was moving the needle, and on the monitor I could see the needle end gently meeting the follicles that contained ova. All of us in the room seemed to be intently watching the »show« on screen. The follicles looked like large fuzzy black holes with whitish grey outlines. It took me a while to »learn« to see them. There were quite a lot of them – many more than I had observed with regular IVF patients in Israel. At the end there was a lot of bleeding, which I had not witnessed before in the many extractions I had seen in Israeli clinics. I could not judge or understand why this was the case now. I was told by the nurses that the operation went well, without any problems. Anna was swiftly wheeled out of the surgery room and back into the recovery room across the corridor.

Post-surgery, when she awoke, Anna continued to bleed quite a bit. She thought perhaps she had started menstruating. Anna began to cry. I didn't realize at the time that the possibility of menstruation would signal for her that she had already ovulated prior to the surgery and would not have had any ova to donate. She would have worried that she'd gone through the whole procedure of month-long injections and general anesthetic for nothing – and also feared having to repay the clinic for the costly injections of hormones it had expended on her. The other women in the communal recovery room told her not to cry, because it would give me a bad impression of them, which I would take with me to Canada. I asked her why she was crying. She told me because »life is hard.« Initially, I thought she meant that her life here in Romania was hard. Yet later I wondered if she may have been crying for other reasons, perhaps to do with how little she was being paid for her eggs. The events that followed suggest that this may have been an accurate assessment of the situation.

When Anna cried, one of the nurses noticed and spoke with her quickly in Romanian, so I did not understand what went on. After this, the clinic staff began to seem more distanced towards me. I felt worried that I had made myself an unwelcome visitor. Perhaps my unconscious guilt over the inequality was making me imagine their hostility. I wondered whether I was enacting a colonialist feminist practice of trying to impose my ideas of »oppression« on others in a situation that might be inappropriate.[29] Anna and I were differently positioned in the global context. Our aspirations were both conflicting and similar. She wanted to become a university student to advance herself. I wanted to finish being a university student, and become a professional academic, in order to financially support myself. I realized that I had more options than she did, and I felt concerned about having replied to her question regarding the payment of donors in other countries.

The following day

Things at the clinic were just getting started at around 10 a.m. the following morning. In the middle of my interview with Elena I was interrupted by a phone call from Israel. It was Dr. Zer (the chief physician and owner of the company) ringing on Nachum's mobile phone. I worried that Dr. Zer might have heard about Anna having been upset the previous day,

29 Aihwa Ong, »Colonialism and Modernity: Feminist Representations of Women in Non-Western Societies«, in: *Inscriptions* 3/4 (October 1984), pp. 79–93.

and that he would put a halt to my research. My instincts were somewhat correct, but he took a different approach. He began by asking me to be »gentler with the girls.« He said he wanted me »not to introduce options that [were] *impossible for them to attain.*« He then informed me that one »girl« (sic) had become upset because I had told her how much money women could get for their eggs in North America. He continued to say that »these women can't afford to fly to the US, so it's unfair to do this to them.« He did not want his clinic to be explicitly linked to the politics of global inequality.

Zer ended by telling me, »I don't interfere with how you conduct your work, so you should not interfere with mine.« He threatened to halt my research at his clinic if I persisted.

However, the more I thought about what Dr. Zer had told me about »options,« being gentle, and the unfairness of telling the clinic's donors how much donors earned elsewhere, the more I disagreed with him. Dr. Zer saw it as his right to pay the donors what he deemed fair. He did not question the »impossibility« of global mobility for the women at his clinic. The research experience made me want to question this global inequality. Afterwards I wished I had had the presence of mind to inform him that he was dealing with highly intelligent women, who were aware of their position in the world: they themselves had articulated the benefits and pitfalls of their situation to me in our discussions and interviews. They were, in a sense, »theorists of reproduction.«[30] Many told me of the financial difficulties of living in Romania, of the changes in reproductive regulations in their country, of differences between themselves and women in wealthier societies. So whilst they often did not know the exact nature of the global markets in ova, they had a deep appreciation for global inequalities in general and a clear picture of the problematic nature of reproduction and inequality in Romania. In an article in *Ha'aretz* newspaper, Dr. Zer was recently quoted arguing that the prices he charged patients had fallen too low, which, of course, reduces his profit margins. At the time of my research, in some countries such as Britain (and Israel) donors were not compensated at all or at most were only compensated for medical and travel expenses. It is not the fact of the payment that is the issue here. But I believe that the Romanian donors should have at least been informed

30 Nahman, »Nodes of Desire«, op. cit. (note 30).

about conventions in other countries. Donors at this clinic got caught up in a system that was not completely transparent to them. They could decide to begin treatment. They did not know where their eggs were going. They could not stop treatment unless they were willing to go into debt to repay the clinic.[31]

Intersecting Aspirations

There are several competing »aspirations,« moralities, and ethics in operation in the practices of ova donation that I have described above.

1. The women who sell their eggs weigh the factors that bear upon their sale of eggs. These factors are often things such as the potential for harm coming to them versus the potential benefits of receiving what amounts to three months' salary for one round of egg donation. They weigh up the danger of being discovered as an egg donor, which involves creating different stories to account for their whereabouts whilst at the clinic.[32]
2. The clinicians, especially the head physician who also co-owns the company, have several considerations. Dr. Zer wants to have a sense that he is helping both women in Israel (reproductively) and women in Romania (financially). His morality does not seem to include the idea (found in some normative Western ethical frameworks) that one should not pay for bodily tissues.

31 There is a much longer discussion to be had regarding »reproductive labour« and the selling of ova, which a number of authors have already begun. Regrettably I do not have the space here to expand on this discussion, but see Charis Thompson, *Making, Parents: The Ontological Choreography of Reproductive Technologies.* (Boston: MIT Press, 2005) and Catherine Waldby and Melinda Cooper, »From Reproductive Work to Regenerative Labour: The Female Body and the Stem Cell Industries«, in: *Journal of Feminist Theory* 11 (2010), 1, pp. 3–22. I have begun to contribute to this discussion by arguing elsewhere that women are *sellers* of ova rather than workers or trafficked slaves (Michal Nahman, »Nodes of Desire: Transnational Egg Sellers as Theorists of Reproduction in a Neo-Liberal Age«, in: *European Journal of Women's Studies* 15 (2008), pp. 65–82.

32 For more on the sellers' perspectives see Nahman, »Nodes of Desire«, op. cit. (note 30).

3. Romanian policy makers have revisited the topic of egg donation. Three years ago they banned the payment of egg donors and thus harmonized national with EU-wide policy in this matter.
4. International non-governmental organizations and women's rights groups, who have campaigned in this area, believe it is morally wrong to sell women's bodily tissues, and feel that the women are voiceless victims who require international support.
5. The ova recipients weigh up the different issues relating to receiving a body part from another person: issues such as medical histories; genetic problems in future children; buying eggs from women poorer than themselves; having children who will not look like themselves, and more.[33]
6. As an anthropologist I have to decide what position to align myself with, or whether to align myself at all. There is the option of simply setting out to »name« the ethical and moral issues.[34] Else, I might try to »change« the practices.[35] Or I could »describe and outline« the power issues evident to me in the ethical dilemmas I witness.[36] I feel it is important to state that I am in tension with those NGOs who have tried to »save« the women who sell their ova.[37] Yet the instances described above, such as Anna's aspiration, do call for some sort of intervention beyond simply witnessing and describing. I not only want to describe what has happened, but to *change it*. Yet how can it be changed? I do not believe the individual physician is at the heart of

33 See Nahman 2005, op. cit. (note 15).

34 Paul Rabinow, *French DNA: Trouble in Purgatory* (Chicago: University of Chicago Press, 1999).

35 Nancy Scheper-Hughes, »Making Anthropology Public«, in: *Anthropology Today* 25 (2009), pp. 1–3.

36 Klaus Hoeyer, »'Ethics Wars': Reflections on the Antagonism between Bioethicists and Social Science Observers of Biomedicine«, in: Human Studies 29 (2006) 2, pp. 203–227; Sarah Franklin and Margaret Lock, *Remaking Life and Death: Towards an Anthropology of the Biosciences* (School of American Research Press, 2003).

37 The mission of *Hands Off Our Ovaries* to call for a global moratorium on the global egg trade failed to take into account the voices of the women actually involved in selling their eggs. This was a group led by Core Ethics for Reproduction, the British-based anti-abortion group. For a fuller discussion of this see Nahman, »Nodes of Desire«, op. cit. (note 30).

the problem. In addition, policies open up new spaces and »opportunities« for new practices to emerge – although some may be worse than what we already have. It seems clear to me from my research that the neo-liberalization of healthcare, together with the persistence of capitalism's incursions into the depths of bodies, is a good place to start when figuring out where to point the finger of blame.

Feminist Intervention?

In recent times the trade in ova has occasionally been referred to as »ova trafficking« rather than donation or selling. The UN protocol against trafficking indicates that there should be an element of deceit, coercion or illicit trade. The deception involved (in terms of how ova donation was presented to the sellers) and coercion (forcing the women to agree to pay the clinic if they decided not to go ahead with treatment, and not permitting them to seek treatment elsewhere should they become ill) both indicate that this particular practice of ova extraction is similar to the UN definition of trafficking. Yet the nomenclature of trafficking also conjures up images of slave laborers and transnational travel. So the language may be inappropriate because, in this case, the only thing that travels is the bodily tissue stored up and cryopreserved in canisters. Further, some of the literature about trafficking seems to imagine a voiceless woman, which the women in my study were not. As I have called them ova sellers, it might seem to make sense to parallel this example with selling sex. However, although there is exploitation and selling in both cases, selling a bodily tissue involves »parting« with some of oneself, whilst selling sex does not. In this case egg selling may be more similar to selling blood. The difference there being that only women can sell ova, and hence selling eggs is part of the wider exploitation made possible by social practices of gendered subordination and oppression of women.[38]

38 Elsewhere I develop the idea of »reverse traffic«: Michal Nahman, »Repromigrations: The Case of Israel and Romania«, in: Special Issue of the *Journal of Reproductive Biomedicine Online*, ed. by Marcia Inhorn and Zeynep B. Gürtin-Broadbent (forthcoming).

Some recent feminist and social scientific work on ovum donation has tried to intervene in the practices of the sale of eggs. This intervention has often been conceptualized within a framework of liberal values of »rights,« »justice,« and »property.«[39] These are culturally specific notions, particular to Western liberalism and of uncertain value when examining ova donation within a broader context of globalization, markets, and social change. Looking historically, these concepts have rarely actually benefitted subalterns and are more about buoying up those in charge.[40] This kind of ideological »propping up,« for example, was seen in the rhetoric used in the lead-up and aftermath of the attacks by the USA and UK on Afghanistan, where the public was told that in addition to fighting American enemies, the aim was also to liberate women in Afghanistan. The outcome of that invasion, we now know, has been a general worsening of their situation.

Some feminists researching in the area of reproductive technologies have argued that what we need is a universal feminist bioethics to protect and preserve against the voracious market for women's bodily tissues.[41] Elsewhere, I began to question the idea that a universal feminist bioethics can be a useful framework from which to take forward a critique of contemporary transnational trade in ova because the concept is laden with such a problematic history.[42] Women have starkly different positions in the world, and simply pointing a finger at physicians will not dissolve the market. This is a bigger problem of the functioning of global capitalism, which creates all sorts of illicit and licit trade in human tissues.

Donna Dickenson, who has written extensively on the topic of what she calls, »body shopping,« suggests that what we need are tougher regulations. However, in 2009 dozens of Israeli doctors were arrested in Romania for continuing to buy women's eggs, despite the illegality of the practice.

So, what can be a useful contribution from anthropology?

---

39 Donna Dickenson, *Body Shopping: The Economy Fuelled By Flesh and Blood* (Oxford: One World, 2008).

40 Ranjana Khanna, »Indignity«, in: *Ethnic and Racial Studies* 30 (2007), 2, pp. 257–280; Nahman, »Nodes of Desire«, op. cit. (note 30).

41 Jyotsna Gupta, »Towards Transnational Feminisms: Some Reflections and Concerns in Relation to the Globalization of Reproductive Technologies«, in: *European Journal of Women's Studies* 13 (2006), pp. 23–38; Carmel Shalev, *Human Being, Nature and Dignity*, paper presented at the Embryonic Hopes workshop (King's College, London, 6 June 2008).

42 Nahman, »Nodes of Desire«, op. cit. (note 30).

Anthropology and Ethics

Nancy Scheper-Hughes has made some very strong arguments for anthropology's duty to play a »public« role, suggesting that human liberation be a central aim. Anthropology »has an opportunity to become an arbiter of emancipatory change not just within the discipline, but for humanity itself.«[43] She recently has become very widely known outside the discipline because she mapped out the vast global networks of the sale (both legal and illegal) of organs. She helped to set up an organization called *Organs Watch*, a medical human rights group attached to Berkeley University comprised of law, journalism, anthropology, and medical students. They conduct ethnographic research around the world to map out the mechanics of the organs market, with a view towards advancing concerns for social justice. Scheper-Hughes has a history of this kind of interventionist or »public« anthropology. Indeed, she has been much critiqued for some of her previous interferences.[44] She has gained much greater support for her more recent interferences. In the quote above, she is suggesting the transformative potential of social scientific investigation.

Actually, what can be thought of as a problem for science and medicine can also be theorized by the social scientist, who may have a historicized and contextualized view of the issues pertaining to what can or should be done in science.[45] Monica Konrad has indicated that anthropologists have useful epistemological tools to offer bioethics by virtue of the fact that anthropology examines the narrative and relational dimensions of bioethics.[46] That is, how people cope with biomedical situations in practice can offer a view to what kind of ethical positions to take. Indeed, questions of bioethics and research ethics overlapped in my research. For instance, a central question that emerged for both the researcher and the research participants alike was: »Should ova donors be paid more to undergo an operation that might affect their future quality of life?« But the

43 Scheper-Hughes, »Making Anthropology Public«, op. cit. (note 34), p. 4.

44 Nancy Scheper-Hughes, *Death without Weeping: The Violence of Everyday Life in Brazil* (California: University of California Press, 1993).

45 Monica Konrad, *Narrating the New Predictive Genetics: Ethics, Ethnography and Science* (London: Cambridge University Press, 2005).

46 Konrad, »*Narrating*«, op. cit. (note 44).

very notion of putting a value on selling a body part simply grants legitimacy to the market, as others have shown.[47]

Also there is no doubt in my mind that some of the encounters retold here are intertwined with my own ambivalence about having once been asked to donate my ova to a woman in exchange for a large sum of money and having said no. After much deliberation I declined, largely because of the power differential and the confusing kinship relations that the exchange of my ova would instantiate between me and the woman who had made the very difficult request. I said no, even though I was deeply saddened by the fact that the woman who had asked me really wanted a child, and I wanted to help her.

By the time I conducted my research in Romania, I was also already deeply moved by the stories I had heard from women in Israel who were trying to have a child. My sense of the profoundly unequal relation between donors and recipients within the global order crystallized in the clinic in Romania. I did not want to counsel women not to sell their ova, sensing that they were part of larger historical and economic processes that went beyond such personal »choices.« Nevertheless, when asked, I provided them with information about payment in other countries that made some of them think twice about donating again in Romania. Others, however, seemed unmoved and held fast to their decisions to sell their ova. In research, we are always in conversation with people who speak, argue back, and develop their own ethical models.

Clearly, then, I do support some intervention in practice. Yet the role of the public anthropologist is far from clear.

Anthropology has a history of assessing the question of making interventions into the lives of the people we research. Colonial anthropologists gathered information from various corners of the British Empire in order to facilitate better rule in the colonies. More recently, a few decades ago, Nancy Scheper-Hughes sparked controversy when working in Brazil and saving the lives of babies who had been left to die. She was critiqued for actually making the lives of women and babies more difficult. According to this argument, people did not have enough resources to take care of these babies, and yet lived in a Catholic society that denied them access to

47 Donna Dickenson, *Body Shopping: The Economy Fuelled by Flesh and Blood* (Oxford: One World, 2008).

contraception: in many ways they did not have a choice but to not help babies who were not thriving.

We have other branches of anthropology interested in salvaging dying cultures. These, too, have been widely criticized for romanticizing the past, for imagining cultures of the »other« as unchanging. This static view is problematic, as it does not take into account the long-standing interferences of colonial, military, and other forces. For instance, recently American anthropology has intervened by taking a position against aiding the US government to fight the war on terror in Iraq. As a result, the American Anthropological Association put together a committee to discuss and debate what the role of anthropologists should be, and the ASA in Britain widely debated the topic on the blogosphere. The recruitment of anthropologists to the contemporary war effort was seen to compromise anthropological integrity by posing a danger to Iraqi people.

Feminism and Ethics

But what can we say about staking a moral position and examining the ethics of a practice in the case of Romanian ova donation?

In the story I have written about Anna, the egg seller, there is clearly much conflict in the aspirations of medical entrepreneurs, young Romanian women who sell their ova, and Israeli ova recipients. This series of encounters in an Israeli ova extraction clinic in Romania show some of the complexities of interfering in research. These encounters between a young ova seller and the anthropologist, between the head physician and the anthropologist, and between the staff of the clinic and the sellers provide a critical space from which to explore the question of what ethnography can actually offer in this controversial and contested zone of politics and practice.

Representational Interference, or Making Feminist Myths as Political Practice

Centrally, then, this research raised questions regarding how academics intervene and interfere in the lives of those they research, and whether they should deliberately intervene. Feminism after all, began as an activist discipline, and anthropology has a long history of intervening, whether as called upon by colonial administrators, or as a more grass-roots, applied intervention in collaboration with its interlocutors.[48]

These are two conflicting kinds of intervention. Both types of intervention have received some criticism from within – for instance, when white Western feminists presume to speak for minoritized women. This is an issue that Western feminists have long had to rethink and have still not resolved.

Whether my telling women in Romania about the global economies of ova helped or hindered their lives is up for debate and may be seen as a relatively insignificant intervention. Unfortunately, groups such as CORE ethics, the pro-life campaigning group that spearheaded the Hands Off Our Ovaries campaign, have far more clout than I and work on much more public platforms such as lobbying the European Parliament, so that their intervention has more effect (including the effect of silencing the actual women in question). Anthropologists who stake a public position by debating their role in the war in Iraq have a significant cultural weight, and this kind of intervention may be seen as a politically useful one at such a time.

With respect to the egg donation story I have been telling I am left wondering what kind of meaningful intervention this research can make. As I said at the start, what if instead of »intervention« we look to »interferences« – or *representational strategies*[49]. That is, what happens if we return to Haraway's (1991) exhortation for feminists to become »cyborg,« embrace fiction as truth-telling? Or put another way, what if we embrace the fantastical, as Marxist science fiction writer China Miéville put it. We may

48 Rylko-Bauer, Singer & Van Willigen, »Reclaiming«, op. cit. (note 9).

49 See John Law & Kevin Hetherington, *Allegory and Interference: Representation in Sociology* (1998), http://www.lancs.ac.uk/fass/sociology/papers/law-hetherington-allegory-interference.pdf [last accessed: 12.11.2010].

get a different sort of outcome than if we »intervene« in practice. True, all writing is always a kind of intervention. But the sense of the allegorical having a place in scholarly production is important for we might not always have had the chance to intervene in a way that is satisfactory, or we might not think that intervention always leads to the best kind of results. Hence, »interferences« and, in this case, writing fiction may be one way to develop an epistemological approach to bringing an emancipatory struggle into academic worlds. This is how I interpret the call to »interfere.« My interference here, at the end of this paper, is more like a question than an answer. The fictional ending I am providing speaks of my regrets about the research, of what I could not accomplish, or of what, at the time, I did not endeavor to achieve. It also speaks of a hope for feminist politics and what it can do. Finally, writing a fictional and hopeful ending here speaks volumes of the direction that some scholars might have to turn to in the current age of UK university restructuring and privatization that will leave many of us without a place to call an intellectual »home.« This kind of allegorical fiction-as-interference is not all we have, but in some instances it may be one powerful front from which to speak as militant anthropologists.[50]

I don't know what happened to Anna or where she ended up. The increasing pressures on researchers to get the job done quickly and publish papers and teach many hours a week meant that my human resources were being spent otherwise than in keeping in touch with research participants. This is something I regret. But in the spirit of feminist myth making, I offer here an imaginary ending:

After Dr. Zer asked me not to interfere in his work, I decided to interfere even more by holding a focus group off the premises with some of the ova sellers. Anna offered to be my paid translator for these focus groups. During these group discussions, Anna not only translated, but gave me deeper insights into cultural references. She offered research questions of her own, helping me to sharpen my investigation and analysis. I paid her for her services out of my research grant. With the money she made from

50 To borrow the phrase from Scheper-Hughes, a militant anthropology is political and morally engaged and active. Nancy Scheper-Hughes, »The Primacy of the Ethical: Propositions for a Militant Anthropology«, in: *Current Anthropology* 36 (June 1995), 3, pp. 409–420.

translating and the funds from selling her ova to the clinic, Anna made enough money to travel to Canada. There, she got a part-time job as a shop assistant, and in her spare time she worked as a language tutor. In her first year in Canada she saw an ad requesting an ova donor just across the border in the United States, where, unlike Canada, egg donation is privatized. She answered the ad, was approved as a donor, and received 30,000 USD for her eggs. With this money she studied for her undergraduate degree in Women's Studies and Public Health. As part of her final year project she decided to travel back home to Romania to talk to some women about their experiences with selling their ova, and this resulted in a campaign to create better regulatory measures for ova donation that would ensure the health and safety of the women in question. They joined together with similar grassroots campaigns across Central and Eastern Europe, and slowly expanded their remit to cover other issues of inequality and health risks in the workplace and broader issues of social justice. The movement has grown to tens of thousands of women and men across Europe. The movement is not without its problems, but it is at least a hopeful beginning.

Resemblance that Matters: On Transnational Anonymized Egg Donation in Two European IVF Clinics

Sven Bergmann

»We are like undercover agents.«[1] Bruno Fischer was talking about the secret trip to Prague he was taking with his wife, Susanne.[2] Neither their family nor their friends or colleagues knew where they were or why they had gone. We were sitting at a coffee table in the cafeteria of Fertilmed, a Czech IVF clinic. The couple from southern Germany was waiting for the outcome of the husband's sperm test, so there was plenty of time for a conversation with me, a researcher from their home country. We talked about their IVF experiences and how they had come to choose the Czech Republic for a cross-border treatment. The Fischers are both in their forties and have been married for over ten years. When they remained childless, they started fertility treatments in 2005. Since that time, Susanne Fischer has had three miscarriages. After the last unsuccessful IVF treatment, their German doctors diagnosed the couple as »low responders« and told them that any other infertility treatment »would be pointless.« Both were struck by the phrase »there is no point in further treatment.« Bruno Fischer repeated this sentence sarcastically throughout the interview. However, the rejection they experienced from the German IVF practitioners did not mark the end of their infertility treatment. It jump-started the couple's activism to search for other possibilities. Using the Internet to research the »low responder« diagnosis, they became aware of the procedure of egg donation, which is practiced outside of Germany.[3] They ended up on the

1 I would like to thank Carola Pohlen, Chris Hayward, and Kareth Schaffer for proofreading different versions of this article and the editors for insightful comments.

2 Names of persons and clinics have been anonymized.

3 Egg donation is prohibited in Germany by the Act for Protection of Embryos (The Embryo Protection Act) [Gesetz zum Schutz von Embryonen (Embryonenschutzgesetz ESchG)] of 13 December 1990: »Anyone will be punished with up to three years imprisonment or a fine, who 1. transfers into a woman an unfertilised egg cell

same Internet platform where my research began, and collected, like I did, information about Spanish and Czech IVF clinics where egg donation is permitted. In the end, the Fischers chose Prague for their treatment for two reasons. Their home town is located close to the Czech border. »Taking the car to Prague is way easier and more comfortable than taking an airplane to Valencia,« Bruno Fischer told me. The five-hour drive was easier to fit into their daily lives. They chose Prague even though they were better acquainted with Spain and its infrastructures from their previous tourist experiences. The second and much more important reason they went to the Czech Republic was the question of supposed resemblance with the donor. Susanne Fischer explained that, because egg donors are legally required to remain unknown to their recipients, they had to trust the clinical selection, but she believed that in Spain there would be only brown-haired and brown-eyed donors – the Fischers both have blond hair and blue eyes. Bruno Fischer described egg donation as a form of »half-sided adoption,« because Susanne would have to somehow give up on passing on her identity,« in their understanding resulting in a »lesser degree of kin relation« with their offspring. To avoid anyone's speculation about the biological-relatedness of a potential child, the couple chose a covert tactic: no one close to them knew about their journey. All of their previous fertility treatments in Germany had been kept hidden, too. They said their family would not accept their decision; Bruno Fischer added that the older generation is very Catholic and would not understand any technological intervention in procreation. In addition to this, Susanne expected that making their problems public would only lead to constant surveillance once she became pregnant. I asked if it was hard to seek treatment in a foreign country. They responded that treatment at home would have been logistically easier because once the fertilized egg cells have begun to divide the embryo transfer in IVF cannot be postponed. However, they added that the biggest step had not been to decide to head abroad for treatment, but rather, that it had been much harder to decide to try

produced by another woman, 2. attempts to fertilise an egg cell artificially for any purpose other than bringing about a pregnancy of the woman from whom the egg cell originated […] http://www.bmj.bund.de/files/-/1147/ESchG%20englisch.pdf [last accessed: 17.6.2010].

IVF with donated eggs and not Susanne's: »Nobody likes to give up on her own genes.«

The Fischer's case illustrates the three topics I will address in this article: (1) the transnational agency of patients searching for reproductive treatments abroad and the demand for egg donors with certain similar phenotypical characteristics such as brown or blue eyes, (2) the recruitment of egg donors whose oocytes contain specific physical criteria for international patients in IVF clinics in Spain and the Czech republic, two of the main European destinations for egg donation, and (3) the cultural project of keeping reproductive technologies hidden through practices of anonymization and the fabrication of phenotypical resemblance and matching in gamete donation.[4] First, I will describe the transnational (covert) agency of patients like the Fischers and their mapping of »phenotypical regions« – patients' imaginations about where different eye and hair colors are »naturally« distributed within Europe. Second, I will compare the different egg donor recruitment strategies used by one Czech and one Spanish clinic. Last, I will examine the roles of anonymization and concealment as vectors for these emerging transnational processes, as well as their effects on kinship as attempts to construct (or pass as) »normal« families.

This article is based on my PhD research »Transnational Economies of Reproduction.«[5] In my fieldwork on gamete donation in Europe, I focus on the routes of patients who travel to circumvent the legal and regulatory

4 I characterize egg donation in Spain and the Czech Republic as anonymized (or »made anonymous«) to point out the asymmetric access to information in this practice. Although Spanish law speaks of »anonymity,« infertility clinics have to collect information about donors and recipients in their databases, so if the law changes or grown children demand this information there still is the possibility of revealing it. Also, by using the active phrasing »making anonymous« I refer to the practice of doing or making non-relatedness: substance is extracted from donors' bodies and alienated from them so that possible kin connections are cut off. However, they remain at least symbolically what Monica Konrad has described as »non-genealogical relations« or »nameless relations.« (Monica Konrad, *Nameless Relations. Anonymity, Melanesia and Reproductive Gift Exchange between British Ova Donors and Recipients* (New York & Oxford: Berghahn, 2005)).

5 This research is funded by the German Research Foundation (DFG) through a scholarship in the Research Training Group »Gender as a Category of Knowledge« at the Center for Transdisciplinary Gender Studies at Humboldt University, Berlin.

frameworks of their own countries, on clinical spaces, and on emergent practices in anonymized egg donation. My comparative and multi-sited ethnography on fertility clinics in Europe led me to understand the clinics as places where medicine, bio-capital, bodies and bodily substances, gamete donors and recipients intertwine. These different actors and domains such as medical knowledge and practice, agency, gender, heteronormativity, kinship, law, ethics, and biopolitics are »ontologically choreographed« [6] in the IVF clinic in practices like coordinating donors and recipients according to physical traits (donor/recipient-matching) or freezing embryos for years, thus calibrating time.

Approaching the Transnational: Ethnography of Cross-Border Treatments

The Fischer's case is a good starting point for an analysis of the spatial and transnational aspects of cross-border IVF in Europe. It alludes to the conflict between what is impossible on the national level and transnational possibilities in reproductive choices. Although some German physicians give patients a hint about egg donation being allowed in other European countries, the Fischers' doctors remained silent about that possibility. Their physician presented the failed IVF as the end of what reproductive technologies had to offer. Internet-based research opened up a whole new array of possibilities for the couple. While they were searching for additional medical information on their infertility diagnosis, they found a website talking about egg donation in countries outside of Germany that permit this treatment. These national differences in applying reproductive technologies have led to a new kind of patient mobility that has been popularized as »reproductive tourism,« »fertility tourism,« or »procreative tourism.«[7] Patients' reasons for taking a reproductive journey are quite diverse: some are circumventing ethical and legal »national containers«

6 Charis M. Thompson, *Making Parents: The Ontological Choreography of Reproductive Technologies* (Cambridge, Massachusetts: MIT, 2005), in particular pp. 8–11.

7 Bartha M. Knoppers & Sonia Le-Bris, »Recent Advances in Medically Assisted Conception: Legal, Ethical and Social Issues«, in: *American Journal of Law & Medicine* 17 (1991), 4, pp. 329–361.

(e.g. egg donation is prohibited in Germany and Italy), others are trying to avoid national waiting lists (e.g. British patients), and still others need to find a way around restrictions for lesbian couples and »single mothers by choice.«[8] In sidestepping ethical, legal, and heteronormative restrictions (among others) in national IVF regulatory schemes (characterized as Europe's »regulatory patchwork«[9]), patients are dealing individually with »moral dilemmas« of the liberal state, where »contradictory elements of western cosmologies collide.«[10] »Reproductive tourism« as a term is controversial. Some authors find the addition of »tourism« in association with a reproductive treatment inadequate and disrespectful. Other terms like »reproductive exile«[11] or »cross-border flow of patients«[12] have been proposed as being more appropriate in a debate initiated by the Belgian ethicist Guido Pennings.[13] During the discussion in the workshop »IVF as Global Form. Ethnographic Knowledge and the Transnationalization of Reproductive Technologies« held in June 2008 in Berlin – the workshop from which this book emanated – Marcia Inhorn pointed out how tourism as a »leisure term« clouds the difficulties and constraints faced by infertile patients traveling for treatment.[14] In my own research, some in-

8 This term was popularized by support groups in the US and a website of the same name, from which the following definition was drawn: »A single mother by choice is a woman who *decided* to have or adopt a child, knowing she would be her child's sole parent, at least at the outset.« <http://www.singlemothersbychoice.com> (21.04.2009)

9 Deborah Spar, »Reproductive Tourism and the Regulatory Map«, in: *New England Journal of Medicine* 352 (2005), 6, pp. 531–533.

10 Stefan Beck, »Globalisierte Reproduktionsregimes: Anmerkungen zur Emergenz biopolitischer Handlungsräume«, in: *Verwandtschaft machen. Reproduktionsmedizin und Adoption in Deutschland und der Türkei*, ed. by Stefan Beck, Nevim Çil, Sabine Hess, Maren Klotz & Michi Knecht (Münster: LIT, Berliner Blätter 42, 2007), pp. 124–151, in particular p. 132 (translation by Sven Bergmann).

11 Roberto Matorras, »Reproductive Exile versus Reproductive Tourism [Letters to the Editor]«, in: *Human Reproduction* 20 (2005), 12, p. 3571.

12 Sirpa Soini et al., »The Interface between Assisted Reproductive Technologies and Genetics: Technical, Social, Ethical and Legal Issues«, in: *European Journal of Human Genetics* 14 (2006), pp. 588–645.

13 Guido Pennings, »Reproductive Tourism as Moral Pluralism in Motion«, in: *Journal of Medical Ethics* 28 (2002), pp. 337–341.

14 See Inhorn, this volume; Marcia C. Inhorn, »Globalization and Reproductive Tourism in the Muslim Middle East: IVF, Islam, and the Middle Eastern State«, in: *Reproduction, Globalization, and the State*, ed. by Carole H. Browner (Durham: Duke University, 2009).

terview partners disliked the term, whereas others thoroughly endorsed it. They found the tourism association quite fitting, pointing out their own pragmatic practice of combining holiday and treatments due to time and money constraints. In this article I will use »cross-border treatment« or »circumvention routes« as working concepts for a *transnational* practice: these concepts characterize both the supply of treatment beyond national borders by IVF clinics and the mobility and agency of patients seeking a treatment abroad.

Across, *beyond*, or *over* are prepositions that indicate the shift toward theorizing the transnational rather than alluding to the (inter-)national or the global. Studies of transnationalism argue against the underlying assumption of international studies that take the nation-state »as the natural social and political form of the world.«[15] They also avoid the vagueness of some globalization approaches that either confound the nation with the state or conceptualize the global as topologically encompassing the nation-state, thereby allowing the latter to vanish like the magician's white rabbit.[16] Trans-national as opposed to inter-national avoids getting stuck in the top-down perspective of »methodological nationalism.«[17] For example, looking for a treatment abroad does not merely depend on push and pull factors like supply and demand; patients' agency is multifaceted and concerned with far more than purely rational economic choice.[18] Eva-Maria Knoll has shown that the process of choosing a clinic depends

15 Andreas Wimmer & Nina Glick Schiller, »Methodological Nationalism and Beyond: Nation-State Building, Migration and the Social Sciences«, in: *Global Networks* 4 (2002), 2, pp. 1470–2266.

16 For a critique of the »vanishing of the state« argument from different perspectives see: Alex Demirovic, »NGOs, the State, and Civil Society: The Transformation of Hegemony«, in: *Rethinking Marxism* 15 (2003), 2, pp. 213–235; Shalini Randeria, »The State of Globalization. Legal Plurality, Overlapping Sovereignties and Ambiguous Alliances between Civil Society and the Cunning State in India«, in: *Theory, Culture & Society* 24 (2007), 19, pp. 1–33.

17 Wimmer & Glick Schiller, »Methodological Nationalism«, op. cit. (note 15).

18 Drawing on anthropological research and theory about transnational migration since the 1990s, I want to emphasize that studies of transnational migration cannot simply be used as blueprints for transnational studies of biomedicine. Although there are some shared characteristics such as tourism, mobility, and sexuality (cf. Inderpal Grewal & Caren Kaplan, »Global Identities: Theorizing Transnational Studies of Sexuality«, in: *GLQ: A Journal of Lesbian and Gay Studies* 7 (2001), pp. 663–679), the regime (or surrounding dispositif) of mobility in biomedicine is quite different.

on a variety of factors, including emotionality and aesthetics.[19] Issues of closeness and distance can be straightforwardly articulated in terms of geographical distance and time of travel, but they also appear as questions of anticipated familiarity with national settings or customs, as well as sympathy towards the staff, clinical ambience, and potential donors. In this article, I will focus on the relation between patients' choices of clinics (and respectively of countries) based on what desired oocytes should contain (phenotypes), as well as on clinics' selections of donors with certain characteristics.[20] My research on gamete donation focuses on the practices of the human and non-human actors I followed across borders and beyond single sites.[21] Doing research in a transnational field, where some actors have been made anonymous by the legal parameters of the clinics (donors) and many others want to remain incognito (receiving patients), poses challenges for ethnographic knowledge production. If actors want to remain anonymous, it becomes difficult to meet and follow them. Although I met patients in the clinics and talked to them, because of practices of anonymization I was not able to ask for a follow-up interview. So in most cases, I never will know if my interview partners' IVF succeeded or if their opinions changed when they became parents. In my research I decided to shift from a more patient-centered perspective focusing on biographical narratives of infertility and kinship to emergent clinical practices in gamete donation such as specializing in treatments for foreign patients,

19 Eva-Maria Knoll, »Transnationale Akteurinnen im Geschäft mit der Hoffnung. Österreichische Momente globaler Verflechtung der In-Vitro-Fertilisation«, in: *Kulturelle Dynamik der Globalisierung. Ost- und Westeuropäische Transformationsprozesse aus sozialanthropologischer Perspektive*, ed. by Johanna Riegler (Vienna: Österreichische Akademie der Wissenschaften, 2005), pp. 201–232.

20 I will only be concerned with donor selection in the context of anonymized donation in Spanish and Czech clinics.

21 Following traces in mobile ethnography means paying attention to cultural practices of crossing borders and the connections between local and translocal actors (see Gisela Welz, »Moving Targets. Feldforschung unter Mobilitätsdruck«, in: *Zeitschrift für Volkskunde* 94 (1998), pp. 177–194.). Multiple research sites not only encompass places and connections, they also span social, cultural, discursive, economic, and political stages (see Regina Römhild, »Ethnographie und Imagination. Das neue europäische Grenzregime als Forschungsfeld«, in: *Grenzen und Differenzen. Zur Macht sozialer und kultureller Grenzziehungen. Tagungsband zum 35. Kongress der deutschen Gesellschaft für Volkskunde in Dresden, September 2005*, ed. by Thomas Hengartner & Johannes Moser (Leipzig: Leipziger Universitätsverlag, 2007).

donor recruitment policies and donor/recipient matching procedures, and challenges for the IVF laboratory. After reading German and English Internet forums, I decided to do my research at two IVF clinics – one in Spain, the other in the Czech Republic – that were named there quite often. Certainly, in an ethnographic investigation of clinical practice with traveling patients who want to stay anonymous, following actors for a long period of time is not possible – although it would be interesting especially in regards to their changing opinions on kinship. For my interviews in IVF clinics where patients were not yet parents, statements about kinship had a speculative dimension: opinions on and practices of concealment and disclosure could and can change.[22] The ongoing comparative-ethnographic research by Stefan Beck, Maren Klotz, Michi Knecht, and Nurhak Polat with its ten-year research design focuses on these long-term effects on doing kinship with IVF and does follow-up interviews with patients in different periods of their treatment and afterwards.[23]

Production of Space: Europe's Phenotypical Landscapes

Allow me to return to the Fischers' infertility story. The Fischers did not choose the Czech Republic for treatment only because of its convenient location close to their home. In fact, the main reason for going to Prague was their assumption that the clinic in Prague could provide them much more easily with a donor whose physical appearance would most closely meet their expectations. Because they wanted to keep the IVF treatment and the egg donation a secret, the question of physical likeness to their offspring was highly important to them. Otherwise, it would be possible

22 In Europe, »reproductive tourism« is still a very recent phenomenon. Several directors and representatives of clinics in Spain as well as in the Czech Republic told me they first noticed patients coming in from abroad around 2000, with the »boom« starting in 2004. On a German Internet forum which started around that time, anonymity is an ongoing discussion topic: while the majority of patients want to conceal their usage of third-party oocytes, some change their minds while raising their child.

23 Especially Maren Klotz's research project on knowledge management in families created through IVF is very interesting in that regard and helpful for balancing out the blank spaces of my ethnography. See Maren Klotz, this volume.

that their project of »completing a family« (modeled upon »natural« procreation with their own biogenetic substance) would be endangered by later comments on the baby's physical resemblance. These comments and queries that express notions of blood relatedness and social legitimacy in identifying similar traits in parents and child are described as »resemblance talk.«[24] Anticipating the intrusion of resemblance talk in their later life, the evaluation of the potential physical characteristics of potential donors in different countries is a constant topic for patients in search of egg donation. Susanne and Bruno Fischers' speculations on whether clinics in Spain or in Eastern Europe would be better providers of blond-haired donors are echoed in Internet forums and online communities of IVF patients. When people discuss phenotypical markers like eye or hair color, knowledge of classic genetics – the heredity of genotypes and phenotypes – is applied and negotiated. In patient interviews and in the research I did in Internet forums, sometimes reference was made to the egg donor as bearer or »genetrix«[25] of these physical traits. At other times these traits were disassociated from the body of the donor and negotiated as a substance or commodity that contained potential phenotypical properties of a future child. In these abstractions, features like blond hair or brown eyes are imagined as resources with a certain regional distribution.

According to Henri Lefebvre, every mode of production produces a certain space, its own space. Therefore, space is an agent of change and plays an active role in the unfolding of events: the »production of space.«[26] In some patients' imaginations of the phenotypical distribution of eye or hair colors, space is constructed and produced according to the dimensions and imaginations of desired physical bodily traits. For example, German couples with blue eyes – in terms of Mendelian laws, both are equipped with the recessive phenotypical marker (allele) for eye color – are preoccupied with finding a blue-eyed donor because donation by a brown-eyed donor could generate a brown-eyed child. This desire to produce a child

24 Gay Becker, Anneliese Butler & Robert D. Nachtigall, »Resemblance Talk: A Challenge for Parents Whose Children were Conceived with Donor Gametes in the US«, in: *Social Science & Medicine* 61 (2005), pp. 1300–1309.

25 »The ›genetrix‹ […] is the woman who is culturally recognized in society as the person contributing female genetic substance.« Konrad, »Nameless Relations«, op. cit. (note 4), in particular p. 104.

26 Henri Lefebvre, *The Production of Space* (Oxford: Blackwell, 1991).

that could pass as one's »own« child with the technique of gamete donation is in most cases not fueled by the idea of creating a child with beautiful looks, but instead by the desire to model one's own family after nature, here after conceptions of genealogical resemblance and blood relations and therefore by the parents' intention of concealing the donation from others. Thus, some of these couples are more oriented towards Middle and Eastern European clinics because they assume it will be much easier to get »blue eyes« (meaning a blue-eyed donor) there. In this assumption, the old »container model«[27] of the nation is represented: a nation contains a city contains a clinic contains donors contains blue eyes: all encompassed by the imagination of a homogeneous ethnic group with low phenotypical variation. European *geno-* and *phenotypical landscapes* are evoked that represent such container models of European nations and regions:[28] an eye-color line of demarcation divides Europe's imaginary landscape into a southern brown-eyed sphere and a north-eastern blue-eyed sphere. Susanne and Bruno Fischer were more familiar with Spain from their tourist experiences, but they chose the Czech Republic for a cross-border treatment because of »considerations about resemblance.« Because they expected a donor in Spain to be brown-eyed, they could not get their »proper« identity markers (blond hair and blue eyes) there. To properly analyze Internet IVF forums and cross-border patient mobility, new spatial understandings beyond center/periphery or virtual/real dichotomies are needed. Imaginations align ethnical fantasies about South and North-East Europe that oscillate between the semiotic and the material. While these images definitely co-constitute recent practices like cross-border IVF, the association between people's fantasies and perceptions about donors' phenotypical markers is at some point disjunctive with the local clinical »production« of oocytes, as I will now show in more detail.

27 Steven Vertovec, »Transnational Challenges to the ›New‹ Multiculturalism«, working paper (Oxford: Transnational Communities Programme, 2001) <http://www.transcomm.ox.ac.uk> [last accessed: 11.4.2009].

28 Drawing on Arjun Appadurai's concept of »techno-scapes,« Marcia Inhorn characterizes these reproductive landscapes as »repro-scapes.« Marcia Inhorn, »Making Muslim Babies: IVF and Gamete Donation in Sunni versus Shi'a Islam«, in: *Culture, Medicine and Psychiatry* 30 (2006), 4, pp. 427–450.

Recruitment of Donors: Spatio-Temporal Fixes in Oocyte Donation

Prague and Barcelona, the locations of the clinics where I did fieldwork, have become »global cities« of reproduction, because (among other reasons) they possess tourism, business, and technology amenities ranging from international airports and telecommunication infrastructures to skilled lab technicians.[29] The production of biotechnological markets like IVF is therefore embedded in actual geographical locations, they rely on »spatial fixes.«[30] With the introduction of the terms »spatial fix« or »spatio-temporal fix« I draw on concepts of critical geography coined by David Harvey and Bob Jessop.[31] The concept of the spatio-temporal fix was introduced to analyze the role of space and location in global capitalism. At first glance, fixes seem to converge with the new mobility of production networks,[32] but in fact, the spatio-temporal structure has been destabilized through the crisis of Fordism.[33] The concept of

29 I am critical of representations which follow media notions that the majority of these clinics are located »at the fringes of Europe« and have no regulations, as stated for example by Cooper and Waldby. Neither Barcelona, Prague nor Brussels are at the margins of Europe. Such depictions are too simple and appear to be stuck in the old methodological nationalism of the center-periphery model. Cf. Catherine Waldby & Melinda Cooper, »The Biopolitics Of Reproduction: Post-Fordist Biotechnology and Women's Clinical Labour«, working paper no. 15 (Global Biopolitics Research Group, 2006) <http://www.kcl.ac.uk/content/1/c6/03/03/65/wp15.pdf> (27.09.2010).

30 Regionalization is part of what Aihwa Ong calls »zones with graduated sovereignty,« cf. Aihwa Ong, *Flexible Citizenship: The Cultural Logics of Transnationality* (Durham: Duke University Press, 1999), in particular pp. 21–24. The regions of Barcelona and Valencia are motors and platforms of biotechnology in Spain. In addition to this, IVF clinics in Barcelona profit from a longstanding tourism platform and the aftereffects of Olympia 1992, one of the starting points of scale-shaping, restructuring, and gentrification of the city.

31 David Harvey, »Globalization and the ›Spatial Fix‹«, in: *Geografische Revue* (2001), 2, pp. 23–30; Bob Jessop, »Spatial Fixes, Temporal Fixes and Spatio-Temporal Fixes«, in: *David Harvey: A Critical Reader*, ed. by Noel Castree & Derek Gregory (Malden: Blackwell, 2006), pp. 142–166.

32 Cf. Mario Candeias, *Neoliberalismus – Hochtechnologie – Hegemonie: Grundrisse einer transnationalen kapitalistischen Produktions- und Lebensweise. Eine Kritik* (Hamburg: Argument, 2004), in particular p. 175.

33 Cf. Jens Wissel, *Die Transnationalisierung von Herrschaftsverhältnissen: Zur Aktualität von Nicos Poulantzas' Staatstheorie* (Baden-Baden: Nomos, 2007), in particular p. 139.

»fix« points to the fact that capitalist production still depends on local infrastructural qualities.

When one begins to analyze the gamete donation economies involved in IVF, the etymological ambiguity of the term »fix« is striking: (1) to put something in place and secure it, and (2) to fix a problem, to repair something. After a donor's follicle puncture in the morning, extracted oocytes are separated from blood and nurturing cells in the IVF laboratory and secured in a Petri dish in the incubator. In the afternoon, they are fertilized either through conventional IVF or (mostly) through ICSI with the sperm of the recipient's husband. They are transferred to the recipient on day 2 or day 3. Egg donation is undertaken as a substitution practice to »fix« the reduced or failed production of oocytes in mostly older recipients. Donors provide the clinics with substance for this oocyte solution »fix.«

Most patients from abroad coming to clinics in Spain or the Czech Republic are looking for a treatment with egg donation. Egg donors provide the clinics with the most indispensable reproductive substance. IVF clinics rely on women living close by who are willing to donate their eggs, because in contrast to sperm donation egg donation is mostly done with freshly donated eggs. In comparing the »reproductive work« of sperm and egg donors, the most salient difference is the potential risks involved in the hormonal stimulation of the egg donor. Contrary to all attempts of appeasement by infertility clinics, no long-term study of side effects has been done. Clinics rely on euphemisms like »collection« or »retrieval« of eggs instead of a more graphic term for the invasive surgical procedure used to detach eggs from the donors' bodies. The different levels of involvement for sperm and egg donors are quite obvious, but there is another difference equally important for the role of time and space in gamete donation.

Sperm as a reproductive substance is much easier to handle: in most cases it can be frozen, stored, shipped, and thawed when it is required. In comparison, results of freezing and thawing unfertilized eggs are still poorer than using fresh donated eggs in an IVF cycle. Although recent years have seen some improvements freezing eggs, during my research only fresh donated eggs were used in IVF cycles while surplus embryos (fertilized eggs) were frozen.[34] While sperm is marketed and exported by leading

34 With more improvements in ova freezing, the spatio-temporal fix of oocyte puncture/embryo transfer could be minimized in the future. Cf. Masahige Kuwayama et

sperm banks as a mass product, the raw material of donated eggs is still bound in time constraints and spatial fixes.

In what follows, I will describe two different clinical models of egg donation. Although suggested in many other reports and in contrast to the practices of sperm banks, no cross-border traffic of oocytes is taking place in these cases; the donors come to the clinics for egg retrieval. Afterwards, micropipettes fix the oocytes in the clinic labs and fuse them with sperm in the very same place. The patients are on the move to receive the gametes or pre-fertilized eggs fixed in incubators held at about 38 °C (100 °F) in Barcelona or Prague.[35] What is indeed striking was the recruitment of different groups of donor by the two clinics.

Barcelona: The »Production« of Donors Just in Time

According to Spanish law, gamete donation has to be strictly anonymized and the clinics are obliged to look for donors with »the most similar phenotypic and immunological match to the recipient woman.«[36] In fact, donor/recipient matching is done by donor and recipient statements as well as the doctor's visual perception of physical characteristics like hair color, eye color, skin color, weight, and height. Spanish clinics try to attract donors from different ethnic groups to provide recipients with a wide range of phenotypical attributes. Transmigrants from Eastern European countries working in Spain, for example, provide the clinics with their

al., »Highly Efficient Vitrification Method for Cryopreservation of Human Oocytes«, in: *Reproductive BioMedicine Online* 11 (2005), 3, pp. 300–308; Lodovico Parmegiani et al., »Freezing within 2 H from Oocyte Retrieval Increases the Efficiency of Human Oocyte Cryopreservation When Using a Slow Freezing/Rapid Thawing Protocol with High Sucrose Concentration«, in: *Human Reproduction* 23 (2008), 8, pp. 1771–1777.

35 Contrary to media claims that donors had been transported to Spain for their follicle puncture, this unbound version of reproductive mobility seems quite unrealistic. The Barcelona clinic where I did my research oversaw the donor's entire cycle: they had to constantly come to the clinic. There are media reports of bringing Ukrainian donors to Cyprus for egg retrieval, cf. Saoulli, »MEP Calls for Action on ›Human Eggs for Cash‹ Claim«, in: *Cyprus Mail*, 4.5.2006.

36 Ley 14/2006, de 26 de mayo, sobre técnicas de reproducción humana assistida, Articulo 6.4. (translation S.B.).

reproductive substances and therefore with »commodities« like blue eyes or blond hair, enabling clinics to meet the requests of non-Mediterranean patients. Assumptions made by patients such as the Fischers about where to get certain phenotypes do not take into account that countries like Spain, which used to experience mostly emigration until the 1980s, have since the 1990s experienced vastly more immigration. In Spain, most egg donors are Spanish and foreign students or migrants from Latin America and Eastern Europe. Dramatic TV images suggest that Africans arriving in makeshift boats at the Canary Islands are the largest immigrant group in Spain; in fact, they form only a small proportion of the country's migrant population. People from Eastern Europe (mainly Poles, Russians, and Romanians) come to Spain to work as seasonal farm laborers and domestic workers. About 50% of the patients at the Instituto Fontana in Barcelona come from various regions of Spain; others come from several European and non-European countries, mainly the UK and Italy. Promotion for donors is done mostly at universities with trendy flyers addressing the reproductive virility, youth, and vitality of both potential sperm and potential egg donors.[37] Whereas other IVF clinics in Spain and Europe have waiting lists for egg donation, in this clinic recipients can immediately start with their cycle. During my fieldwork in Instituto Fontana, I was quite surprised by the clinic's offer to start an IVF treatment with egg donation at whatever time fit their patients' schedules. At a patient's first consultation, one of the doctor's last questions usually was, »So when was your last period? Will you start your treatment with the beginning of the next?« Víctor, a gynecologist and a joint partner of the clinic, explained to me the temporal constraints and fixes in synchronizing IVF cycles with patients from abroad. I asked what happened in case of travel problems.[38] Víctor mentioned the airport strike in summer 2006, »when there was the chaos at Barcelona airport,« to illustrate that even under circumstances like that there was still the possibility of shifting the embryo transfer from preferred day 2 to day 4 or even day 5. But these are the limits for a fresh

37 At Instituto Fontana, donors get paid 900 euros for a successful donation. An IVF with egg donation costs about 10,000 euros in 2006.

38 Shortly before conducting fieldwork in September 2006 there had been serious air traffic problems for patients from the UK: because of rumors of a terrorist attack on Heathrow airport, new rules were immediately enforced, causing lengthy delays and inconveniences for passengers.

cycle. After that, the clinic will match the donor's eggs with another recipient couple. Víctor added, »This is a very dynamic process. Many people intervene […] and sometimes the donor doesn't respond to the stimulation so well. In those cases, we have to look quickly for a donor with the same characteristics. That's what we call a back-up donor [donante de reserva].« In other words: donor/recipient matching and synchronization can only work so well and steadily because donors and recipients are always in line. Once on the birth control pill, donor/recipient cycles can be synchronized. Whereas other clinics first match recipients to donors and then start synchronization, here donors can start immediately with their hormonal stimulation and the clinical team assigns a fitting recipient with the same cycle. If a donor cycle has to be canceled, there will be a back-up donor to fix a fresh cycle: this is the clinic's primary solution to the temporal fix in coordinating IVF cycles. The second option is to halt time by freezing fertilized eggs if sperm is available in the clinic. The reproductive spatio-temporal fix of the clinic is, first, to always fix donors waiting in line and, second, to have the option of fixing or circumventing a donor's failed response by having a second donor in line. Cross-border mobility problems are expected and taken care of: transfer can be delayed for two or three days and the embryos can be cryopreserved.

Prague: The »Production« of Low-Risk Rural Donors

Fertilmed in Prague is a private clinic mostly visited by patients from the Czech Republic, from the former Yugoslavia, or from German-speaking countries.[39] International patients started coming to the clinic a couple of years ago. When I did my research in 2007, the average waiting time for an IVF with egg donation was 10–12 months. This was due to the fact that the clinic was very busy with the patients it was already treating. The

39 Czech health insurance covers three IVF treatments for heterosexual couples under the age of forty, international patients have to pay the treatment by themselves. In Fertilmed an IVF with egg donation cost 3500 euros in 2007. In the same year the clinic had opened a new branch in Prague for German patients only, where treatment was more expensive (5500 euros) but without waiting lists. Donors received 1000 euros for a successful donation.

Czech clinic attracted its donors in different ways than the Spanish clinic. Although Prague's inner center is loaded with tourists, expatriates, and exchange students from around the world, in comparison with other European countries the Czech immigration rate is lower. Besides so-called minority groups (Slovaks, Hungarians, and Roma), the largest migrant groups in the Czech Republic come from other Slavic speaking countries like Ukraine and Russia, and additionally from former socialist partner countries like Vietnam. In contrast to the situation in Spain, where there is a lot of marketing for donors in universities and through advertisements in free magazines and on the radio, I did not see any advertisements for egg donation in Prague. During my second week in the Prague clinic, the gynecologist Lucie Novakova invited me to attend two consultations with potential egg donors. Both donors (aged 27 and 29) came from a little town in the Sudety Mountains, had two children, and were planning on donating for the first time.[40] After taking the patients' information, Dr. Novakova said about one of the women, »She is the ideal donor. She is beautiful, young, and already has two children.«[41] I asked Dr. Novakova how the clinics advertise for donors. She told me she works with a network of gynecologists in the rural, mostly northeastern regions of the Czech Republic where she grew up. These physicians send the donors for a first screening to the clinic in Prague, where later the follicle puncture is also done. The stimulation check-up during the hormonal cycle, as well as routine ultrasounds, are both done at the local, countryside practices. Afterwards, word-of-mouth advertising produces more donors. The amount the clinic pays for egg donation is almost the double average monthly income of women in these poorer rural regions of the Czech Republic, which is why Lucie Novakova is sure the donors are doing it because of the money. The eastern regions of the Czech Republic are poorer, but

40 It is hard to avoid the historical and genealogical irony of young Czech women from villages in the Sudety Mountains donating their eggs to German patients and thereby helping to reproduce German babies, while at the same time revisionist and revanchist »German Expellees Organizations« [Vertriebenen-Verbände] still claim the former »Sudetenland« as their homeland.

41 The clinic prefers donors between 18 and 35 years old who already have children. There are two reasons for this: 1) if donors already have children of their own, prospective claims towards the children are more unlikely, 2) children are the most definite test for fertility (a past abortion would also indicate that there is no primary infertility).

they are inhabited by »normal« social groups, she added. I asked her if the clinic recruits donors from Prague at all. Dr. Novakova explained they prefer working with donors from the countryside, because in Prague donation would attract potential donors from »other social classes and gypsies« and told me: »No one wants a gypsy donor.«[42] Antiziganism (racism directed at Romani people) is as common in the Czech Republic as it is in most European countries.[43] The Czech physician used it to demarcate a line between »us« and »them« articulated in terms of the »normal« (White Czech Central European), who is differentiated into different social classes but absolutely opposed to the essentialized »other.«[44] Later, when I asked Dr. Novakova if women from other countries are opting to donate, she answered that the clinic could recruit foreign donors, but their internal policy is not to do it and she referred immediately to the high prevalence of HIV among Ukrainians.

Donor recruitment policies differ between Barcelona and Prague: Fertilmed sticks to something I would call a »back-door policy,« while Instituto Fontana has a »front-door policy«: the clinic in Barcelona pragmatically addresses all women living in the Catalan agglomeration between 18 and 35 as donors, but in Prague there is a pre-selection of donors at work, triggered by recruitment through networks of doctors. Fertilmed avoids straightforward promotion in the urban space. One articulated reason for this is the wish to exclude populations epidemiologically stigmatized as risky. Second, it is meant to exclude minority groups like Roma and Sinti and poorer urban classes from donation. In any case, danger is related to the city, whereas the countryside is imagined as ethnically homogenous and immune to global risks. Different exclusion strategies are embedded and intersect in the recruitment of donors:

42 Romani people live in several places in the Czech Republic, mostly in the industrial cities in the north of Bohemia as well as in the southeast (Moravia). The eastern Bohemian towns in the Sudety Mountains are populated by a relatively homogenous white Czech population. Czech Sinti who survived the Holocaust have since 1945 been made mostly invisible by way of various assimilation strategies.

43 See Miranda Vuolasranta, »Roma und Sinti – Europäische Identitäten. Antiziganismus muss erkannt und bekämpft werden«, in: *Europäische Roma – Roma in Europa,* ed. by Reetta Toivanen & Michi Knecht (Berlin: LIT, Berliner Blätter 39, 2006), pp. 20–24.

44 Because the racial category white is universal, the »white gaze« constructs the »other« but never challenges its own premises and constructions. See Frantz Fanon, Black Skin, White Masks (London: Pluto, 1996).

potential donors are excluded through racism (antiziganism), classism (exclusion of »dangerous« urban populations), and nationalism (exclusion of migrants).

Different Economies of Reproduction

Without having such established donor systems, the Spanish and the Czech clinics would not be such important IVF destinations. Patients' imaginary landscapes, fixes, and circumvention routes form the places and spaces of reproductive technologies in Europe. Trajectories and routes of human and non-human actors, body parts, knowledge, know-how, work flow, and biocapital are their connecting agents. Combining fixes and mobility may sound like an oxymoron, but mobility should not only be understood as contradictory to fixes. It also forms a link between imagined spaces and the fixed localities actually made by patients on their circumvention routes. I want to suggest thinking of these (inter-)connections as intertwining trajectories. The choreography of a fresh IVF cycle (with egg donation) across national borders and long distances, as shown in the Barcelona case, is an example of flexible practices. Storing technologies like cryopreservation can circumvent the temporal fix of egg fertilization and embryo transfer in IVF. Freezing can expand biotechnological time-compression and bodily limits.

Both clinics differ in their specific way of establishing their *oocyte commodity chain.* While the clinic in Spain relies on a centralized network scheme, the Czech clinic is working with a decentralized one. Donors at Instituto Fontana have to live close to the metropolitan region of Barcelona, but their national origin does not matter because an ethnic diversity of donors is desired. The donors must visit the clinic several times, because the entire hormonal cycle is supervised by the clinic's egg donor coordinators. In Prague, donors come to the Fertilmed clinic only twice: for their first consultation and, later, for the egg retrieval operation. The treatment required between these two appointments is delegated to the donors' gynecologists at home. While cooperation between public and private sectors seems to be pretty common in the Czech Republic, there is much more competition between clinics in Spain. Whereas the Prague clinic relies on a platform of donor (re-)production through networks in the rural regions, the clinic in Barcelona has established a stand-by donor system with a fancy donation campaign featuring a young urban woman with a piercing and tattoos. In contrast to this, the network recruitment scheme in Prague can be read as a representation of exclusion of cosmopolitan lifestyles that are labeled as potentially risky behavior. Most importantly, certain racialized donors are clearly unwanted: Romani people, Ukrainian immigrants, and the poorer urban classes.

As I have shown, two different donor recruitment systems are at work: the ethno-national-purified donor system of Fertilmed and the pragmatic-cosmopolitan donor system of the Instituto Fontana. Both establish a spatial fix for the high demand of egg donors. The clinic in Prague caters to three groups of patients in particular: Czechs, Germans, and patients from the former Yugoslavian Republics. They provide an ethnically more homogeneous pool of donors with mostly Central European characteristics. Donation takes place between a national (Czech) donor and a foreign recipient, and can thus be termed more inter-national: foreign and non-white donors are excluded in Prague. In comparison, the Barcelona case can be considered more trans-national because donor recruitment and female migration align with each other: Instituto Fontana recruits a more diverse donor pool. Not only do the patients come from quite different regions, the donors in Barcelona are nationally and ethnically quite diverse as well. Donors and patients are matched and assigned to each other along certain phenotypical parameters. Perhaps a blue-eyed Spanish donor will be synchronized with a German recipient, a Latin American donor with an Italian recipient, or a Russian donor with an Irish couple. The clinic insists on matching patients and donors according to Spanish law, but it seems like clinic and patient enact these matching categories in co-productive performative practices. One day I observed a consultation with a Scottish couple who was determined to get a »non-Mediterranean donor,« while on another day, an English woman was flattered by the doctor's offer to match her with a Mediterranean donor because of her intense suntan. In contrast to the non-anonymized donation situation in the US described by Charis Thompson, in the two European cases preoccupation with physical resemblance (represented by a handful of phenotypical parameters) predominates over matching »identity properties« such as nationality, ethnicity, or religion.[45]

Genes & Analogies: Passing for Kinship

Ethnographic studies have shown that IVF patients connect to their children »whether ›blood related‹ or not throughout the process of becoming parents, because ›genealogical traces‹ are also embodied in non-substantive ways.«[46] What Jeanette Edwards described for Northwest England is mirrored in my encounter with Silja and Raul Kramer, another German couple I interviewed in Prague. They did not believe that genes embody social categories; they told me that these are always the result of the child's upbringing and education. Still, they emphasized that physical appearance »is in fact not a social category«: they did not have the option of influencing the looks of their child. They considered bodily appearance to be contained inside the donated oocyte. Therefore, the Kramers hoped for a good phenotypical matching. There seemed to be anxiety about the uncertainties of physical resemblance with the offspring when the couple talked about having no »social« influence on their child's physical appearance. This makes sense when thinking about the concealment practices of couples who use reproductive technologies to conceive. They are often afraid of family members, neighbors, or even unknown people on the street who start their »resemblance talk« after the birth of a child.[47] People want to (be able to) identify certain physical criteria in the child, following the cultural assumptions that children resemble their ancestors in terms of at least some of their physical criteria.[48] The Kramers separate the social from the natural; in their conception kinship is mostly construed as a social re-

45 Thompson, »Making Parents«, op. cit. (note 6), in particular pp. 145–178.

46 Jeanette Edwards, »›Make-up‹: Personhood through the Lens of Biotechnology«, in: *Ethnos* 70 (2005), 3, pp. 413–431, in particular pp. 424–426.

47 Becker et al., »Resemblance Talk«, op. cit. (note 24).

48 »It is in this particular sense of having already drawn a cognitive-visual map of relations as genotypical cross-relatedness, that the arrival of new persons is anticipated well before the physiological event of birth itself.« Konrad, »Nameless Relations«, op. cit. (note 4), p. 142.

lation of being there for the child. However, in this conception of kinship – which would also be attainable by adoption – what is missing is a biological relation which is in turn marked by biogenetic resemblance. The construction of family as a model beyond comparison is underscored by physical resemblance between parents and children.

In the perception of Susanne and Bruno Fischer, kinship and substance overlap, they contain each other. They lament a loss of identity when they state, »Nobody likes to give up on his own genes.« They feel a loss of consanguinity and a lack of resemblance ties and traits which is mediated through their understanding of genetics. For the Fischers, it does not seem too dramatic to cross the border for a treatment that is prohibited in Germany, because they consider German law to be wrong and outdated. Opting for an egg donation has been a much more significant »border-crossing« because they understand it as a »half-sided adoption,« as a loss of identity and kinship for the mother. When the Fischers describe themselves as »undercover agents,« they do not only refer to their practice of circumventing prohibitive laws, but moreover to their practices of clandestine family-building. They want to hide from their social surroundings their substitution of genetic kinship with an egg donation. Phenotypical matching allows for a form of conventional kinship by offering incorporated physical traits in the donated substance; it helps them to look like a »natural« family. I characterize these effects as »passing for kinship«: whereas procreation can be modelled in the laboratory, relatedness should still be modelled »after nature.«[49] Donor recruitment according to phenotypical criteria and anonymization are the factors that help to achieve this. Monica Konrad writes that anonymity in egg donation is »recruited here into the service of conventional kinship and this is undeniably a cultural project.«[50]

Most of the German patients I asked were afraid of being rejected by their environment and also by their prospective children. That is why they were opting for anonymization and against disclosure. In this article I portrayed people like the Fischers who, at the moment I met them in the field (before IVF succeeded), were very much occupied with resemblance

49 Marilyn Strathern, *After Nature. English Kinship in the Late Twentieth Century* (Cambridge: University Press, 1992).

50 Konrad, »Nameless Relations«, op. cit. (note 4), in particular p. 144.

to their potential offspring. Indeed, I also met others who did not think about these consequences before entering the clinic or had other views like the Kramers. Moreover, because in the first instance they all want to have a child, not all patients are obsessed with a good matching. Not all intend to conceal the use of IVF from a future child — but often they do wish to conceal it from their familial or societal surroundings.[51]

Doing kinship here is an attempt to construct or to pass for a normal family under the supervision of resemblance talk. Judith Butler's work is helpful in conceptualizing these identification processes as something other than a performance of a single subject.[52] Kin resemblance identifications are enacted by a number of people (family members, friends, neighbors, and nosy strangers), who repeat these norms by looking at the baby in the buggy and commenting on its looks. Most of the German patients I asked expressed anxiety about being rejected by their environment as well as by their prospective children. That is why they were opting for anonymized gamete donation and against disclosure. Maybe their attitudes will change if they become parents. Some discussions in IVF Internet forums allude to this possibility.[53] Some of the British patients I spoke to in the Spanish clinic were much more open about disclosure, a reflection of the discourse concerning prospective children's rights and the governmental withdrawal of anonymization in the UK.[54] In fact, cultural projects of doing kinship the »conventional way« (through concealment) are contested by children's rights lobbyists, who demand disclosure and promote educational campaigns on how to tell children about donation and practices that displace hegemonic family definitions through »queer reproduction.«[55] On the one hand, performativity in kin-making with reproductive technologies offers opportunities for more open cultures of relating. It cre-

51 See Joan Bestard Camps, *Tras la Biología: La Moralidad del Parentesco y las Nuevas Tecnologías de Reproducción* (Barcelona: Universitat de Barcelona, 2004), in particular pp. 69–83.

52 Judith Butler, *Bodies that Matter: On the Discursive Limits of »Sex«* (New York: Routledge, 1993), in particular p. 15.

53 Cf. Maren Klotz, op. cit. (note 23) for management of kinship knowledge in families created through IVF.

54 Sarah Franklin & Celia Roberts, *Born and Made. An Ethnography of Preimplantation Genetic Diagnosis* (Princeton: University Press, 2006), in particular p. 70.

55 Laura Mamo, *Queering Reproduction: Achieving Pregnancy in the Age of Technoscience* (Durham, NC: Duke University, 2007), in particular pp. 123–127.

ates new options for less reductionist understandings of kinship as »affinity ties«[56] and conceiving genealogical traces in »a non-substantive way.«[57] On the other hand, IVF regulations that require anonymization, thus severing genetic kinship, are mostly used to stabilize the heterosexual nuclear family model.

Anonymization as a Vector in Transnational Gamete Donation

In Spain and the Czech Republic the anonymization of gamete donation is required by national law. All clinicians I talked to favored anonymization – most of them argued that this would facilitate keeping the donation a secret after the birth of a child. Patients I talked to were much more ambivalent about secrecy or disclosure towards their intended children. Anonymized donation severs the genetic relation between the donor and her reproductive substance, while IVF with egg donation establishes a new kin-relation between recipient and the embryo. Marilyn Strathern characterizes anonymized donation as a form of *non-genealogical relatedness* that »may not have relatives, but it does have signifying others,«[58] that is to say the images of donors as the third parties in these processes. Michi Knecht asks how forms of prospective and potential kinship could be mapped, and how we could chart the role of a willingness not to know when doing kinship using reproductive technologies. As of now, the spatial dimension of kinship has never been represented in ethnological genealogy diagrams.[59] So how can such »relatedness without relatives« and anonymization in gamete donation be described using the concept of transnational spaces? In

56 Mamo, »Queering Reproduction«, op. cit. (note 55), in particular pp. 190–223.

57 Edwards, »Make-up«, op. cit. (note 46).

58 Marilyn Strathern, *Kinship, Law and the Unexpected: Relatives Are Always a Surprise* (New York, NY: Cambridge University Press, 2005), in particular p. 76 (referring to Monica Konrad's study of egg donation in the UK before the withdrawal of anonymity by the HFEA).

59 Michi Knecht, »Spätmoderne Genealogien: Praxen und Konzepte verwandtschaftlicher Bindung und Abstammung«, in: *Verwandtschaft machen. Reproduktionsmedizin und Adoption in Deutschland und der Türkei*, ed. by Stefan Beck, Nevim Çil, Sabine Hess, Maren Klotz & Michi Knecht (Münster: LIT, Berliner Blätter 42, 2007), pp. 92–108, in particular p. 96 and p. 105.

terms of enacting anonymized and concealed knowledge about origins, I prefer to use the prefix trans- rather than inter-, because international donation would better describe open donor systems where the donor exists *between* knowing parties and can be physically located. Transnational donation points towards the ambiguity of an anonymized donor system, where knowledge about the donor is *beyond* all realms. *Trans* literally means beyond: it leaves traces, not fixed relations. Genealogically and spatially it is »terra incognita.« In terms of genealogical tracings concerned with places of origin, this »space beyond« seems to represent a negative ontology. Recipients will know a little bit about what their future child might look like (phenotypical parameters), but nothing about where the donor is and where she comes from. My comparison of egg donor recruitment in two European clinics shows how – in the Spanish case – egg donation emerges as a form of (re-)productive work for migrant women. While future donor tracking would be very difficult in the national donor recruitment system in the Czech case, it would be even more difficult in locations like Barcelona, where transnational migration and gamete donation intersect.[60] The prefix *trans* in transnational entails a supplementary element or effect, as Aihwa Ong remarks: »Trans denotes both moving through space or across lines, as well as changing the nature of something.«[61] It is thrilling to relate Ong's argument about nature-changing to the practice of black-boxing genealogical knowledge in the process of anonymized donation mediated by IVF clinics. In the case of gamete donation, anonymization challenges »natural« assumptions about kinship and assumptions about kinship as »natural.« The supplementary dimensions of transnational anonymized donation changes »natural« ideas of where we are from. Anonymization therefore operates as a vector. Vec-

60 Transnational gamete donation can potentially lead to the genealogical tracking of children conceived through gamete donation. Anticipating potential networks around the non-traceable, Monica Konrad calls this kind of tracking »conception-related ›detective work‹,« (Konrad, »Nameless Relations«, op. cit. (note 4), in particular p. 216). If data records are collected by clinics and regulative institutions like the Catalan Ministry of Health and if we take into account the growing role of the law, a demonstration of donor offspring in front of the clinic in Valencia or the Czech Ministry of Health demanding the opening of the archives might be a possible scenario in the near future. The children conceived by egg donation addressed in this article are as of now still too young.

61 Ong, »Flexible Citizenship«, op. cit. (note 30), in particular p. 4.

tors are etymologically able to carry, to pull, and to transport something. Regarding the high performativity in doing kinship with IVF, anonymization must not necessarily lead to concealment practices, but it does serve as a facilitator in severing or hiding knowledge about origins and genitors. Another vector that stabilizes this culture of disguise is the fabrication of resemblance guaranteed by infertility clinics. The comparison of two distinct European clinics has shown how clinics operationalize this problem by recruiting (in the Barcelona case) a heterogeneous donor group or (as in the Prague case) a more homogenous donor group to serve the phenotypical needs of patients. The case of the Fischers has shown that through imaginations about the dissemination of phenotypes in Europe, the Fischers reconstruct homogenous spaces of inhabitation which are indeed challenged by mobility and migration. For them, the resemblance question was the most important factor in choosing a clinic abroad because they wanted to conceal their decision. A donor with similar bodily markers would help them later install social legitimacy: resemblance serves as a vector for the conception of how a family should look like.[62] A combination of anonymized donor selection, phenotypical donor matching, and (transnational) distance stabilizes a culture of disguise in which resemblance (mediated through genes) still matters. Even though other bodily substances can be transferred to another body without establishing a kin connection, gametes endow genetic information and thus also bio-genetic relatedness: at least, as long as Euro-American kinship is conceptualized as originating through substance, whether blood, genes, or chromosomes.

62 Caroline Jones, »Looking like a Family: Negotiating Bio-Genetic Continuity in British Lesbian Families Using Licensed Donor Insemination«, in: *Sexualities* 8 (2005), 2, pp. 221–237.

Biomedical Mobilities: Transnational Lab-Benches and Other Space-Effects

Stefan Beck

The following article sets out to explore a challenge posed by recent developments in late modernity that for some time has been constituting a predicament for the social sciences and especially for socio-cultural anthropology: The intertwined questions of how to conceptualize and of how to make methodologically accessible the new spatiotemporal arrangements, the new modes of ordering or structuring institutional as well as vernacular practices that are commonly labeled as *transnational* or *global.* The following article will analyze instances of – what tentatively will be called – *biomedical mobilities* in the domain of in vitro fertilization and reproductive medicine as a prominent example of these developments; and it will suggest some theoretical and methodological adaptations which will allow to take these transformations into account. The perspective suggested here does not focus on the state as a unit of analysis or on changing modes of governing. Instead, it proposes to analyze practices characterized by *biomedical mobilities,* »civil« as well as »scientific« practices in the medical domain that *do relations* beyond the boundaries of states, societies or institutions by moving people, knowledge, ideas as well as biomedical »things.« This approach can be seen as an ethno- or praxeographic twin to the »methodological cosmopolitism« suggested by Ulrich Beck and Edgar Grande, a perspective that takes »variations of modernity and its global interdependencies as a point of departure for theoretical reflection and empirical inquiry.«[1]

1 Ulrich Beck and Edgar Grande, »Jenseits des methodologischen Nationalismus. Außereuropäische und europäische Variationen der Zweiten Moderne«, in: *Soziale Welt* 61 (2010), 3/4, pp. 187–216. (transl. SB)

A Praxeographic Perspective on Biomedical Mobilities

I borrow the concept of *mobilities* from John Urry who coined the term to indicate that in late modern societies not only migration or transnational media, but technological infrastructures, knowledge or environmental hazards, among other features of emerging global and moral economies, undermine state-bound instruments of governance. As he points out, ideas, objects, people are »criss-crossing societal borders in strikingly new temporal-spatial patterns« that question existing notions of society and citizenship.[2] Here, I use the term *biomedical mobilities* to analyze three examples of these emerging patterns in the domain of biomedicine; the term *mobilities* underlines the heterogeneity of elements set in motion: people, knowledge, ideas as well as things are mobilized to travel beyond borders.[3] As will be argued in the following, biomedical platforms[4] as they are in operation in reproductive medicine afford an opportunity structure for new types of mobilities and new transnational practices that are in conflict with established regimes of governing a territory and a population demarcated by well defined national borders: (1) Biomedical platforms make cells and tissues »bioavailable«[5] on an increasingly global scale through the procurement, purification, genotypic classification and subsequent »bio-banking« of human cells. (2) In the field of IVF, the mobilization of gametes and patients seeking treatment beyond national borders weakens national bioethical or legal regulation – an erosion of the national encompassment of biopolitical regimes.[6] (3) The emergence of

2 John Urry, *Sociology beyond Societies: Mobilities for the Twenty-first Century* (London, New York: Routledge, 2000), p. 4f.

3 For a fuller account on the notion of *medical mobilities* and their potential *sub-political effects* cf. Stefan Beck, »Staging Bone Marrow Donation as a Ballot. Reconfiguring the Social and the Political Using Biomedicine in Cyprus«, Special Issue „Medical Migrations», *Body & Society* 2011, in print.

4 Peter Keating and Alberto Cambrosio, *Biomedical Platforms: Realigning the Normal and the Pathological in Late-Twentieth Century Medicine* (Cambridge, Mass.: MIT Press, 2003).

5 Lawrence Cohen, »Operability, Bioavailability, and Exception«, in: *Global Assemblages. Technology, Politics, and Ethics as Anthropological Problems*, ed. by Aihwa Ong and Stephen J. Collier (Malden & Oxford: Blackwell Publishing, 2005), pp. 79–90.

6 Guido Pennings, »Legal Harmonization and Reproductive Tourism in Europe (reprinted from *Human Reproduction* 19, pp. 2689–94, 2004)«, in: *Reproductive Health Matters* 13 (2005), 25, pp. 120–128.

a global system of distribution and consumption of »reproductive medical services« – in part market-driven, in part characterized by altruistic exchange – is accelerated through the highly dynamic dissemination of medical knowledge, laboratory equipment, and the installation of commercial biobanks. (4) In addition, national regulatory regimes are under pressure to produce legitimacy through the implementation of internationally accepted legal and ethical »best practices.«[7] However, in spite of this accommodation, national differences in regulation remain in place to some extent due to the »path dependency« of welfare state regimes,[8] »local« experiences,[9] or historically contingent legal conditions – e.g. the ban of preimplantation diagnosis and embryo selection in Germany due to a legislation that reflects inhuman euthanasia practices during the Nazi rule.[10] (5) But where, like in Germany, gametes or fertilized eggs are de-mobilized by restrictive national regulations, patients or donors try to evade implemented legal regimes and travel instead – what often is misleadingly discussed under the label of medical »tourism.«[11] (6) These mobilities and the introduction of regulations that aim at controlling these movements are a case in point where a dialectic of weakening and strengthening of national forms of governance can be observed in oper-

7 European Union, »Directive 2004/23/EC of the European Parliament and of the Council of 31 March 2004 on setting standards of quality and safety for the donation, procurement, testing, processing, preservation, storage and distribution of human tissues and cells«, in: *Official Journal of the European Union*, L102 (2004), pp. 48–58.

8 Peter Baldwin, *Contagion and the State in Europe 1830–1930* (Cambridge: Cambridge University Press, 1999), Martin Lengwiler and Jeanette Madarász, »Präventionsgeschichte als Kulturgeschichte der Gesundheitspolitik«, in: *Das präventive Selbst. Eine Kulturgeschichte moderner Gesundheitspolitik*, ed. by Martin Lengwiler and Jeanette Madarász (Bielefeld: transcript, 2010), pp. 11–30.

9 Martin Lengwiler and Stefan Beck, »Historizität, Materialität und Hybridität von Wissenspraktiken. Die Entwicklung europäischer Präventionsregime im 20. Jahrhundert«, in: *Geschichte und Gesellschaft* 33 (2008), 4, pp. 489–523.

10 Regine Kollek, *Präimplantationsdiagnostik: Embryonenselektion, weibliche Autonomie und Recht* (Tübingen: 2000).

11 Cf. Andrea Whittaker, Lenore Manderson and Elizabeth Cartwright, »Patients without Borders: Understanding Medical Travel«, in: *Medical Anthropology: Cross-Cultural Studies in Health and Illness*, 29 (2010), 4, pp. 336 – 343. For a discussion of the terminology refering to medical travel in the field of reproductive medicine see Knoll and Inhorn in this volume.

ation.[12] In sum, biomedical platforms afford not only the mobilization of cells, patients, medical equipment and knowledge, but also of moral convictions, of imaginations, of desires, and of feelings of solidarity that travel beyond borders. This mobilization of material-discursive »things,« these new relations between discursive practices and material phenomena, these entanglements of human and non-human forms of agency,[13] threaten to escape attempts of »national encompassment,«[14] giving rise to a dialectic of globalization and attempts at re-localization.

From a praxeographic perspective, what is at issue here are conflicting, pragmatic regimes that align an equipped or furnished humanity: they attempt to delimit understandings of what is good and legitimate and they suggest forms of activity that require reflective argumentation, because they are contestable morally but also because they are dependent on scientific knowledge and »progress.« Pragmatic regimes make equipment – technologies, infrastructures, »things« – available practically as well as normatively through defining »rational forms of use.«[15] These pragmatic regimes – understood as »ways of engaging the world« – are »social devices which govern our way of engaging with our environment inasmuch as they articulate two notions: (a) an orientation towards some kind of good; (b) a mode of access to reality«[16] – in the examples discussed below the morally acceptable use of a biomedical platform to alleviate suffering, to make connections, and to transform social positions.

The emergence of these conflicting, rapidly changing pragmatic regimes pose several problems for ethnography, a discipline that was long content in restricting its studies to units of analysis that were assumed to be securely demarcated by local, regional or national containers (vil-

12 Cf. Joy Yueyue Zhang, »The Cosmopolitanization of Science. Experience from Chinese Stem Cell Scientists«, in: *Soziale Welt* 61 (2010), 3/4, pp. 257–276.

13 Cf. Karen Barad, »Posthumanist Performativity: Toward an Understanding of How Matter Comes to Matter«, in: *Signs* 28 (2003), 3, pp. 801–831.

14 James Ferguson and Akhil Gupta, »Spatializing States: Toward an Ethnography of Neoliberal Governmentality«, in: *American Ethnologist* 29 (2002), 4, pp. 981–1002.

15 Cf. Joseph Rouse, »Two Concepts of Practices«, in: *The Practice Turn in Contemporary Theory*, ed. by Theodore R. Schatzki, Karin Knorr-Cetina and Eike von Savigny (New York: Routledge, 2001), pp. 189–198.

16 Laurent Thévenot, »Pragmatic Regimes of Governing the Engagement with the World«, in: *The Practice Turn*, ed. by Schatzki, Knorr-Cetina and von Savigny, op. cit. (note 15), pp. 56–73, p. 67.

lages, islands, remote regions and more often than not marginal states). How can these transnational phenomena be made observable? What are appropriate concepts to come to terms with these highly dynamic and fleeting processes? And how can path-dependencies and idiosyncrasies in pragmatic regimes be taken into account? Or to phrase the problem differently: To what extent the close observation of situated, concrete practices will afford the reconstruction of abstract processes and dynamics – i.e. globalization, Europeanization, transnational entanglements – that eschew direct perception in the observational mode of ethnography? How can we conceptualize the interrelation of highly localized practices on the one hand and thoroughly globalized practices on the other? While this puzzle is not new in principle, the epistemological problem in the current situation, where, among other old certainties the »state of the state« has become questionable, concerns the reconstruction of the specific dynamic created by the processes of dis-embedding and re-embedding that are characteristic for late modernity – to use the vocabulary of Anthony Giddens[17] – and to invent adequate modes of description.

Usually this problem is tackled by focusing on the role of the state as a unit of analysis. Anthropologist Aihwa Ong, for example, points to an acute deficit in empirical studies of late modern statehood and suggests as a remedy that »it would be useful to understand how states in practice actually manage a range of transnational networks that variously integrate them into the global market and political community.«[18] Ong proposes to analyze what she calls the »graduated sovereignty« of late modern states by paying close attention to the new modes of control, surveillance, and regulation states try to implement vis-à-vis markets, populations, and external agencies. While Ong follows a Foucauldian line of thought, anthropologists James Ferguson and Akhil Gupta suggest to analyze new modes of spatialization that are applied by states in reaction to challenges posed by current socio-political transformations. They characterize modern states as »powerful sites of symbolic and cultural production« that – among other things and thoughts – would create a »commonsense topography« of levels

17 Anthony Giddens, *The Consequences of Modernity* (Stanford, Calif.: Stanford University Press, 1990).

18 Cf. Aihwa Ong, »Graduated Sovereignty in South-East Asia«, in: *Theory, Culture & Society* 17 (2000), 4, pp. 55–75.

of sociality: beginning from individuals to families to communities to society, the state usually is imagined as the top-layer of a neatly stacked social cake, its practices of governance characterized by *vertical encompassment*[19]. Ferguson and Gupta argue that this imaginary of a vertical topography of power created by the modern state also structured the taken for granted battle order of modern political conflicts: the state emerges as a *naturalized* sovereign over a territory and a population; consequently he is the logical addressee of political demands, expostulations, thorough critique as well as the obvious object of protest and revolutions.

But as I will argue: this metaphor of sociality, depicted as a layered cake, neatly covered by an icing that is decorated with the well established insignia of sovereignty, a metaphor that in one version or another has dominated and is still dominating the social imaginary of Western modernities, tends to prevent an adequate analysis of the nature of connections that are labeled transnational but that are not channeled *through* the state – nor are these connections necessarily moderated *by* the state. As a consequence, new conceptual frames or metaphors are needed in order to address these constellations adequately: I suggest the playful metaphor of *wormholes* or *hyperspaces* to address configurations that allow actors in separate states to link up via a host of networked mechanisms in order to join forces, to pursue their common interests, while happily or grudgingly ignoring their respective states and the borders they attempt to draw around »their« populations. These practices create a *networked topography* that is transnational not in the commonsensical notion of »above« or »beyond« the state, as the notion is often applied by political practitioners or social scientists analyzing transnational or global dynamics, but in the sense of a dimensional shift, connecting diverse localities and exploding the cake(-metaphor). These practices of citizens that reject or bypass national state power – such as the »new« social movements – participate intentionally or unintentionally in the erosion of state-power. Likewise anthropologist Michel-Rolph Trouillot points to the apparent contradiction that while »the routinizations of governmental presence in the lives

19 Ferguson and Gupta, »Spatializing States«, op. cit. (note 14).

of citizens abound everywhere,« governmental power is at the same time challenged, diverted, or simply giving way to supranational institutions.[20]

It is this fluctuating constellation that is of interest here. What has to be addressed is the specific spaciality of late modernity as it emerges out of the dynamic of knowledge societies.[21] The field of reproductive medicine may serve as a prime *Versuchsanordnung* (an experimental *cum* experiential system »in the wild,« outside of controlled laboratory settings) where the progressing decline of direct government, the neoliberal privatization of health care systems, the availability of new technologies of the self and claims to individual autonomy – »choice« in the consumerist American, *Selbstbestimmung* (»self-determination«) in the existentialist German frame of mind – can be observed producing new subjectivities, new moralities and social obligations, as well as new relations.

The methodological *cum* theoretical question of how to grasp the topo*logy* of late modernity should be answered by socio-cultural anthropology by closely analyzing exemplary topo*practices* through adequate topo*graphical methods*. The obvious methodological recipe are »multi-sited observations« of practices (G. Marcus) and flows (A. Appadurai) or empirical explorations in actor-networks (B. Latour), in socio-technical assemblages (P. Rabinow; M. DeLanda) and analyses of material-discursive practices (A. Mol).[22] Privileging practices as the observational unit –

20 Michel-Rolph Trouillot, »The Anthropology of the State in the Age of Globalization. Close Encounters of the Deceptive Kind«, in: *Current Anthropology* 42 (2001), 1, pp. 125–38, especially p. 125.

21 Cf. for a fuller account Stefan Beck, »Globalisierte Reproduktionsregimes: Anmerkungen zur Emergenz biopolitischer Handlungsräume«, in: *Verwandtschaft machen. Reproduktionsmedizin und Adoption in Deutschland und der Türkei*, ed. by Stefan Beck, Nevim Çil, Sabine Hess, Maren Klotz and Michi Knecht (Münster, Hamburg, Berlin, London: Lit, 2007), pp. 124–151.

22 George E. Marcus, »Ethnography in/of the the World System: The Emergence of Multi-Sited Ethnography«, in: *Annual Review of Anthropology* 24 (1995), pp. 95–117; Arjun Appadurai, »Fieldwork in the Era of Globalization«, in: *Anthropology and Humanism* 22 (1997), 1, pp. 115–118; Bruno Latour, *Reassembling the Social. An Introduction to Actor-network-theory* (Oxford: Oxford University Press, 2005); Paul Rabinow, George E. Marcus, James D. Faubion and Tobias Rees, *Designs for an Anthropology of the Contemporary* (Durham: Duke University Press, 2008); Manuel DeLanda, *A New Philosophy of Society. Assemblage Theory and Social Complexity* (London, New York: Continuum, 2006); Annemarie Mol, »I Eat an Apple. On Theorizing Subjectivities«, in: *Subjectivity* 22 (2008), pp. 28–37.

rather than states, regions, or localities that are conceptualized to »encompass« socialities – implies a radical re-conceptualization of space. As Michel de Certeau analyzed in his book *Arts de faire*, using the city scape as an example, modern concepts of space are characterized by purity (suppressing all physical and political contaminations), by timelessness (i.e. the establishment of a pervasive present and the suppression of »tradition«), and by the creation of an universal subject as inhabitant. In contrast, de Certeau suggests not to analyze this idealized space but to observe the trajectories of actors, their concrete appropriations of spatial arrangements, their »rhetoric« of use. Through their practices – as de Certeau interprets it – *ideal space is realized as concrete, lived, highly interconnected places.*[23] And realization of space here has two connotations: to make space real and to make it perceptible. Likewise, but applying the conceptual frame of actor-network-theory, Michael Schillmeier and Wiebke Pohler, taking the »SARS epidemic« of 2002 as their example in a recent paper, analyze what they call *»the practiced space«* created by an heterogeneous assemblage of pathogens, their vectors, health institutions like the WHO and national health services and their respective knowledge practices.[24]

In the following, I will present three examples of different actors *realizing space* – again: realization in its double sense – as a rather unintended consequence of their practices in the field of biomedicine. In all three examples personal or situated *experiences* are transformed into types of knowledge that *travel* and that in traveling redefine a specific space. I will arrange the examples according to what I call – borrowing from Arjun Appadurai – their *scape effects*, that is their potential to reorder practices in space-time. I will come back to the concept after the presentation of my cases.

23 Cf. Michel de Certeau, *The Practice of Everyday Life* (Berkeley: University of California Press, 1984).

24 Michael Schillmeier and Wiebke Pohler, »Kosmo-politische Ereignisse. Zur sozialen Topologie von SARS«, in: *Soziale Welt* 4 (2006), pp. 331–349.

First Example: Mobilizing a Biomedical Platform and Stabilizing Expertise

At first sight, the department of reproductive medicine of Ege University Clinic in Izmir, on the Aegean coast of Turkey, resembles a glittering, outlandish spacecraft after a messed up emergency landing, being inseparably interlocked with a crumbling, ugly concrete building urgently in need of refurbishment. Reaching the department, located on the second floor of the state-run policlinic, via worn-out stairs, passing through overcrowded waiting areas, where patients and their accompanying family members wait in different states of nervousness, along corridors with flaked off grey paint, one suddenly stands in front of an automatic plate glass door that – with a soft hum – opens to a calm, brightly lit and air-conditioned reception area: several nurses welcome visitors from behind a front desk that is dominated by an aquarium where colorful exotic fish swim their rounds. The walls of the clinic are covered with expensively framed paintings, among them a big oil painting representing the late founder of the gynecological clinic in Izmir who was an influential patron in the 1980s, supporting the establishment of *in vitro fertilization* in his clinic.

In fact, Ege University was the first clinic in Turkey to offer *in vitro fertilization* (IVF) to its patients. In the mid 1980s, Erol Tavmergen and his sister Ege returned from Germany where they had been trained as gynecologists, specializing with a PhD in reproductive medicine at the medical school of Kiel University. Erol even completed his *Habilitation*, qualifying for a professorship in reproductive medicine in the German university system; doing so, Erol followed in the footsteps of his father who also had studied medicine and habilitated in gynecology in Munich. And, as their father had done, both his children decided to return to their hometown Izmir together. Here, Erol and Ege Tavmergen pioneered the field of reproductive medicine in Turkey – as Erol recalls:

»We were trained in the relevant techniques in Kiel and we brought in vitro fertilization to Turkey in the mid 1980s. At this time the field of reproductive medicine in Turkey was not developed at all. So we had to bring everything from Germany and had to train the laboratory personnel and the nurses. We brought mice for tests and training purposes from Kiel, four females and three males of the strain

CB6 F1. We transported them in our hand luggage in the plane when we came back from Germany.«[25]

Apart from the animals, they also had to import all lab equipment, materials and necessary chemical substances from Germany since these were not available in Turkey in the mid 1980s. In doing so, they could rely on their professional contacts to colleagues in Germany.

Erol: »We conducted around 3500 training cycles with the staff before officially founding the Ege Laboratory for the Human Being [...] We were very proud that we succeeded to introduce healthy pregnancies in two from our first seven patients. Given the time and the available technology, this was a very good outcome. The first IVF-baby in Turkey was born by one of these seven patients; also the first twins were produced here – at that time it was perceived as a sensation! One year after our big successes here, the second IVF-clinic opened in Istanbul in a private clinic, and after that a clinic in Ankara was opened.«
Stefan: »When you opened the clinic, was there already a demand for fertility treatment in Izmir? Were patients traveling abroad for treatment?«
Erol: »Yes – for example the couple with our first IVF-baby, they had tried it in England before, in Hammersmith Hospital in London. The woman knew through a former diagnosis that she had a tubular restriction caused by a past Tuberculosis infection. Since the treatment in London was not successful, she came to us. We had five cycles and then we introduced a successful pregnancy. We were very happy, because – the Hammersmith Hospital is a very good clinic, it still is. They did not succeed, but we did [he and his sister laugh]. The public reaction here was remarkable. There was demand then but in the last ten years demand grew rapidly: In the second half of the 1980s five centers were opened in Turkey, in the late 1990s already 30 centers were operating, and now, in 2005, more than 60 centers are offering IVF treatments in Turkey.«

For many years now, Erol Tavmergen has been involved in the Turkish association of reproductive medicine in leading positions and was influential in creating a favorable political environment for the new technique locally as well as nationally. Therefore, he is quite proud about the expansion of his field: »In 2002 and 2003 the overall number of treatment cycles was about 12.000 per year, in 2004 the figure doubled already, and in 2005 it will be about 30.000 cycles in Turkey.«

25 The interview was conducted in 2005 with Erol and Ege Tavmergen in their clinic in Izmir.

The clinic in Izmir's Ege University is special for several reasons. It is quite large – 45 people work here as nurses, embryologists, gynecologists and anesthesiologists. And it is a public-private hybrid: since the clinic also financially supports its own administrative and nursing staff, it is economically, administratively and scientifically independent from the surrounding policlinic while firmly integrated with the gynecological department of the public hospital. In contrast to the private, commercial IVF-centers in Turkey, the Tavmergens' clinic is also involved in research and recruits PhD-students from the university. The clinic is cooperating on a regular basis with a psychologist who is also responsible for the internal evaluation of services and surveys regarding patient satisfaction. It is remarkable that many employees have been working in the clinic since its foundation, a mutual loyalty crucial to both the Tavmergens and – as they see it – an important means to enhance the professional standards and success-rates of their clinic.

The quasi autonomous status of the clinic in the public health care system is seen by Erol and Ege as an important achievement that could only be realized after endless struggles with the clinic bureaucracy and diverse authorities in the health care and political system. They were successful not at least because they managed to secure financial and political support from private donors – the local mother's associations, the Rotary Club and influential businessmen in the Izmir region. As Ege Tavmergen stresses, only their economically as well as administratively semi-independent status enabled them to equip their clinic with the newest technologies, to hire qualified specialists, and to refurbish the old hospital rooms in *their* realm.

Their success, in turn, generated positive coverage in the national press and public attention that helped secure the status of the clinic against bureaucratic indifference. Erol and Ege Tavmergen are ingenuous in playing this card: Years ago, they thought that it would be comforting for the families of IVF-children to exchange experiences and views. So they created a yearly event, a small celebration, where former IVF-patients and their families are invited to participate. This gathering also provided them with the opportunity to stay in touch with their patients and to bring in touch families with older and younger IVF-children as well as with would-be

IVF-parents. And of course, these celebrations were also intended to promote public relations.

In the mid 1980s, Erol and Ege Tavmergen not only established a medical technology in Izmir by – quite literally – moving expertise and equipment from the »center« (in this case: Germany) to the »periphery« (then: Turkey), their initiative was also influential in shaping the entire sector of reproductive medicine in Turkey. From the start, they saw their clinical department as competing with successful clinics in Britain, Germany, or the US, and they took on this challenge. Accordingly, they struggled to gain independence from – as they felt – bureaucratic shortcomings, financial constraints and legal restrictions imposed upon them from local or national authorities that hindered their scientific and clinical progress. They successfully won a high degree of scientific as well as financial independence from »their« hospital and the Turkish medical system – not least because they successfully mobilized »local« support from patients[26] to gain legitimacy and sponsors to receive additional funding for transforming their department into a respectable player in the international community of reproductive medicine. The long-term spatial effects are obvious: Ege and Erol Tavmergen were influential in the transformation of a former medical periphery into one of several European IVF-hubs where increasingly patients from other countries seek treatment. Through mobilizing their professional contacts to German colleagues they put Izmir and, successively, Turkey on the map of internationally competitive reproductive medical services.

Second Example: Transnational Prevention Regimes – Grassroots-Style

The second example will also elucidate the potential of »local« actors to enter the transnational stage. It stems from my ongoing fieldwork in Cyprus, a former British colony that was released into independence in 1960.

26 For an analysis of the work of ÇİDER, the highly influential patient organization in the field of reproductive technologies in Turkey, see Nurhak Polat's contribution in this volume.

What is remarkable is that in Cyprus a host of highly successful patient groups are operating. One of the many groups, the Thalassaemia International Foundation – TIF for short – is especially successful internationally: It was founded in 1986 as a »spin-off« from the Cypriot patient organization for sufferers of Thalassaemia, a severe hereditary hemoglobin disorder that results in an early and painful death. This organization was – in close collaboration with hematologists and with support from the Orthodox Church – one of the key actors in implementing the most successful prevention program against a genetically caused disease world-wide. This program involves a population wide educational campaign, the early diagnosis of carrier status and the recommendation for carriers not to marry. I will not touch upon the ethical critique this scheme provoked in the international bioethics community;[27] what is central to the argument here is only that the program was highly successful in reducing the number of children born with Thalassaemia in Cyprus from an average of 150 per year to nearly zero. What is more, this »local« success had a significant impact on the British and the Australian health care system respectively where Cypriot migrants requested carrier screening and prenatal diagnosis in hematological clinics and thus put Thalassaemia on the medical agenda in these countries for the first time.[28]

However, the founders of TIF – all of them had direct experience of the severity of the disease either as family members or physicians – were of the conviction that their recipe for success should be made available to other developing countries where Thalassaemia was an even greater public health problem than in Cyprus. So they went global: Now, 20 years after its foundation, Thalassaemia International provides political, educational, logistical, and financial support for 98 national Thalassaemia associations from over 60 countries across the world, e.g. Malaysia, Iran, Bangladesh,

27 For an account of these issues cf. Stefan Beck and Jörg Niewöhner, »Localising Genetic Testing and Screening in Cyprus and Germany. Contingencies, continuities, ordering effects and bio-cultural intimacy«, in: *The Handbook of Genetics and Society: Mapping the New Genomic Era*, ed. by Paul Atkinson, Peter Glasner and Margaret Lock (London: Routledge, 2009), pp. 76–93.

28 Bernadette Modell, Maren Khan, Matthew Darlison, »Survival in ß-Thalassaemia major in the UK: Data from the UK Thalassaemia Register«, in: *The Lancet* 355 (2000), June 10, pp. 2051–2052. Paramjit S. Gill, Bernadette Modell, »Thalassaemia in Britain: a Tale of Two Communities. Births are Rising among British Asians But Falling in Cypriots«, in: *British Medical Journal* 317 (1998), pp. 761–762.

and Thailand. The organization is involved in training medical practitioners and nurses, it lobbies for the introduction of prevention programs in developing countries, runs information campaigns and collects funds for training medical staff in close collaboration with the World Health Organization.[29]

TIF is exemplary for a postcolonial legacy: it is an organization that understands how to act from a position of marginality and institutional weakness, that pragmatically draws together available resources and sees its priorities in education and the change of conduct. Since TIF knows that first class medical care will be unavailable for most people in developing countries, they pragmatically take recourse to cheap, effective *social interventions*: they propagate a rationality of risk management through changing marriage practices, the mantra being: two diagnosed carriers of the Thalassaemia trait should simply not marry. However, since costs for IVF-treatments have dropped dramatically and success-rates have been constantly increasing in recent years, the organization lobbies to make IVF and pre-implantation diagnosis available also in poorer countries. Again, experiences from Cyprus are decisive here: Against the backdrop of advances in reproductive medicine, Cypriots who are diagnosed as carriers of the Thalassaemia trait do not strictly follow the recommendation not to marry or not to have children any more. As soon as prenatal diagnosis became more reliable in the 1990s, they used amniocentesis and eventually abortion to preclude giving birth to a thalassaemic child; and since preimplantation diagnosis is readily available now, two carriers of Thalassaemia have the option to plan healthy pregnancies – and many do, while common sense in Cyprus still assumes that it is better not to take risks and that therefore two carriers should not marry. TIF successfully translated individual and local experiences in Cyprus into the *formulation of best practices* easily applicable in other socio-cultural contexts. Doing that, TIF is a truly global actor in that it systematically bypasses national health policies in cooperating with grass-roots initiatives as well as with global agencies like WHO to create new preventive regimes in the field of reproductive practices. The NGO is propagating a *pragmatic regime* for managing Thalassaemia rationally – and it connects sufferers, medical professionals and activists in a grass-roots-style. TIF acts in a geographical space that is fore-

29 Cf. http://www.thalassaemia.org.cy/.

most defined by the world distribution of the Thalassaemia trait; while population history matters, national, social, cultural or economical borders come into view as mere obstacles in trying to implement rational policies.

Third Example: Knowledge Franchising and Transnational Lab-Benches

In 2004, the most influential Turkish charity opened a hypermodern clinic south of Istanbul in cooperation with Johns Hopkins Medicine in Baltimore. The new clinic aspires to serve its patients »with world-class health care«; as the advertising on the homepage makes clear, the target group for the medical services consists of affluent patients from Turkey as well as from the middle east, who might encounter visa-problems traveling to the USA or feel more comfortable bringing their families along to a Muslim country.[30] To quote from the corporate mission statement: »In the midst of rapid and global change, where the traditional boundaries of time, place and expertise are no longer obstacles to meet patients' needs, we take pride in providing outstanding service to patients from abroad.« Already during planning and construction the foundation and its architects cooperated intensely with their counterparts in Baltimore regarding the design of operation rooms, the acquisition of equipment for diagnosis or treatment, and, most crucially, the complete setup of laboratories.

This cooperation did not stop after the opening ceremony but rather intensified during normal operations. For the department of reproductive medicine, this intimate collaboration is one of their most valuable assets, as director Aytuğ Kolankaya explained to me in 2006: Since the equipment for diagnosis and IVF-treatments is identical with the clinic in Baltimore and staff follows the same protocols or standardized procedures and applies the same pharmaceutical substances, a direct comparison of success-rates is possible. In fact, the work of IVF-teams in both facilities is constantly monitored according to identical evaluation protocols. As soon as a significant deviation in success-rates emerges, team members will exchange

30 Cf. http://www.anadolumedicalcenter.com/.

experiences via tele-conferences or even will be »sent over« for training to profit directly from *local* experiences and specific workmanship.

What is created by the close collaboration is a seamless transnational lab-bench and a single, globally extended examination room where patients are subjected to the same knowledge practices; however, it is a space that produces unintended overflows – for example: Turkish patients are subjected to the same informed-consent-procedures as their US-American counterparts disregarding different conceptions of conception, dissimilar, culturally grounded expectations of the doctor-patient-relationship, distinct moral obligations in relation to their respective families, and the need to comply with different legal and economic conditions due to their integration in national health-care systems. These evidence-based practices tend to co-produce a universal, naturalized body whose gold-standard are patients in the US. The same also applies to other IVF-clinics in Turkey which collaborate with medical centers in Europe: the clinic Eurofertil in Istanbul, for example, is intimately linked to a hospital in Düsseldorf, Germany, via a constant flow of money, expertise and personnel. It is here that the metaphor of the wormhole fully applies: By entering the facilities in Istanbul, patients enter a space created by globalized reproductive practices that at the same time – if only for reasons of advertising – transmits a certain aura of German or American locality. While these IVF-clinics in Boston, Istanbul or Düsseldorf are subject to state regulations, most crucial for their operation are practices that are defined in a space marked by universalizing knowledge practices, namely the scientific standards of biomedicine and internationally acceptable ethical regulations.

Bodies Cosmo-Politic?

What all three examples have in common is that they point to practices where *situated experiences* are *abstracted* from individual and local contexts and transformed so that they will travel. These generalizing or universalizing practices travel well beyond the container provided by modern nation states, they only partially address constituencies of specific nation states, and they create resources for a public domain that is not bound by national boundaries. Some use these resources self-interestedly – as medical entrepreneurs –, some altruistically – as scientists – or cosmopolitically – as NGO activists; but these distinctions blur. The protagonists are a highly diverse lot: »lay«-people as well as scientists are involved in like intellectual practices that have the potential to participate in the development of a new politics of life where the good old modern state is only one of many actors. All participate – intentionally or unintentionally – in the creation of a trans-national space where exchange, multiple translations and mutual learning are possible.

In these examples, patient groups and experts in the field of reproductive medicine are inadvertently joining their resources to create a new type of »body politic«[31]: *a body cosmo-politic*. In doing so, they often feel that they have to confront the »old«, state-centered type of biopolitics that still tries to hold on to its sovereignty over its citizens in the domain of health, allowing certain reproductive interventions or banning others, establishing *national ethics committees* and propagating *national health policies* that try to regulate reproductive choice or *Selbstbestimmung* (self-determination) of its citizens. I suggest conceptualizing this antagonism between states and the new biopolitical entrepreneurs as *»gegenstrebige Fügung«* – a notion coined by the liberal German-Jewish philosopher Jakob Taubes.[32] Taubes uses the notion *gegenstrebige Fügung* to characterize his antagonistic relationship to Carl Schmitt, the right-wing theoretician of modern state-sovereignty, whose ideas where – among others – adopted by US neo-cons like Leo Strauss et al. *Gegenstrebig* alludes to two struts working in opposite direction (=Streben) but also to opposite aspirations (=anstreben). And *Fügung* means »coalescence« as well as »foreordination.« Out of this antagonistic relation emerge not only challenges to claims of sovereignty over the reproduction of a territorially bound population as it is still affirmed by modern states via legislation and bioethical regulations about legitimate uses of reproductive medicine. But the new biopolitical entrepreneurs help to bring into existence or to stabilize material-discursive practices that define and demarcate a transnational sphere of exchange,

---

31 Cf. Nancy Scheper-Hughes and Margaret Lock, »The Mindful Body: A Prolegomenon for Future Work in Medical Anthropology«, in: *Medical Anthropology Quarterly* 1 (1987), 1, pp. 6–41.

32 Jacob Taubes, *Ad Carl Schmitt. Gegenstrebige Fügung* (Berlin: Merve, 1987).

commerce, competition, communication, and interaction that provides the infrastructure for cosmopolitical action and reflection – an emergent biopolitical sphere located beyond national containers.

Notes on Contributors

Stefan Beck is professor of European Ethnology at Humboldt-University at Berlin. His research focuses on the anthropology of the life sciences, knowledge, and technology in a comparative perspective. Publications include: »Staging Bone Marrow Donation as a Balott: Reconfiguring the Sociel and the Political Using Biomedicin in Cyprus« (in: *Body & Society* 17, 2011); (with Jörg Niewöhner) »Somatographic Investigations across Levels of Complexity« (in: *BioSocieties* 1, 2006); (with Andreas Roepstorff and Jörg Niewöhner) »Enculturing Brains through Patterned Practices, in: *Special Issue of Neural Networks on Social Cognition: From Babies to Robots*, 23, 2010, and »Translating Experience into Biomedical Assemblages. Observations on European Forms of (Imagined) Participatory Agency in Healthcare« (in: *Health Promotion and Prevention Programmes in Practice*, Münster, 2010).

Sven Bergmann is a cultural anthropologist and a PhD student at the Department of European Ethnology, Humboldt University at Berlin. He holds a scholarship in the German Research Foundation (DFG) research training group »Gender as a Category of Knowledge« at the Center for Transdisciplinary Gender Studies, Humboldt University of Berlin. His dissertation project is concerned with the ethnographic research of the economics, significances, and practices of gamete donation in Europe. Other research interests include: transnational migration, urban ethnography, STS, and surveillance technologies. He is member of the newly founded DFG-network »Economies of Reproduction.«

Aditya Bharadwaj is a lecturer at the School of Social and Political Studies, University of Edinburgh. His principal research interest is in the area of new reproductive, genetic, and stem cell biotechnologies, and their rapid spread in diverse global locales ranging from South Asia to the United Kingdom. His interests also include medical sociology, anthropology of India, globalization, science and technology studies, and ethnographic research and design. Aditya Bharadwaj has published in peer-reviewed journals such as *Social Science and Medicine*, *Anthropology and Medicine*, *Health, Risk and Society*, and *Culture, Medicine and Psychiatry*. He has contributed several book chapters in edited and University Press collections in the UK and the USA. He is the co-author of *Risky Relations: Family, Kinship and the New Genetics* (Berg, 2005); and lead author of *Local Cells, Global Science: The Rise of Embryonic Stem Cell Research in India* (Routledge, 2009). He is currently completing a research monograph titled *Conceptions: Infertility and Technologies of Procreation in India (*Berghahn Books, 2011).

Sarah Franklin is professor of Sociology at the University of Cambridge. Her research focuses on IVF, cloning, embryo research, and stem cells, combining traditional anthropological approaches like kinship theory and ethnographic methods with more recent approaches from science studies, gender theory, and cultural studies. She has written and edited 15 books on reproductive and genetic technologies, as well as more than 100 articles, chapters, and reports. Among her recent publications are *Biological Relatives: IVF, Stem Cells and the Future of Kinship* (Duke, in press); (with Johnson, Hopwood, and Cottingham) »Why the Medical Research Council Refused Robert Edwards
indexEdwards, RobertindexEdwards, Jeanetteand Patrick Steptoe Support for Research on Human Conception in 1971« (in: *Human Reproduction* 25, 2010); *Dolly Mixtures* (Duke, 2007); and (with Roberts) *Born and Made* (Princeton, 2006).

Zeynep B. Gürtin is a research fellow at the Centre for Family Research, University of Cambridge and convener of the Cambridge Interdisciplinary Reproduction Forum (CIRF). Her academic interests revolve around the social, psychological, and bioethical questions surrounding the use of assisted reproductive technologies (ARTs). Her research is primarily focused on the three areas of gamete donation, reproductive »tourism,« and ARTs in developing countries. Her PhD thesis details the socio-cultural constructions of IVF in Turkey, examining both its representation in public discourses and its impact on private lives. She is currently working on a project examining ten years of egg-sharing in the UK, investigating the experiences of women who have participated as donors and recipients, and reviewing the ethical debates surrounding such schemes. Zeynep B. Gürtin lectures and supervises for several departments in Cambridge, and is on the Editorial Advisory Board of the Journal of Middle East Women's Studies. Recent publications include »Anything to Become a Mother« (in: *Marginalized production*, Earthscan, 2009); and »Assisted Reproductive Technology in Secular Turkey« (in: *Islam and the Biotechnologies of Human Life*, Berghahn books, in press).

Viola Hörbst, anthropologist, is an assistant researcher at the ISCTE-IUL, Lisbon University Institute, with the CEA, Centro de Estudos Africanos. She has carried out fieldwork in Mesoamerica (Mexico), Germany, and West Africa (Mali, Togo), where she has conducted long-term fieldwork on infertility and assisted reproductive technologies. Further research interests include the transfer of medical technologies, hospital ethnography, processes of globalization and transnationalism in medicine, Islam and health, and urban health. Among her recent publications are (together with Schuster) »Reproductive Disruptions: African Perspectives« (Thematic Issue, *Curare*, 2006); »Focusing Male Infertility in Mali: Impacts on Gender Relations and Biomedical Practice in Bamako« (in: *Muslim Medical Ethics*, University of South Carolina Press, 2007); and »Male Perspectives on Infertility and Assisted Reproductive Technologies (ART) in sub-Saharan Contexts« (in: *Social Aspects of Accessible Infertility Care in Developing Countries*, *ObGyn*, 2010).

Marcia C. Inhorn is the William K. Lanman Jr. Professor of Anthropology and International Affairs at Yale University, where she also directs the Council on Middle East Studies. A specialist on Middle Eastern gender and health issues, Inhorn is the author of four books on infertility and assisted reproductive technologies in the Arab world, including *Reconceiving Middle Eastern Manhood* (Princeton University Press, forthcoming); *Local Babies, Global Science* (Routledge, 2003); *Infertility and Patriarchy* (University of Pennsylvania Press, 1996); and *Quest for Conception: Gender, Infertility, and Egyptian Medical Traditions* (University of Pennsylvania Press, 1994), which have won the AAA's Eileen Basker Prize and the Diana Forsythe Prize for outstanding feminist anthropological research in the areas of gender, health, science, technology, and biomedicine. She is also an editor of eight volumes, including *Medical Anthropology at the Intersections* (Duke University Press, forthcoming), as well as founding editor of the *Journal of Middle East Women's Studies* and co-editor of the Berghahn Book series on »Fertility, Sexuality and Reproduction.« In Fall 2010, she was the inaugural Diane Middlebrook and Carl Djerassi Visiting Professor at the University of Cambridge's Centre for Gender Studies.

Maren Klotz is a research fellow and PhD candidate at the Department of European Ethnology, Humboldt University at Berlin. She works at the intersection of anthropological kinship studies and science and technology studies. Her ethnographic research focuses on the familial and institutional knowledge practices involved in gamete donation in the UK and in Germany. She has studied ethnology and science and technology studies in Berlin and Exeter, and her PhD is part of a joint supervision program (co-tutelle) between the Humboldt University and the University of Exeter. She is an associate member of the »Kinship-Cultures« research project and co-organizer of the »IVF as Global Form« workshop from which this volume originated. Among her recent publications are (with Michi Knecht) »Wissenswege lokal – global: Zur Ethnographie von Wissenspraxen und Regulierungsformen im Umgang mit Reproduktionstechnologien« [»Local and Global Knowledge Pathways: On the Ethnography of Knowledge-Practices and the Regulation of Reproductive Technologies«] (in: *Zum Profil einer volkskundlichen Kulturwissenschaft*, LIT Verlag, 2009); and »Verwandtschaft wissen. Familiäres und regulatives ›Wissensmanagement‹ im Bereich assistierter Reproduktion« [»Knowing Kinship. Familial and Regulatory ›Knowledge-Management‹ in the Realm of Assisted Reproduction«] (in: *Bilder, Bücher, Bytes – Zur Medialität des Alltags,* Waxman, 2009).

Michi Knecht is a researcher and lecturer at the Department of European Ethnology, Humboldt University at Berlin. She is the principle investigator in a comparative research project in Istanbul and Berlin, »Kinship as Representation of Social Order and Practice in the Context of Social and Technological Change,« which is part of the collaborative research cluster SFB 640, »Representations of Changing Social Order – Intertemporal and Intercultural Comparisons« (with Stefan Beck and Nurhak Polat), a co-founder of the Research Network »Economies of Reproduction,« and the *Collaboratory Social Anthropology and Life Sciences*. Her main areas of research and publication address reflexive medicalization, new kinship, economies of reproduction, Christian fundamentalist movements, poverty, and urban spectacles of difference. Recent publications include: (ed. with Feuchter and Bock) *Religion and Its Other: Secular and Sacral Concepts and Practices in Interaction* (Campus Publishers and Chicago University Press, 2008); »*Samenbanken – Samenspender. Ethnographische und historische Perspektiven auf Männlichkeiten in der Reproduktionsmedizin*« [»Sperm Banks – Sperm Donors. Ethnographic and Historiographic Perspectives on Maleness in reproductive medicine«] (ed. with Heinitz, Burghardt und Mohr, LIT, 2010); »Reproduktionstechnologien und die Biomedikalisierung von Verwandtschaft« [»Reproductive Technologies and the Biomedicalization of Kinship«] (in: *Das Argument* 275, 2008).

Eva-Maria Knoll is a researcher at the Austrian Academy of Sciences, Social Anthropology Research Unit. Her main research interests include tourism, science and technology, gender relations, medicine, and body concepts. She has co-edited *Ritualisierungen von Geschlecht* [»Ritualizations of Gender«] (Wiener Universitätsverlag, 2006) and *Lexikon der Globalisierung* [»Handbook Globalization«] (transkript 2011). Recent publications include »Fortpflanzungsmedizin ohne Sexualität als gesellschaftliche Irritation« [»Reproductive Medicine without Sexuality as a Societal Irritation«] (in: *Sexualität als Experiment* Campus, 2008), and »So weit gehen für ein Kind: Reproduktionstourismus als grenzüberschreitender Umweg,« [»Going so far for a child: reproductive tourism as a border-crossing detour«] (in: *Umwege zum eigenen Kind. Ethische und rechtliche Herausforderungen an die Reproduktionsmedizin 30 Jahre nach Louise Brown* Universitätsverlag Göttingen, 2008).

Michal Nahman is senior visiting fellow at the BIOS Centre for the Study of Bioscience, Biomedicine, Biotechnology and Society at the London School of Economics, and senior lecturer in sociology and criminology at the University of the West of England. She has conducted ethnographic research into gender and sexuality online; and into practices, experiences and discourses of the extraction, exchange and implantation of womens eggs transnationally. Her recent publications include: »Materialising Israeliness« (in: *Science as Culture* 15, 2006); »Nodes of Desire« (in: *European Journal of Women's Studies* 15, 2008); »Embryos are our Baby« (in: *Technologized Images, Technologized Bodies,* Berghahn Books 2010) and »Synecdochic Ricochets« (in: *Genetics, Biosociality and the Social Sciences. Making Biologies and Identities*, Routledge, 2007).

Nurhak Polat is a social anthropologist and a PhD candidate at the Department of European Ethnology, Humboldt University at Berlin. She is also a fellow researcher at the research project »Kinship as Representation of Social Order and Practice in the Context of Social and Technological Change,« which is conducted comparatively in Istanbul and Berlin as a part of the Collaborative Research Centre 640 »Representations of Changing Social Order – Intertemporal and Intercultural Comparisons« (with Stefan Beck and Michi Knecht). Her current ethnographic research focuses on knowledge, regulation, and kinship in the field of reproductive technologies in Turkey. In her PhD project she works on a case study of a Turkish concerned group and on the multiple forms of knowledge production and management in reproductive technologies. Her main research interests include studies in migration, gender, kinship, knowledge, and technology.

Bob Simpson is a professor of anthropology at Durham University. Since 2001 he has been carrying out research into the reception of new reproductive and genetic technologies in developing world contexts. His work has focused particularly on the encounter between challenging technological developments and local systems of values and beliefs in Sri Lanka. In 2003 he completed a 15-month Wellcome Trust Fellowship in biomedical ethics to develop this research. The Sri Lankan research is now part of a larger project that explores the relationship between science, ethics, and culture across South Asia. This project investigates international science collaborations and their relationship with bioethics. Recent publications include »A ›Therapeutic Gap‹« (in: *Predictive Testing and the Social Sciences,* University of Amsterdam Press, 2010); »We Have Always Been Modern« (in: Special edition of *Culture and Religion* 10, 2009); »›Please Give a Drop of Blood‹« (in: Special issue of *Body and Society* 15, 2009).

Index of Names and Places